LACHMAN'S CASE STUDIES IN ANATOMY

Lachman's Case Studies in Anatomy

FIFTH EDITION

REVISED BY David Seiden
AND Siobhan A. Corbett

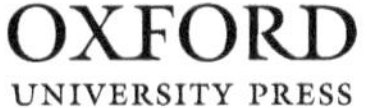

OXFORD UNIVERSITY PRESS

OXFORD
UNIVERSITY PRESS

Oxford University Press is a department of the University of Oxford.
It furthers the University's objective of excellence in research, scholarship,
and education by publishing worldwide

Oxford New York
Auckland Cape Town Dar es Salaam Hong Kong Karachi
Kuala Lumpur Madrid Melbourne Mexico City Nairobi
New Delhi Shanghai Taipei Toronto

With offices in
Argentina Austria Brazil Chile Czech Republic France Greece
Guatemala Hungary Italy Japan Poland Portugal Singapore
South Korea Switzerland Thailand Turkey Ukraine Vietnam

Oxford is a registered trademark of Oxford University Press in the UK
and certain other countries

Published in the United States of America by
Oxford University Press
198 Madison Avenue, New York, New York 10016

Library of Congress Cataloging-in-Publication Data
Seiden, David.Lachman's case studies in anatomy. – 5th ed. / rev. by David Seiden,
Siobhan A. Corbett.
p. ; cm.
Case studies in anatomy
Includes bibliographical references and index.
ISBN 978-0-19-984608-5 (pbk. : alk. paper)
I. Corbett, Siobhan A. II. Lachman, Ernest, 1901–1979. III. Title.
IV. Title: Case studies in anatomy.
[DNLM: 1. Anatomy, Regional. 2. Pathologic Processes. QZ 4]616'.09—dc23
2012022535

CONTENTS

UNIT TWO—BACK

UNIT THREE—THORAX

UNIT FOUR—ABDOMEN

UNIT SEVEN—LOWER LIMB

PREFACE

We are pleased and honored to have been asked to update this iconic book, first published by Ernest Lachman almost 5 decades ago. We have completely revised and modernized the existing patient presentations to make them even more useful to the student of anatomy and deleted those we felt were no longer pertinent to current medical practice. In addition, we have written 19 entirely new cases drawn from our own experiences as medical educators. Our goal was to provide scenarios commonly encountered in clinical practice that illustrate important clinical anatomy that is being stressed in most medical schools. Whenever possible, we have used patient examples that represent clinical encounters required in clerkship curricula. This should allow students to draw from this book throughout their 4 years in medical school. Finally, we have expanded the scope of the book to include embryological development by incorporating three new cases of developmental abnormalities: tracheoesophageal fistula, tetralogy of Fallot, and omphalocele.

We have maintained the original format of the book. Each chapter starts with a clinical case presentation, followed by diagnosis and therapy and then an extensive discussion of the anatomy that is relevant to the case. We have modified the format of the patient presentations to make the history and physical examination findings consistent with the standard format that students will utilize in clinical training. Diagnostic and therapeutic procedures that are discussed have been brought up-to-date and are consistent with current medical practice. We have added many new figures and have included many diagnostic images including radiographs, computed tomography scans, magnetic resonance images, and ultrasound scans. To help the reader feel confident that the major anatomical points have been mastered, we have added review questions and answers at the end of each unit.

We are grateful to George W. Mulheron, PhD, and to Jeffrey A. Seiden, MD, who read, corrected, and commented on every chapter. However, any shortcomings or errors in this book are our responsibility. We thank Ruth Baygell and Kaplan Health for giving permission for us to use several illustrations from the Kaplan USMLE series. We thank Dr. Donald R. Cahill for his excellent preparation of the fourth edition of this book and for entrusting the preparation of the fifth edition to us. We have been fortunate to work with Andrea Seils, Kurt Roediger, and the entire team at Oxford University Press. We extend our sincere thanks to Annie Grace and Emily Perry for their excellent editorial assistance. Lastly, we thank our spouses, Norine R. Seiden and Kevin S. Corbett, for their encouragement and support throughout the preparation of this book and, indeed, throughout our careers.

This book is dedicated to our mentors who have been so instrumental in shaping our careers.

I (DS) am eternally grateful to Carson D. Schneck, MD, PhD, who taught me anatomy and showed me, by example, how to make the teaching of clinically relevant anatomy engaging and effective. His wisdom and talents guided my career and shaped my own style of teaching. I owe him a debt of gratitude for the joyful career that I have enjoyed.

I (SC) dedicate this book to the late Stephen F. Lowry, MD, MBA, FACS, FRCS (hon), the consummate surgeon, educator, researcher, and mentor. His support and friendship was the foundation for my career in academic surgery. Dr. Lowry was absolutely dedicated to medical student education and would have loved that a surgeon brought a unique perspective to this text. He is missed by all who had the pleasure of working with him.

New Brunswick, NJ D.S.
June, 2012 S.C.

PREFACE TO THE FIRST EDITION

In the teaching program in Gross Anatomy we face the well-known dilemma that at the time the student has to master a large body of anatomical information he is not aware of its application to clinical medicine. On the other hand, when he is ready to utilize his knowledge at the bedside, he has forgotten a substantial part of this material. Yet the importance of anatomical reasoning and the application of anatomical principles in the explanation of clinical signs and events and in the design of therapeutic procedures can be exemplified almost from the first week of the basic course. This will strengthen the student's motivation for learning and satisfy his thirst for information relating to clinical medicine. We cannot afford to stifle this basic interest which has brought a large proportion of our students to medicine. The student can be made to realize from the beginning that his day-by-day learning is meaningful in terms of his future work as a physician.

Thus, the case studies presented in this book are directed specifically to the first and second year medical student for collateral reading either in the basic anatomy course or in advanced courses in the field. Elective courses in the clinical years can readily be based on the exercises presented here, particularly if they are supplemented by pertinent and specialized dissections, executed by the student himself. Residents may find these case reports useful in their review studies, particularly for board examinations.

In each case a short history, physical findings, diagnosis, therapy, and further course are given. This is followed by a discussion of the material from the anatomical viewpoint, generally in the form of questions posed and answers given. The underlying anatomy is illustrated by drawings. This presentation lends itself to self-study since all questions formulated are answered in detail and in a comprehensive discussion of the subject matter.

The individual exercises are based on case histories chosen from the literature and from the author's experience and present a composite picture that exemplifies the characteristic anatomical features of the problem under discussion. In a few instances the history is taken from one of the classical collections of masterfully composed case studies available in the literature, such as the works of Hertzler, Cabot, or Kanavel. This type of presentation should call the student's attention to a stimulating form of medical instruction. In this connection it may be worth noting that in law classes in American universities the case method has been utilized for many years, even in the freshman year, whereby principles of law are illustrated by actual cases and real-life legal problems.

All case histories contained in this book have appeared previously in *The New Physician,* but in many instances their format has been changed, and a large number have been revised and amplified.

Grateful acknowledgement is made to *The New Physician* and its editorial staff for permission to utilize these case histories.

Permission was also granted by the C. V. Mosby Company to use part of two case histories from Hertzler's *Clinical Surgery by Case Histories;* by the W. B. Saunders Company to utilize a portion of one case history published in Volume I of Cabot's *Differential Diagnosis;* by Lea and Febiger to use a case history from Kanavel's *Infections of the Hands;* by Doctors R. D. Duncan and M. E. Myers, Dr. L. B. Rose, and Dr. D. H. O'Donoghue to utilize material from individual case histories published by them. To these publishers and authors I express my grateful appreciation.

Thanks are due to the artists Mr. E. F. Hiser and Dr. J. E. Allison for their fine co-operation in executing the drawings, and to Frank Romano.

I am greatly indebted to Doctors G. H. Daron and K. K. Faulkner for many thoughtful suggestions.

Especially warm thanks are rendered to Mrs. Pat Friedel, our department secretary, whose tireless efforts were so helpful in bringing the work to speedy completion.

Oklahoma City E. L.
October 1964

UNIT I

Head and Neck

1

Facial Paralysis (Bell's Palsy)

A 36-year-old woman awoke one morning with a feeling of numbness on the right side of her face. On arising and examining herself in the mirror, she noticed that her face was distorted and deformed, and she could not close her right eye. She had some difficulty in speaking, eating, and drinking. Food seemed to collect between her teeth and right cheek. Saliva and liquids that she tried to drink ran out of the right corner of her mouth, although she had no difficulty swallowing. She became apprehensive that she had suffered a stroke and immediately consulted her primary physician.

Evaluation

With further questioning, the patient reports no recent rashes, arthralgias, or fevers and no changes in her hearing. She has not had any trauma to the area, although she reports a history of mild aching pain behind the right ear for the past 2 days, for which she had taken acetaminophen with mild relief. She has not received the influenza vaccine, taken any new medications, or had any recent dental work. She reports an occasional cold sore and had chicken pox as a child. She is not an "outdoors" person and reports no recent tick bites. On physical examination, the right side of the patient's face appears immobile and without expression. All wrinkles have disappeared from the right side of her forehead; the right nasolabial fold is less distinct than the left. The right eyebrow droops, and the right lower eyelid sags. She is emotional, and although both eyes exhibit tearing, tears run down only the right side of her face. Her mouth and nose seem deviated toward the left side, and the right corner of her mouth is sagging.

On further examination, many facial movements appear to be affected. The patient cannot smile on the right side when asked to do so. When she attempts to shut her eyes, the right eye does not close completely. She cannot purse her lips tightly, whistle, or puff out her cheeks. Asked to show her teeth, she uncovers them only on the left side, and her lips seem to be drawn to the left side. When she attempts to laugh, the distortion of her face becomes considerably more noticeable and disfiguring. The corneal reflex is absent on the right. Examinations of the parotid gland, ear canal, tympanic membrane, and oropharynx are normal. She has no cervical, posterior auricular, or occipital lymphadenopathy. The remainder of the physical examination, including the neurological examination, is within normal limits. She is embarrassed by her appearance and does not want anyone to see her in this condition.

Diagnosis

All signs and symptoms point to a facial palsy. The fact that the forehead muscles as well as the lower face muscles are affected indicates that the lesion is a peripheral lesion of the facial nerve rather than an upper motor neuron lesion in the central nervous system. Facial nerve paralysis may occur at birth, from a neoplastic lesion, or as a result of infection (e.g., Lyme disease), trauma, or iatrogenic causes. However, the most common cause of unilateral facial nerve paralysis in adults is Bell's palsy, named for Charles Bell, the British anatomist and surgeon who first described the disease in 1821. In this instance, there is no clearly identifiable cause for the facial nerve paralysis, although an inflammatory process, possibly viral in origin, is believed to be at fault.

Therapy and Further Course

The patient is given a prescription for prednisolone, an oral corticosteroid, to reduce facial nerve inflammation. A patch is placed over her right eye, and she is provided with artificial tears to lubricate the eye and protect it from corneal ulceration until recovery occurs. After 5 weeks, the patient has almost completely recovered, and only traces of the previous paralysis, particularly around the mouth, can be demonstrated.

Discussion

Bell's palsy is believed to be caused by inflammation and swelling of the facial nerve within the facial canal (Fig. 1.1). The etiology of the inflammation is uncertain, but several researchers believe that Bell's palsy may be caused by a prior viral infection, with the herpes simplex virus (HSV-1) being the primary culprit. Besides HSV, possible infectious causes of Bell's palsy include *Borrelia* bacteria (etiologic agent of Lyme disease), herpes zoster virus (chicken pox), Epstein-Barr virus (mononucleosis), and cytomegalovirus.

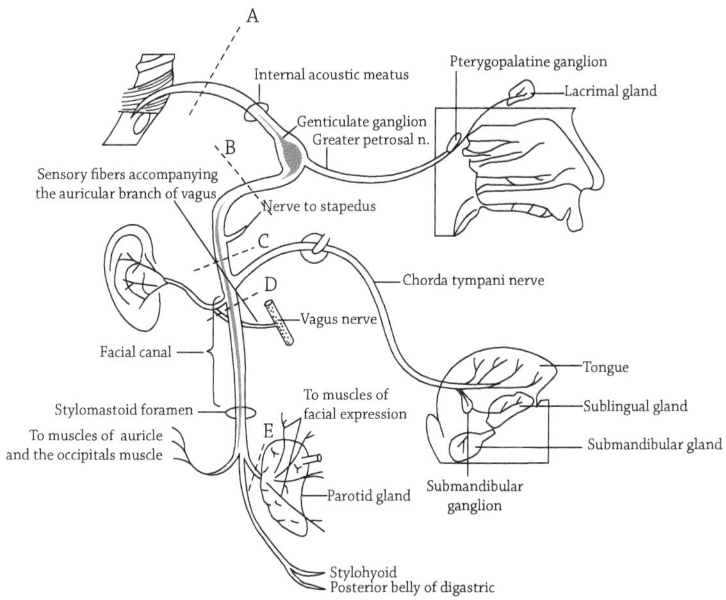

FIGURE 1.1

Schematic of the facial nerve. Refer to Table 1.1 for sites of lesions.

The facial nerve courses within the facial canal of the petrous portion of the temporal bone, where even slight swelling of the nerve within its tight-fitting bony surroundings would subject the nerve to destructive pressure. The facial nerve emerges from the skull at the end of the facial canal through the stylomastoid foramen. At this point, the nerve passes through the parotid gland and gives rise to multiple branches that supply all of the muscles of facial expression.

Effects of Paralysis on Facial Muscles

The motor deficiencies in this case demonstrate the actions of the muscles of facial expression innervated by the seventh cranial nerve. These muscles are responsible for voluntary movements of the face and for emotional expression. Because some of the creases and folds of the skin are brought about by muscular activity (e.g., on the forehead in frowning, around the eyes in squinting), many of these are decreased or disappear with facial palsy.

Among the muscles innervated by the facial nerve is the orbicularis oculi. Paralysis of this muscle prevents the patient from closing her eye in squinting, but more importantly it prevents blinking. Blinking distributes tears over the cornea, which is necessary to keep it moist and to prevent drying and consequent ulceration, the most serious complication of facial paralysis. The sagging of the lower lid, caused by loss of muscle tone, results in its eversion and the spilling of tears, as in this case. Normally, tears remain in the conjunctival sac and then drain through the nasolacrimal duct which opens into the inferior meatus of the nasal cavity.

The muscle responsible for opening the eye is the levator palpebrae superioris. This muscle has a skeletal muscle portion, which is innervated by the oculomotor nerve, and a smooth muscle portion, which is innervated by sympathetic nerve fibers from the superior cervical ganglion. Because both of these nerve innervations are unaffected in facial palsy, the eye in patients with facial paralysis remains partially open due to the unopposed pull of the levator palpebrae superioris against the paralyzed orbicularis oculi.

Education of patients involves teaching them to use droplets of artificial tears during the day and to apply ointment and tape the eyes shut at night to prevent desiccation of the cornea. The use of an eye patch, such as in this patient, is often recommended until there is recovery of facial muscle function.

Why is the patient's face distorted (asymmetrical) in appearance, particularly when she is smiling? The distortion results partially from a shift of her face toward the side that remains innervated, which is caused by the unopposed pull of the innervated muscles.

The corneal reflex is absent in this patient. This reflex is tested by having the physician stimulate the cornea by lightly stroking it with a wisp of cotton. This should evoke a responsive blink. The pathways for this reflex include a sensory limb that is carried by the ophthalmic division of the trigeminal nerve, central connections located in the pons and midbrain, and a motor pathway carried by the facial nerve. Paralysis of the facial nerve in this patient interrupted the motor limb of the corneal reflex. Normally, stimulation of one cornea causes both eyes to blink. Blinking of the eye that is stimulated is called the *direct blink reflex*; blinking of the contralateral eye is called the *consensual blink reflex*. This allows the examiner to distinguish between a facial nerve injury and a trigeminal nerve injury when the blink reflex is impaired. In this patient, when either the right or left cornea is stimulated, only the left eye blinks. This means that the trigeminal nerves on both sides are intact but the facial nerve on the right is lesioned. If the trigeminal nerve on the right were lesioned, neither eye would blink after stimulation of the right cornea.

The buccinator muscle is another important facial muscle that is innervated by the facial nerve. The buccinator has the essential function of maintaining the tension of the cheek and keeping food from passing between the cheek and the teeth. It also prevents the mucous membrane of the cheek from being caught between the teeth in the act of mastication. Paralysis of this muscle allows food to collect between the teeth and the cheek, making it difficult to chew the food.

The inability to purse the lips or to show the teeth of the affected side is caused by paralysis of the orbicularis oris, which through its action as a whole or in parts can either protrude the lips as in pouting or draw them against the teeth. Contraction of this muscle is necessary for making a tight seal of the lips to retain food and saliva in the oral cavity. Patients with Bell's palsy often have saliva and other liquids drip from the mouth on the affected side. The resulting embarrassment often impedes social interactions of patients with Bell's palsy. Our patient's inability to whistle is attributable to the paralysis of this muscle as well as the buccinator.

The absence of smiling is the result of the dysfunction of numerous small facial muscles, all of which have in common a superficial subcutaneous location, the absence of a muscle fascia, insertion into the skin, and innervation by the facial nerve. Their paralysis is responsible for the previously mentioned characteristic feature of Bell's palsy: loss, on the paralyzed side, of the expression of emotion.

Movements of the scalp muscles (frontalis and occipitalis), the extrinsic muscles of the ear, the stylohyoid, and the posterior belly of the digastric muscle, all of which are innervated by the facial nerve, are difficult to demonstrate.

The facial nerve also contains sensory nerve fibers whose cell bodies are in the geniculate ganglion. Some of these sensory fibers enter the posterior auricular branch of the facial nerve, a branch that arises immediately distal to the emergence of the facial nerve from the stylomastoid foramen. The posterior auricular nerve provides sensory innervation to the region posterior to the external ear and also to the posterior portion of the external ear canal. The pain experienced by this patient in this region is probably attributable to compression of these sensory nerve fibers within the facial canal.

The chorda tympani is a branch of the facial nerve that emerges from the nerve within the temporal bone and then passes through the middle ear cavity and emerges through the petrotympanic fissure to enter the infratemporal fossa. The chorda tympani contains preganglionic parasympathetic nerve fibers that synapse in the submandibular ganglion. Postganglionic fibers from this ganglion innervate the submandibular and sublingual glands, two salivary glands in the floor of the mouth. Because the parotid gland, the largest of the salivary glands, is not innervated by the facial nerve (but rather by the glossopharyngeal nerve), patients with Bell's palsy typically do not complain of dry mouth. Additionally, the chorda tympani contains sensory fibers for taste from the anterior two-thirds of the tongue. However, because there are alternative pathways that allow taste sensation to reach the brain, only about half of Bell's palsy patients report a change in taste.

The facial nerve also provides motor innervation to the stapedius muscle in the middle ear. The function of this muscle is to attenuate the amplitude of vibration of the stapes and thereby attenuate the perceived sound entering the inner ear at the oval window. If the stapedius muscle is paralyzed, the patient may report that sounds seem louder than normal (*hyperacusis*). The patient in this case did not report any change in hearing.

Localization of the Lesion

An analysis of which functions are retained and which are lost or impaired, along with an understanding of the location of the nerve pathways responsible for these functions, allows us to determine the site of the nerve injury (Table 1.1). Because the patient produced tears during the examination in apparently similar amounts from both eyes, we can conclude that the nerve pathway for lacrimation is functioning normally. This pathway includes the greater petrosal nerve, a branch of the facial nerve that carries preganglionic parasympathetic fibers to the pterygopalatine ganglia. From there, postganglionic parasympathetic fibers innervate the lacrimal gland. Thus, we can conclude that the injury to the facial nerve is distal to the emergence of the greater petrosal nerve, which is at the geniculate ganglion.

The absence of hyperacusis suggests that the lesion is distal to the emergence of the nerve to the stapedius. The absence of any change in taste or salivation suggests that the lesion is distal to the origin of the chorda tympani. The paralysis of the facial muscles and

TABLE 1.1 Sites of Lesions in Bell's Palsy

Lesion	*Location*	*Clinical Findings*
A	Proximal to geniculate ganglion	Loss of facial muscle function Sensory abnormality behind ear Reduction of salivation Reduction of taste Hyperacusis Reduced lacrimation
B	Between geniculate ganglion and stapedius	Loss of facial muscle function Sensory abnormality behind ear Reduction of salivation Reduction of taste Hyperacusis
C	Between stapedius and chorda tympani	Loss of facial muscle function Sensory abnormality behind ear Reduction of salivation Reduction of taste
D	Between chorda tympani and stylomastoid foramen	Loss of facial muscle function Sensory abnormality behind ear
E	Within parotid gland	Loss of facial muscle function

the sensory disturbance in the region of the external ear suggests that the lesion is proximal to the emergence of the facial nerve from the stylomastoid foramen. Thus, we can conclude that the compression of the facial nerve is in the distal region of the facial canal, distal to the emergence of the chorda tympani and proximal to the stylomastoid foramen.

2

Trigeminal Neuralgia

A 55-year-old woman has suffered attacks of sharp, stabbing pain on the right side of her nose and cheek and the right upper lip for more than 1 year. These paroxysms (sudden attacks) of pain last only a few seconds but are so unbearable that they cause the patient to seek immediate help. She reports that when the pain started it was less intense, occurred less often, and was felt only at the side of the nose rather than in the larger area where it is now located. She also states that the pain ceased for a period of 4 months but then returned in greater intensity and frequency. Because it was believed that a maxillary tooth infection could be the cause of the pain, she had significant dental work done. However, the episodic pain persisted. Attacks may be brought on by chewing, drinking, washing, drying her face, or blowing her nose. A light touch to the side of the nose often precipitates a paroxysm of pain. The patient protects her face against touch and drafts with a scarf. On questioning, she states that the pain is always confined to her right side and never crosses the midline.

Examination

During the examination, an attack is observed during which the patient winces and contorts her face in a tic-like fashion. Because of difficulties in eating and drinking, she has lost 15 pounds and appears dehydrated. On neurological examination, no motor defects or interference with any modality of sensation on the face can be discovered. A complete cranial nerve examination is also negative. Except for the patient's appearing anxious and tense, the physical examination is noncontributory.

Diagnosis

The diagnosis is neuralgia (tic douloureux) of the maxillary division of the trigeminal nerve.

Therapy and Further Course

A magnetic resonance imaging (MRI) study of the head is ordered to determine whether there is an identifiable cause to the trigeminal neuralgia (TN). Intravascular contrast material is used to assist in identifying any vascular anomalies. Sometimes an intracranial tumor (e.g., meningioma) compresses the trigeminal nerve. Although this accounts for only about 5% of TN cases, it must be ruled out before proceeding with a therapeutic plan. The MRI is negative for any tumor. It is also negative for multiple sclerosis. Although TN is fairly rare, it is substantially more common in patients with multiple sclerosis than in the remainder of the population. A more common cause of TN is compression of the nerve by a blood vessel in the region. The MRI with contrast revealed a suggestion of an artery in contact with the trigeminal nerve immediately after its exit from the brain stem.

The possible courses of action are discussed with the patient. It is decided to try a medical approach to addressing the pain. The patient is prescribed carbamazepine (Tegretol), an antiseizure medication that has been shown to be effective in many patients in relieving the pain of TN. The patient is seen regularly, but treatment gives only temporary relief. When the pain returns, she requests surgical measures. The various surgical options are discussed with the patient, including percutaneous approaches to the trigeminal nerve, Gamma Knife radiosurgery, and open microvascular decompression. It is decided to use Gamma Knife radiosurgery because it is the least invasive option and has a reasonably good likelihood of being effective. On follow-up visits, the patient reports that within about 3 weeks after the procedure she started to notice a diminution in the pain and a decrease in the frequency of pain; after 3 months she was pain free and continued to be so 1 year later.

Discussion

General Definition of Trigeminal Neuralgia

This patient suffered from TN involving the maxillary division (second division, V_2, also called the maxillary nerve) of the trigeminal nerve. The patient was typical in terms of age, sex, and the involved division of the trigeminal nerve. The disease is more common in women than in men. Incidence increases with age, and patients are typically more than 50 years old. Although it is not fatal, TN represents one of the most catastrophic afflictions of humans; the pain can be so intense that before effective therapies were available, it was known to drive some sufferers to suicide. Fortunately, the patient in this case was cured by radiosurgery.

The neuralgia consists of paroxysmal attacks of pain that involve the sensory distribution of one or more divisions of the trigeminal nerve. The attacks are characterized by their short duration, by intervals of relief from pain, by their unilaterality, by the absence of objective neurological findings, and by the frequent presence of trigger zones in the face or the mucosa. These zones, when lightly touched, may induce an attack. As in this patient, it is not unusual for patients to be seen by dentists before a correct diagnosis is made, and frequently patients have had one or more teeth extracted in the belief that the pain has its origin in a diseased tooth.

Trigeminal neuralgia previously was known as tic douloureux (painful twitch). This is a somewhat misleading term in that it might be deduced that a muscular spasm is the cause of the pain. Actually, the sequence is reversed: It is the excruciating pain that causes the patient to wince and grimace by contorting the facial muscles.

Course and Distribution of the Maxillary Nerve

The only division involved in this case is the maxillary division (V_2) of the trigeminal nerve. The maxillary nerve, as this division is frequently called, runs from the middle portion of the trigeminal ganglion along the lateral wall of the cavernous sinus. It leaves the middle cranial fossa through the foramen rotundum to enter the pterygopalatine fossa. As it passes through the pterygopalatine fossa, it is accessible by passing a needle from the cheek, through the infratemporal fossa, and through the pterygomaxillary fissure into the pterygopalatine fossa. In years past, this accessibility was used to advantage in patients with TN to inject alcohol into the nerve, which damaged the nerve and thereby blocked the pain. This procedure has since been replaced by more effective therapies.

While passing through the pterygopalatine fossa, the maxillary nerve gives off branches that enter the nasal cavity, oral cavity, orbit, and infratemporal fossa. These branches continue on to reach skin and mucosal surfaces that are supplied with sensory innervations. These branches include the nasopalatine nerve, which passes through the sphenopalatine foramen and enters the nasal cavity to supply the mucosa of the lateral and septal walls of the nasal cavity; the greater and lesser palatine nerves, which pass through the greater palatine canal and enter the oral cavity to supply the mucosa of the hard and soft palates; the zygomatic nerve, which enters the orbit through the inferior orbital fissure and continues through the orbit to reach the skin of the face in the temporal and zygomatic regions; and the infraorbital nerve, which enters the orbit through the inferior orbital fissure and continues through the orbit in the infraorbital canal to reach the face, supplying the skin and conjunctiva of the lower eyelid, the skin below the orbit and above the mouth, the skin and mucosa of the upper lip, and the skin of the lateral surface of the nose.

As the infraorbital nerve passes along the floor of the orbit, it gives rise to nerves that innervate the mucosa of the maxillary sinus and all of the maxillary teeth (Figs. 2.1, 2.2, and 2.3). It is because of the latter innervations that it is often suspected, as in this patient, that the pain a patient with TN is experiencing is arising from the maxillary teeth or maxillary sinus. The distribution of the sensory innervation of the maxillary nerve corresponds to the regions where pain is perceived by patients with TN of the maxillary division.

Intracranial Anatomy of the Trigeminal Nerve

The trigeminal nerve emerges from the brain stem at the anterolateral surface of the pons. There are two roots of the nerve, the larger

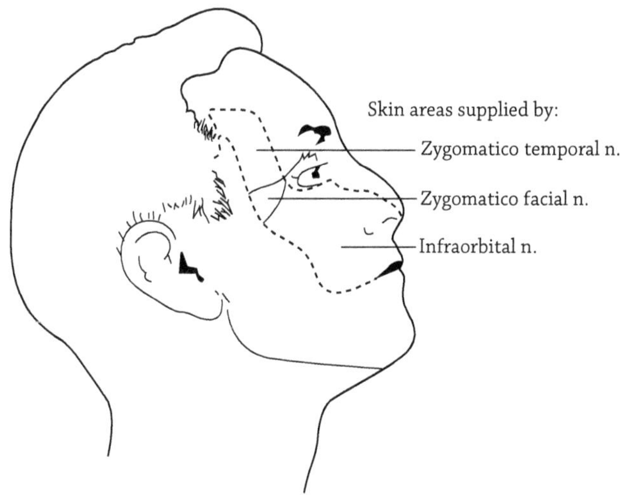

FIGURE 2.1

Skin areas supplied by the maxillary division of the trigeminal nerve.

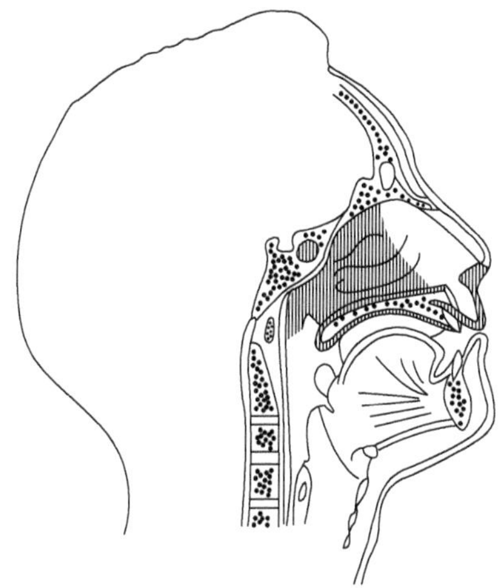

FIGURE 2.2

Mucosal areas supplied by the maxillary division of the trigeminal nerve (*shaded*).

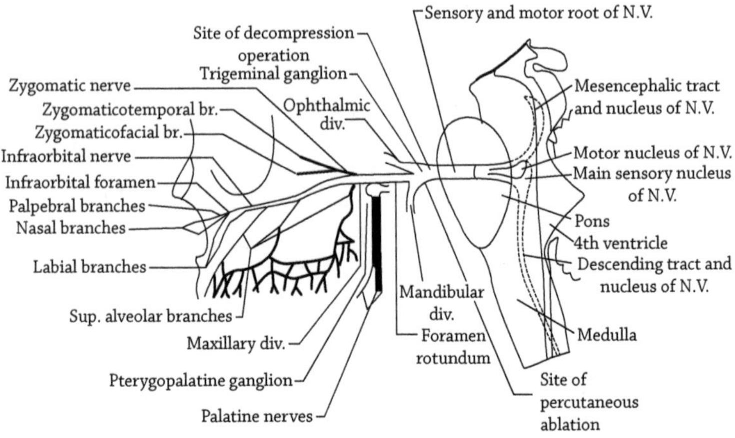

FIGURE 2.3

Trigeminal nuclei and tracts; root, ganglion, and divisions of the trigeminal nerve; and distribution area of maxillary division. Notice the sites of surgical intervention for decompression and percutaneous ablation. br., branch; div., division; N.V, cranial nerve V.

sensory root and the smaller motor root. Just after the sensory root passes over the petrous ridge of the temporal bone to pass from the posterior cranial fossa to the middle cranial fossa, it reaches the trigeminal ganglion, the site for the cell bodies of the sensory neurons in the trigeminal nerve. Distal to the trigeminal ganglion, the nerve divides into three divisions: ophthalmic, maxillary, and mandibular. The ophthalmic division passes within the lateral wall of the cavernous sinus to reach the superior orbital fissure, through which it passes to reach the orbit. Branches from the ophthalmic division provide sensory innervations to the skin and mucosal surfaces from the level of the lateral angle of the eye up to the interauricular line (the line connecting one external auditory meatus to the other) on the scalp. This includes the skin of the forehead and the anterior portion of the scalp, the skin and conjunctiva of the upper eyelid, and the mucosa of the frontal sinus. The dorsum of the nose also receives its sensory innervations from a branch of the ophthalmic division.

The maxillary division passes within the lateral wall of the cavernous sinus to reach the foramen rotundum, which it traverses and then follows the course described earlier. The mandibular division passes through a dural recess (Meckel's cave) to reach the foramen ovale, which it traverses to enter the infratemporal fossa. It then gives rise to branches that innervate the skin overlying the mandible, the mandibular teeth and gums, the mucosa of the floor of the mouth, the anterior two-thirds of the tongue, and the mucosa and skin of the cheek.

The motor root of the trigeminal nerve passes the trigeminal ganglion without going through it and then joins the mandibular division to enter the infratemporal fossa. It provides motor innervations to the four muscles of mastication as well as the mylohyoid, the anterior belly of the digastric muscle, the tensor palati, and the tensor tympani.

Applied Anatomy of Surgical Approaches to the Trigeminal Nerve

After medical treatment did not provide relief to our patient, she chose to use Gamma Knife radiosurgery to address the problem. In this procedure, many small beams of radiation (approximately 200 beams) are directed at the trigeminal nerve from multiple directions. MRI and computer guidance are used to aim these beams. The energy level of each beam is low enough so as not to damage the tissue through which it passes. However, all of the beams converge at the trigeminal nerve, proximal to the trigeminal ganglion, to provide an energy level high enough to damage the nerve fibers that are carrying the pain associated with TN. This relieves the patient's symptoms and in most cases does not interfere with other sensory modalities, although some patients report areas of numbness after the treatment.

Another surgical option that is available is percutaneous lysis of the trigeminal ganglion. In this procedure, a needle is introduced through the patient's cheek, lateral to the corner of the mouth, and, under fluoroscopic observation, the needle is advanced to and through the foramen ovale to the trigeminal ganglion. With the needle in place, ablation of pain-transmitting sensory neurons in the ganglion can be accomplished by the introduction of glycerol through the needle. An alternative method is to pass a radiofrequency current through the needle to heat it and cause a thermal ablation of the pain-conducting nerve fibers. The risks associated with these percutaneous procedures are related to the possible misplacement of the needle and consequent introduction of glycerol or application of a thermal insult to an unintended region.

There is also an open surgical approach of microvascular decompression that can be used to treat many cases of TN caused by compression of the trigeminal nerve by a nearby artery. This method is reported to have the highest success rate in effecting permanent pain relief, but it is the most invasive procedure and carries with it the associated risks of open surgery. An incision and craniotomy are made behind the ear, and the trigeminal nerve is approached as it exits the pons. Any blood vessel that is in contact with the trigeminal nerve is identified, and a Teflon sponge is put into place to cushion the nerve from the blood vessel. Because this is an open surgical procedure, a hospital stay of several days and a longer recovery period are needed. Gamma Knife radiosurgery and percutaneous ablation of the trigeminal ganglion are outpatient procedures with very short recovery periods.

Regardless of the procedure used to treat TN, it is most important to preserve the fibers of the ophthalmic division, if at all possible, because destruction of the sensory fibers from the cornea leads to loss of the protective corneal reflex. The absence of this reflex makes the cornea susceptible to inflammation and ulceration as a result of desiccation and trauma. Serious keratitis and possible loss of eyesight on the injured side may follow denervation of the ophthalmic division. The other portion of the trigeminal nerve that needs to be spared is the motor root, which is not too difficult to separate from the sensory root. The motor root runs along the undersurface of the sensory root, from medial to lateral, then joins the mandibular nerve (division), with which it passes through the foramen ovale, as described earlier.

3

Septic Thrombosis of the Cavernous Sinus

A 32-year-old business executive returned from a hunting trip, where living conditions had been rather primitive, and presented to the emergency room with a 3-day history of fever, chills, and severe headaches. He relates that about 6 days earlier he developed a boil (furuncle) on the right upper lip, which resulted from a cut while shaving. He squeezed the boil to try to resolve it, but rather than improve, it has become increasingly painful and enlarged. Associated with the boil, he developed severe headaches about 3 days ago, lateralized to the right frontal region. The headaches have increased in severity and are described as sharp and constant. He also reports pressure behind the right eye and recent onset (5 hours) of double vision. He also notices tingling and burning (paresthesia) of the right forehead, the right side of his nose, and the upper portion of his face. He is nauseated and has vomited once.

Examination

On physical examination, the patient is ill-appearing and restless. His temperature is 102.8° F. Marked rigidity of his neck muscles, a clinical sign of meningeal irritation, is noted. His upper lip is hard, markedly swollen to about twice its normal size, and dusky red. Some dark crusts cover the right side of the upper lip, and some pus oozes from several points. The right cheek and right side of his nose are swollen and hard. The right upper and lower eyelids are swollen, as are the palpebral and bulbar conjunctivae. The right eyeball protrudes farther than the left (exophthalmos).

Examination of the right eye shows swelling of the eyelids and dilation of the pupil. Chemosis (fluid in the conjunctiva) is also noted. Fundoscopic examination shows engorgement of the retinal veins and some edema of the optic nerve at the papilla. All voluntary movements of the right ocular muscles, including the superior oblique and lateral rectus muscles, are absent. There seems to be some hardening along the course of the right facial vein. Computed tomography imaging of the head is ordered and reveals intracranial extension of the infection into the cavernous sinus.

On subsequent examination, there is some swelling of the left eyelid with protrusion of the left eyeball and inability to abduct the left eye completely. Repeated blood cultures are positive for *Staphylococcus aureus*. The patient has marked leukocytosis (increase of leukocytes in the bloodstream). His differential blood count also indicates the presence of an acute infection.

Diagnosis

The patient is diagnosed as having a severe staphylococcal infection of the subcutaneous tissue of the upper lip (carbuncle), infectious cavernous sinus thrombosis on the right, and beginning cavernous sinus thrombosis on the left, with right-sided paralysis of all ocular muscles (ophthalmoplegia), abducens paralysis on the left, and staphylococcal bacteremia.

Therapy

The patient is admitted to the intensive care unit and immediately started on broad-spectrum intravenous antibiotics, including coverage for gram-positive, gram-negative, and anaerobic organisms, pending the results of the blood cultures. Once *S. aureus* is identified as the infectious agent, intravenous antibiotics directed at this organism are continued, including vancomycin to treat a possible methicillin-resistant *S. aureus* (MRSA) infection. Local warm, moist dressings are applied to both eyes and to the right side of his face, and narcotics are given for the pain.

The patient responds only slowly to the antibiotic treatment. He remains febrile for several days and then gradually improves. There is some sloughing of the subcutaneous tissue of the upper lip. Ocular function improves gradually but finally returns to normal. Antibiotic treatment is continued on an outpatient basis for 4 weeks.

Discussion

Infectious cavernous sinus thrombosis is a condition that is almost invariably fatal if not diagnosed and treated properly. The infection in this patient began as an innocuous-appearing boil in the hair follicles of the upper lip, a rather common occurrence. Because there is a rich venous plexus of labial veins superficial to the main muscle mass of the lips, the orbicularis oris, it was possible for the infection to spread through the venous system. Squeezing of the boil and the never-ceasing motion of the labial muscles, which are traversed by numerous veins, led to propagation of infected material. It passed first through the finer venules, then through the smaller and larger veins draining the lips, with resulting infectious thrombosis of these veins (thrombophlebitis).

The Facial Vein, Its Tributaries and Communications

The labial veins are tributaries of the facial vein, which usually terminates in the internal jugular vein. The facial vein was thrombosed and could be felt as a hardened cord. It runs posterolateral to the facial artery in front of the masseter muscle, where it passes across the lower border of the mandible. More important for the spread of the disease is the communication of the beginning of the facial vein, the angular vein, with the superior ophthalmic vein, and through it with the cavernous sinus (Fig. 3.1). The infection may spread by means of an embolus (detached clot) from the face via the facial and angular veins and through the superior ophthalmic vein into the cavernous sinus, or by an infectious thrombosis extending through the same vascular channels. The end result is a septic thrombosis of the cavernous sinus.

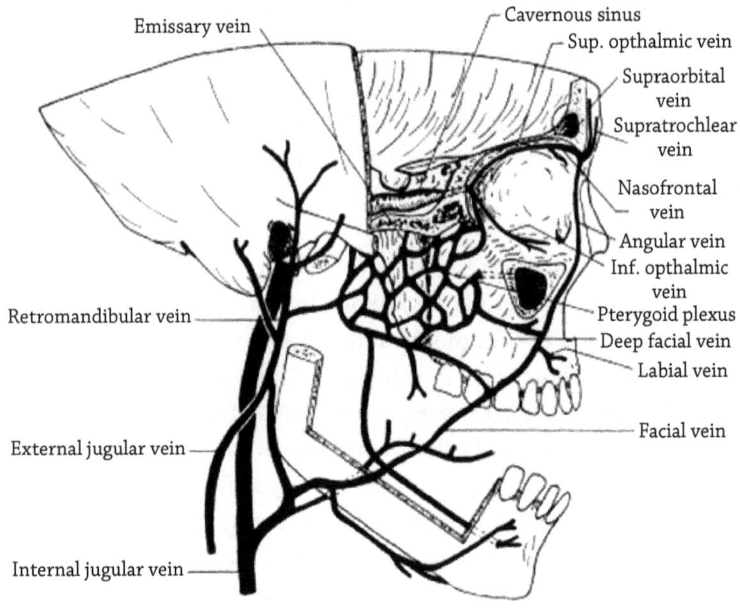

FIGURE 3.1

Communications of the facial vein and pterygoid plexus with the cavernous sinus. Inf., inferior; Sup., superior.

An important anatomical feature is the absence of valves in the veins of the face, which makes it possible for the venous blood to flow in either direction—toward the neck and the internal jugular vein or in the opposite direction, toward the beginning of the facial vein at the inner angle of the eye. The supratrochlear and supraorbital veins descend from the forehead to unite at the upper medial corner of the orbit to form the angular vein, which then continues across the face as the facial vein, receiving tributaries from the eyelids, the side of the nose, and the lips. It is the important communication of the angular vein with the superior ophthalmic vein that is responsible for the serious outcome that is seen when, as in this patient, there is infection in the area drained by the facial vein (Fig. 3.1).

Because the muscles of facial expression are located in the subcutaneous tissue and are intimately connected with the skin, they lack the covering of deep fascia and fascial septa that other muscles have, which could limit the spread of infection. On the contrary, the contraction of these muscles, as in speaking or eating, tends to milk infectious material along the venous channels.

Even if flow through the facial vein is obstructed, for example by ligation or thrombosis, there are other pathways that can allow venous flow from the face to the cavernous sinus. There is a large communication from the facial vein via the deep facial vein to the pterygoid plexus. The latter anastomoses with the cavernous sinus by means of emissary veins that pass through foramina in the base of the skull. It is important to note that opening of the carbuncle on the upper lip is not indicated. Cutting through infected tissues may spread the infection and generally results in worsening of the condition.

The upper lip is not the only area from which infection can be propagated to the cavernous sinus. Any portion of the skin of the face that is drained by the facial vein can serve as the site of a primary focus. Boils of the nasal cavity and cellulitis of the cheeks, eyelids, eyebrows, forehead, and lower lip have at times been the source of this dangerous complication.

Emissary Veins

In addition to the face, there are other regions of the head and neck that can serve as a primary site of infection that spreads to the cavernous sinus. Anatomically, any region with veins that communicate with the cavernous sinus can serve as such a site. The pharyngeal and pterygoid plexuses communicate with the cavernous sinus by way of emissary veins that pass through the foramen ovale and adjacent foramina. The pterygoid plexus also anastomoses with the inferior ophthalmic vein by a vein traversing the inferior orbital fissure. The inferior ophthalmic vein is a direct or indirect tributary of the cavernous sinus (Fig. 3.1). All of the aforementioned veins, as well as the previously discussed superior ophthalmic vein, drain important regions of the head that frequently harbor infection. Thus, tonsillar and paratonsillar abscesses, dental infections (particularly after extractions), infections of the paranasal sinuses and the orbit, and posttraumatic infections of the face, the maxilla, and the frontal bone all may lead to infectious cavernous sinus thrombosis.

Emissary veins are communications between intracranial dural venous sinuses and extracranial veins. They are thin-walled, valveless vessels that pass through cranial openings generally termed *emissary foramina*. Blood in these veins may flow in either direction. Their presence represents a safety mechanism that comes into play when there is an increase in intracranial venous pressure that might otherwise endanger the brain. On the other hand, the blood flow may be reversed, passing from the outside to the dural sinuses, if there is an obstruction in the extracranial veins, as in our case of thrombosis of the facial vein. Ophthalmic veins establish a communication between the facial veins and the cavernous sinus and can be regarded as emissary veins. Again, the blood flow can be in either direction, toward the cavernous sinus or toward the facial veins, depending on the ever-changing venous pressure conditions.

Cavernous Sinus

The superior ophthalmic vein is the main tributary of the cavernous sinus. It enters the anterior end of the sinus at the superior orbital fissure. The cavernous sinus is continuous posteriorly at the apex of the petrous bone with the superior and inferior petrosal sinuses. The cavernous sinus drains its blood into the superior and inferior petrosal sinuses and through them into the transverse sinus and the internal jugular vein, respectively. Retrograde spread of infection from the ear via the petrosal sinuses represents an additional and important route leading to cavernous sinus thrombosis. If one keeps in mind that cerebral and meningeal veins also drain into the cavernous sinus, other serious complications, such as brain abscess and spreading meningitis, can be understood on the basis of retrograde spread. Signs of meningeal irritation, such as rigidity of the neck and headache, were also present in this patient.

Like other dural venous sinuses, the cavernous sinus is located between two layers of dura, is lined by endothelium, and lacks a muscular coat. It differs from other dural sinuses, however, in that it is traversed by numerous dural trabeculae, which give it a spongelike appearance. This arrangement makes it more susceptible to stasis and thrombosis. Embedded in its lateral wall are the oculomotor nerve, the trochlear nerve, and the first and second divisions of the trigeminal nerve; the internal carotid artery, with its sympathetic plexus and the abducens nerve, courses through its lumen (Fig. 3.2).

Eye Signs in Cavernous Sinus Thrombosis

Our patient has swelling of the eyelids and conjunctiva, exophthalmos, congestion of the retinal vessels, and edema of the optic nerve. All these signs are caused by interference with the blood flow in the cavernous sinus and connecting veins as a result of the thrombosis. The latter causes retrograde congestion of the ocular veins and edema (swelling) of the orbital structures. Detailed examination pertaining to the function of individual eye muscles was difficult in our patient because of swelling of the right eye and the patient's poor condition, but it was found that all voluntary movements of the eyeball were abolished.

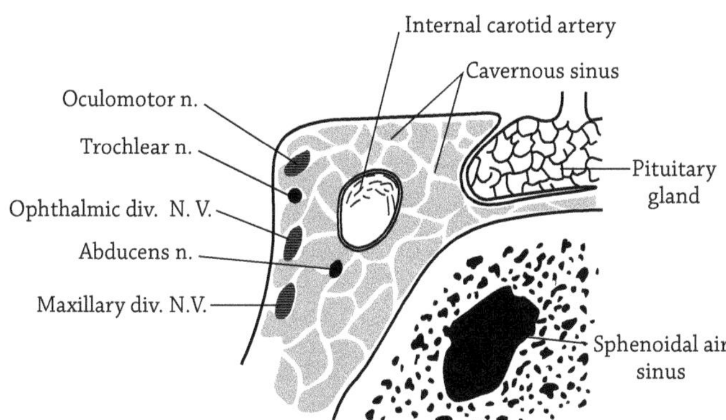

FIGURE 3.2

Frontal section of the left cavernous sinus showing its important nerve and arterial contents (viewed from behind). div., division; n., nerve; N. V., cranial nerve V (trigeminal).

The oculomotor nerve supplies all muscles moving the eyeball with the exception of the superior oblique and lateral rectus muscles, which are innervated by the trochlear and abducens nerves, respectively. How would you test the functions of these two muscles? If the superior oblique is paralyzed as a result of involvement of the fourth cranial nerve, there is loss of downward movement of the eyeball from the adducted position. In the case of paralysis of the lateral rectus, there is loss of full abduction of the eyeball. Both of these motions were abolished in this patient. The impairment of vision in the right eye can be explained on the basis of edema of the optic nerve with congestion of the central vein of the retina, which drains into the superior ophthalmic vein.

As mentioned previously, retinal congestion was observed in this patient. Blindness is a definite possibility and will occur if the thrombosis completely blocks flow in the superior ophthalmic vein, because the central vein of the retina does not anastomose with other veins. There are clinical indications that the upper two divisions of the trigeminal nerve, which lie in the wall of the sinus, are also involved. There are sensory disturbances (paresthesias) in the face along the distribution of these two divisions.

Later protrusion and swelling of the left eye with abducens paralysis indicates involvement of the left cavernous sinus also. There are anatomical pathways for the spread of the infection from the right to the left sinus. The two cavernous sinuses are connected by anterior and posterior intercavernous sinuses, which may readily spread infection from one sinus to the other. The abducens nerve, being in a more exposed position within the sinus, is often the first of the nerves supplying the eye muscles to be involved in cavernous sinus thrombosis.

The presence of positive blood cultures in this case indicates that the infection had spread beyond the confines of the cranium. The final happy outcome of the case is gratifying. Before effective antibiotic therapy became available, the mortality rate from septic cavernous sinus thrombosis was almost 100%. Now, in areas where aggressive antibiotic therapy is available, the mortality rate has dropped to about 25%. Even among the survivors, there remains a significant morbidity, with visual impairment and impairment of function related to the cranial nerves that traverse the cavernous sinus being most common. Early identification and aggressive treatment of infections that can spread to the cavernous sinus is the most effective prevention of this serious condition.

4

Orbital Floor Fracture

The patient is a 14-year-old female, with no significant past medical history, who presents to the emergency department complaining of facial pain and double vision (diplopia). The patient was well until 1 hour ago, when she was struck in the face by a softball, in the area of the right eye. She was taken from the ball field, and an ice pack was immediately applied. Despite the first aid, her parents reported rapid swelling and bruising around the eye. She also had a nosebleed that subsided spontaneously. The patient reported to her parents that her vision in the affected eye seemed fine, but that she had double vision, especially when attempting upward gaze. For this reason, her parents brought her to the emergency department. She reports no loss of consciousness. Her parents state that the patient was found to have 20/20 vision at her most recent visual acuity check. She is up-to-date on all her vaccinations and has met all developmental milestones. She is currently in eighth grade, doing well in school.

Examination

The patient's vital signs are stable and she is afebrile. On inspection, there is right periorbital ecchymosis and edema. No proptosis (outward bulging of the eye) or enophthalmos (recession of the globe within the orbit) is noted. With retraction of the eyelids, the right eye can be more easily visualized. The pupils are equal in size, round, and reactive to light and accommodation. (*There is an accepted and commonly used abbreviation for this series of findings on physical examination: PERRLA—Pupils Equal, Round, Reactive to Light and Accommodation*).

There is minimal conjunctival hemorrhage in the right eye. Her visual acuity is checked with a card and is found to be similar in both eyes. There is no ocular misalignment. However, when her extraocular muscles are examined, there is limited upward movement of the right eye compared to the left. Slit-lamp evaluation and tonometry are performed and found to be normal. Palpation of the right infraorbital rim reveals a step-off, consistent with a fracture. However, there is no subcutaneous emphysema overlying the fracture site. There is numbness over her right cheek; otherwise cranial nerves II through XII are intact.

The remainder of her physical examination is within normal limits.

Diagnosis

The diagnosis is orbital floor fracture with possible extraocular muscle entrapment and infraorbital nerve injury.

Therapy and Further Course

Computed axial tomography of the head was performed to visualize the facial bones and confirmed the diagnosis of an orbital floor fracture. The inferior oblique muscle was found to be round and inferiorly displaced, indicating that it had prolapsed into the orbital floor defect, causing entrapment. Although repair of an orbital floor fracture is typically performed electively to allow the facial swelling to subside, entrapment of the extraocular muscle is an indication for immediate intervention due to concern about ischemia of the muscle. For this reason, the patient was admitted to the hospital and scheduled for surgery the following day.

With the patient under general anesthesia, a transconjunctival incision was used to expose the orbital floor. The fracture site was explored to identify and remove any bony fragments. Inspection of the soft tissue was then performed. The inferior oblique muscle was identified and freed from its entrapment. The defect in the floor of the orbit was reinforced with prosthetic material, and the incision was closed. Postoperatively, the patient's extraocular muscle function was intact and the numbness resolved.

Discussion

The Bony Orbit

The orbit is the cavity within the skull that contains the eyeball and associated structures. The orbit is pyramidal in shape, with four walls and an apex. The roof of the orbit is formed mostly by the frontal bone and is related to the frontal sinus and the anterior cranial fossa. The floor is formed mostly by the maxilla and is related to the maxillary sinus. The medial wall is formed mostly by the ethmoid and sphenoid bones and is related to the ethmoid air cells and the nasal cavity. The lateral wall is formed mostly by the zygoma and sphenoid bones and is related to the temporal fossa and middle cranial fossa.

The apex is posteriorly positioned and includes several openings: the optic canal, the superior orbital fissure, and the inferior orbital fissure (Fig. 4.1). The optic canal communicates with the middle cranial fossa and conveys the optic nerve and ophthalmic artery. The superior orbital fissure communicates with the middle cranial fossa and conveys the superior ophthalmic vein (to the cavernous sinus) as well as cranial nerves III, IV, VI, and the ophthalmic division of cranial nerve V. The inferior orbital fissure communicates with the infratemporal fossa and the pterygopalatine fossa and conveys the inferior ophthalmic vein, the infraorbital nerve, and the zygomatic nerve. On the anterior surface of the orbit are the supraorbital and infraorbital foramina. The supraorbital foramen conveys the supraorbital nerve, artery, and vein. The infraorbital foramen is the anterior opening of the infraorbital groove and canal in the floor of the orbit and conveys the infraorbital nerve, artery, and vein. The supratrochlear nerve and infratrochlear nerve also exit from the front of the orbit but do not have any associated foramina.

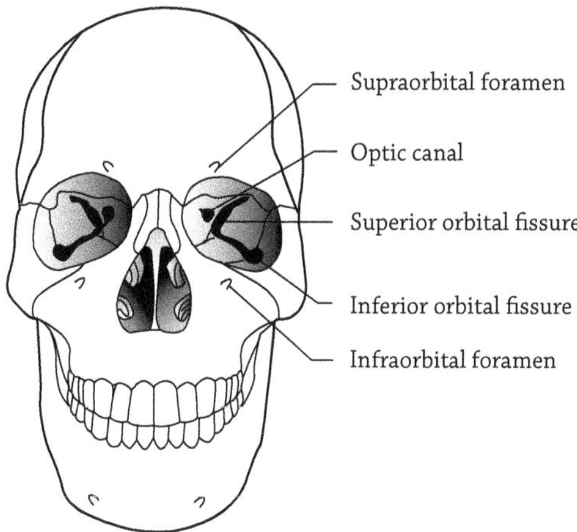

FIGURE 4.1

The bony orbit.

Extraocular Muscles

There are seven extraocular muscles: One, the levator palpebrae superioris, attaches to the upper eyelid, and six attach to the eyeball. Of these six, four have their origins on a common ring tendon in the posterior part of the orbit. These are the superior rectus, inferior rectus, lateral rectus, and medial rectus muscles. The other two have independent origins from the wall of the orbit, the superior oblique near the back of the orbit and the inferior oblique near the front of the orbit (Fig. 4.2). Notice that the site of origin of the inferior oblique muscle is the anteromedial portion of the floor of the orbit. This is the site of the fracture suffered by this patient and accounts for the entrapment of the muscle.

The four rectus muscles insert on the front half of the eyeball and the two oblique muscles on the back half of the eyeball. The tendon of the superior oblique passes through a fibrocartilaginous pulley, the trochlea, before turning to reach the back of the eyeball. The lateral rectus is innervated by the abducens nerve (VI). The superior oblique is innervated by the trochlear nerve (IV). The remaining muscles are innervated by the oculomotor nerve (III). The functions of these muscles are summarized as follows:

Muscle	*Function*
Levator palpebrae superioris	Elevation of the upper eyelid
Superior rectus	Elevation and adduction of eye
Inferior oblique	Elevation and abduction of eye
Inferior rectus	Depression and adduction of eye
Superior oblique	Depression and abduction of eye
Lateral rectus	Abduction of eye
Medial rectus	Adduction of eye

When the superior rectus and inferior oblique contract together, pure elevation results. Similarly, when the inferior rectus and the superior oblique contract together, pure depression results:

Muscles	*Combined Function*
Superior rectus + Inferior oblique	Elevation
Inferior rectus + Superior oblique	Depression

The patient had an entrapment of the inferior oblique muscle in the fracture of the floor of the orbit. This entrapment interfered with the function of the muscle as an elevator of the eyeball. When she attempted an upward gaze, the right eye did not elevate along with the left, and diplopia resulted.

The Infraorbital Nerve

The infraorbital nerve is a branch of the maxillary division of the trigeminal nerve. It enters the orbit through the inferior orbital fissure and then runs along the floor of the orbit. In the posterior portion of the orbit, the infraorbital nerve and vessels lie within the infraorbital groove on the orbital floor. In the anterior part of the orbit, this

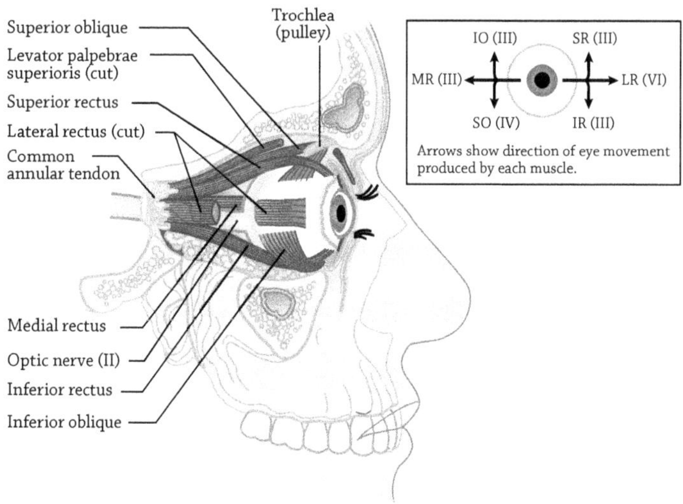

FIGURE 4.2

The extraocular muscles. III (oculomotor), IV (trochlear), and VI (abducens) indicate the cranial nerves supplying these muscles. IO, inferior oblique; IR, inferior rectus; LR, lateral rectus; MR, medial rectus; SO, superior oblique; SR, superior rectus. (Courtesy of Kaplan Medical.)

groove closes over to become the infraorbital canal, and the infraorbital nerve and vessels continue into this canal. At the anterior end of the orbit, the infraorbital canal opens onto the face at the infraorbital foramen. The infraorbital nerve and vessels reach the face through this foramen. The infraorbital nerve provides sensory innervation to the skin of the face below the orbit. This patient experienced an area of numbness in the region innervated by the infraorbital nerve. Presumably, this was caused by compression of the infraorbital nerve as it runs along the floor of the orbit in the region of the fracture.

The Maxillary Sinus

There are four pairs of paranasal sinuses, air filled cavities within the skull that communicate with the nasal cavity. Three of these pairs of sinuses are related to the walls of the orbit. The frontal sinus is superior to the orbit; the roof of the orbit separates the orbit from the sinus. The ethmoid air cells are medial to the orbit and are separated from it by the orbit's medial wall. The maxillary sinus is inferior to the orbit; the floor of the orbit is the roof of the sinus. Therefore, the fracture in the floor of the orbit is a fracture in the roof of the maxillary sinus.

It is likely that the nosebleed suffered by the patient was related to bleeding from the disrupted maxillary sinus mucosa. The blood in the maxillary sinus can enter the nasal cavity through the ostium of the maxillary sinus. Branches of the infraorbital nerve descend from the floor of the orbit to innervate the mucosa of the maxillary sinus. Similarly, branches of the infraorbital artery provide blood supply to the maxillary sinus. Many of these neural and arterial branches continue through the maxillary sinus to reach the maxillary teeth and gums. For this reason, inflammation of the maxillary sinus often presents clinically as pain referred to the maxillary teeth. The fact that this patient did not have subcutaneous emphysema on physical examination indicates that air did not escape from the sinus into the soft tissue. Therefore, it would appear that there was no significant disruption of the maxillary sinus wall.

5

Bilateral Dislocation of the Temporomandibular Joint

About 45 minutes before being brought to the emergency department, a 22-year-old college student took a large bite of an apple. She immediately experienced sharp, severe pain on both sides of her face just in front of the ear. Since that moment, she has been unable to close her mouth completely or speak clearly and has had difficulty swallowing. She also complains of pain in both temporomandibular joints (TMJs) when she tries to open or close her mouth. The pain radiates to the ear and the skin above it. She has no prior history of injury to the jaw or mouth. The remainder of her history is noncontributory.

Examination

On examination, the patient appears to have a severe malocclusion, with her lower jaw protruding beyond her upper jaw (prognathism). She is unable to bring her upper and lower teeth together when she tries to close her mouth. On both sides there is an obvious dimpling of the skin and a depression in the preauricular area that corresponds to the mandibular fossa. She has no evidence of gingival lacerations. Examination of the cranial nerves reveals no deficits. The remainder of the physical examination is within normal limits.

Diagnosis

The diagnosis is bilateral anterior dislocation of the mandible.

Therapy and Further Course

Intravenous medication is given to induce analgesia, sedation, and relaxation. This may be supplemented by injection of a local anesthetic (e.g., lidocaine) directly into the TMJ space at the site of the preauricular depression. It may then be possible to perform a closed reduction of the mandible by applying downward bimanual pressure on the lower molar teeth, followed by a backward push of the mandible. The mandible is grasped by the physician with the thumbs inside the mouth. The mandible is pressed down with the thumbs and then slid backward to return the condyle of the mandible into the mandibular fossa. Because the patient's mandible will close forcibly when the dislocation is reduced, the physician's thumbs are padded with gauze for protection. To obviate the possibility of recurrence of the dislocation after recovery from the anesthesia and the muscle relaxant, the patient is advised to avoid wide mouth-opening for the next 2 weeks. She is given a follow-up referral to an oral maxillofacial surgeon. One year later, the patient reports that no further incidents of dislocation have occurred.

Discussion

The TMJ is the only synovial joint in the skull, with the exception of those between the ear ossicles. It is also the only joint in the body where a dislocation can occur spontaneously by exaggerated but otherwise normal movements in articulation. Most often this happens during yawning, but it can also occur while laughing, singing, or biting into an apple or in a dentist's chair when the mouth is opened too widely. Traumatic dislocation is not as common as the spontaneous variety.

The Temporomandibular Joint

Bones, Cartilage, and Capsule

To understand the readiness with which dislocations occur, we must look at the anatomy of this somewhat complex joint. The uninitiated observer may assume that the TMJ is a simple hinge joint,

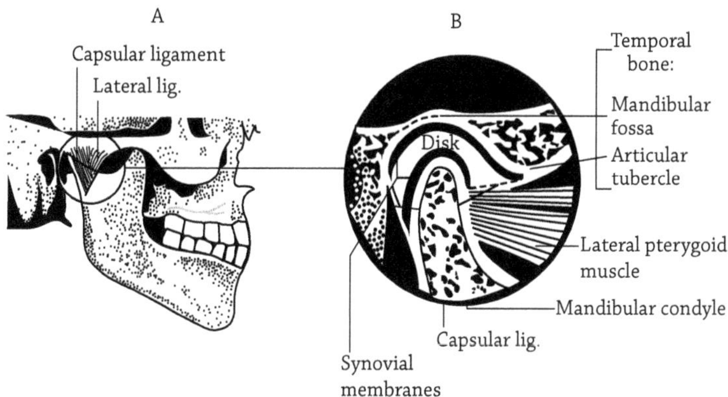

FIGURE 5.1

A, Lateral view of the articular capsule of the temporomandibular joint. B, Sagittal section through the temporomandibular joint. Notice the fibrocartilaginous disk and attachments of the lateral pterygoid muscle.

with the upward and downward movements of the jaw taking place around a horizontal axis laid through the joint. Actually, the joint has two compartments, an upper and a lower, which are completely separated by an articular disk composed of dense fibrous connective tissue and areas of fibrocartilage (Fig. 5.1). Superiorly, the bony articular surface consists of the anterior portion of the mandibular fossa and the downward-protruding articular tubercle (eminence); both are parts of the temporal bone. Below, the bony articular surface is formed by the condylar head of the mandible. In contrast to other freely movable joints, in which the articulating surfaces are covered by hyaline cartilage, avascular fibrocartilage covers all parts of the articular bony portions.

Superiorly, the disk is convex over the mandibular fossa and concave over the articular tubercle. Inferiorly, it is concave for the convex head of the mandible, thus harmonizing the two bony surfaces. The disk also acts as a shock absorber. It is thicker at the periphery, where it attaches to the joint capsule. The capsule, which is lined by synovial membrane, is rather loose and attaches above and below to the margins of the bony parts of the joint.

The articular disk of the TMJ may commonly become displaced. This can become evident in two ways. Some patients hear a "snap" in the ear on opening the mouth, followed by a "click" every time they open the mouth. Other patients suffer occasional attacks of locking and salivation. The disk must be reduced by a dentist or physician, or it may reduce itself. When this occurs, the discomfort and pain cease.

Ligaments

The tonus of the muscles responsible for joint movement is of major importance in stabilizing the joint. The ligaments play only an ancillary role in maintaining the position of the mandible, but they aid in limiting exaggerated movements (Fig. 5.2). The most important of these ligaments is the lateral (temporomandibular) ligament, which extends from the zygoma (zygomatic process of the temporal bone) to the lateral and posterior parts of the neck of the mandible and restrains mainly the backward movement of the jaw. The two ligaments on the medial side of the mandible, the sphenomandibular and stylomandibular ligaments, are not very significant for the function of the joint.

Movements of the Joint

The expected hinge action takes place in the lower compartment, between the inferior surface of the disk and the condyle of the mandible, but opening of the mouth is always accompanied by a forward gliding motion of the disk and condyle of the mandible onto the articular tubercle. Because the summit of the articular tubercle reaches more inferiorly than the inferior surface of the mandibular fossa, the forward movement of the mandible in itself results in a separation of the teeth. Thus, the motion of opening the mouth actually takes place in both compartments, with the axis of the combined motion running transversely through the mandibular foramina located on the medial sides of the two mandibular rami, approximately at their center. This location prevents the unnecessary stretching of the

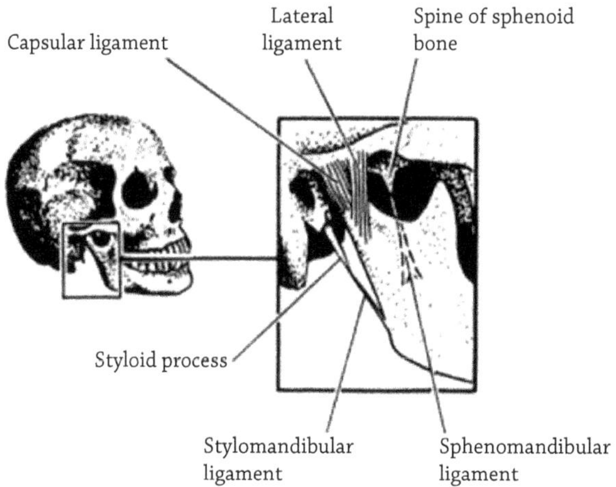

FIGURE 5.2

Lateral view of the ligaments of the temporomandibular joint.

alveolar nerves and blood vessels at their points of entrance into the mandible when the mouth is opened. A reverse series of motions takes place in all parts of the joint when the mouth is closed. Other movements of the joint, such as protrusion (protraction), retrusion (retraction), and grinding (side-to-side motion), and the muscles that execute them are discussed in the following section.

Muscles Controlling the Movements

All motions of the jaw are the result of highly integrated and closely coordinated actions of the muscles listed here, but it should not be forgotten that the finer and more complex movements are individually attuned to the shape and position of the teeth and differ from one person to another.

The muscles of the two sides act either in unison (as in depression, elevation, protrusion, and retrusion of the mandible) or alternately on the two sides (as in the side-to-side gliding motion that occurs with grinding the teeth or chewing).

As stated previously, movement of the mandible in opening the mouth consists of a simultaneous forward gliding of the mandible with its disk onto the articular tubercle and depression of the mandible as a result of the hinge action within the lower compartment of the joint. The forward motion is effectuated by the lateral pterygoid muscle, which runs horizontally backward from its origin in the infratemporal fossa to its attachment on the disk of the TMJ and the neck of the mandible (Fig. 5.1). The right and left lateral pterygoid muscles function together to cause symmetrical anterior movement of the mandible. If one of the lateral pterygoid muscles is paralyzed, there is asymmetrical movement of the mandible, and the jaw deviates toward the side of the paralyzed muscle. The mandible is depressed by contraction of the digastric and mylohyoid muscles and the infrahyoid muscles (thyrohyoid, sternothyoid, and sternohyoid).The digastric and mylohyoid muscles are linked inferiorly to the sternum through the infrahyoid muscles by their common attachments to the hyoid bone.

The opposite action of elevation of the jaw in closing the mouth is brought about by the powerful contractions of the masseter, temporalis, and medial pterygoid muscles. These muscles arise from the bones of the lateral side of the skull. The temporalis muscle arises from the temporal fossa of the temporal bone and inserts onto the coronoid process and the anterior border of the ramus of the mandible. The medial pterygoid muscle arises from the medial surface of the lateral pterygoid plate of the sphenoid bone and inserts on the medial surface of the mandible near its angle. The masseter muscle arises from the zygomatic arch and inserts onto the lateral surface of the mandible near its angle. (See Chapter 7, "Fracture of the Mandible.")

Protrusion of the chin is brought about by muscles that arise anterior to the joint and course backward, such as the lateral pterygoid muscle and, to a lesser extent, the medial pterygoid muscle. The opposite motion of retraction takes place mainly when the postero-inferior portion of the temporalis muscle contracts. In grinding and chewing (side-to-side) motions, the movements of the two sides are coordinated, but the right and left lateral pterygoid muscles act in alternating contraction.

Causes, Clinical Signs, and Symptoms of Dislocation

Almost all TMJ dislocations consist of an abnormal anterior displacement of the mandible, which takes place when a blow to the chin or an exaggerated opening of the mouth causes the articular disk and condyles of the mandible to be pulled over the summits of the articular tubercles (Fig. 5.3). This movement is due mainly to forcible involuntary contraction of the lateral pterygoid muscles. Spasm of the superioinferiorly directed muscles (such as the temporalis, the medial pterygoid, and the deep part of the masseter) keep the jaw arrested in the infratemporal fossa with the mouth half open.

In some disease states, such as tetanus, the patient cannot open the mouth because of muscular spasm of these masticatory muscles. This muscular spasm, called *trismus*, is often very painful. It may be relieved by muscle relaxants or general anesthesia.

During the examination of the patient, the heads of the mandible could not be palpated from within the external acoustic meatuses. This is a common diagnostic procedure in examination of the TMJ, because the joint lies directly in front of the external meatus. The examiner lets the tip of a finger slide over the tragus of the external ear into the meatus. The examiner then can analyze by palpation the movements of the mandibular heads on opening and closing of the mouth, in protrusion and retraction of the chin, and during grinding motions. In this case, the absence of the heads from the articular fossae was easily diagnosed and confirmed by the depression and dimpling of the skin that could be felt and seen in front of the ears.

The patient also rather typically complained of pain in the joint that radiated into the external ear and the temporal region. The nerve that is mainly responsible for the sensory supply of the joint, including its capsule, is the auriculotemporal branch from the mandibular division of the trigeminal nerve (V_3). It courses immediately behind the joint and in front of the ear and then ascends over the temple, posterior to the superficial temporal artery. Along this course it supplies, in addition to the joint, the external acoustic meatus, the outer surface of the tympanic membrane, and the lower

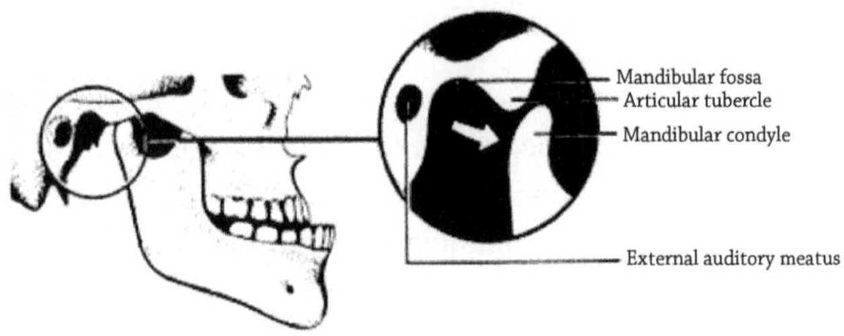

FIGURE 5.3

Lateral view of dislocation of the temporomandibular joint. Notice the overriding of the articular tubercle by the mandibular condyle.

lateral region of the scalp. This explains the radiation of the pain to the ear and temporal region. It also confirms Hilton's law: "A joint is supplied by the same nerve trunk that supplies the skin over the joint and also the muscles crossing the joint." In the latter connection, it is interesting that the nerves to the masseter and temporalis muscles from V_3 also provide sensory branches to the temporomandibular joint.

Clinically, it must be realized that once bilateral dislocation has occurred, it can easily happen again, and people afflicted with this condition are known as *chronic dislocators*. Some are asymptomatic, but others suffer a great deal of pain in the area of the TMJ. For relief of the latter group, the height of the articular tubercle may be surgically reduced to allow unrestricted anterior movement of the mandibular condyles and to eliminate the pain associated with dislocation. This surgery may cause dislocation to occur more frequently, however.

6

Tracheoesophageal Fistula

A newborn baby boy is noted to have excessive salivation within the first 12 hours after birth. Copious secretions are seen at the mouth and nose. The secretions are cleared by suction, but the problem recurs despite repeated suctioning. Episodes of coughing and mild cyanosis are noted. This problem is exacerbated when feeding is attempted. This full-term baby had a birth weight of 5 pounds 12 ounces. The mother reports that she did not have access to prenatal care. She reports that her abdomen was unusually large during most of her pregnancy and that she was surprised by the low birth weight of the baby.

Examination

Examination of this infant reveals excessive secretions in the mouth and nose. The abdomen is moderately distended, and there are normal bowel sounds. An attempt to pass a nasogastric tube to decompress the stomach is not successful. Radiographic examination reveals that the nasogastric tube is coiled in the thoracic portion of the esophagus, indicative of esophageal atresia. Meconium has been passed, and examination of the anal region indicates normal patency of the anal canal. Auscultation of the chest reveals normal heart sounds and noticeable gurgling in the lung fields. A thorough examination of the baby reveals no other obvious congenital defects.

Diagnosis

The diagnosis is esophageal atresia with associated tracheoesophageal fistula (TEF).

Therapy and Further Course

The baby is scheduled for surgery the next day. To minimize the risk of aspiration, continuous suction of the upper pouch of the esophagus is applied and the infant is positioned with the head elevated. Nutrition and fluids are administered intravenously. Because of the risk of aspiration pneumonia, prophylactic antibiotic therapy is initiated. Cardiac and renal ultrasound studies are performed to rule out congenital defects of these organs.

Surgical repair is performed through a right thoracotomy in the posterolateral fourth intercostal space. A retropleural approach to the mediastinum is used. The azygos vein is identified and divided. The right vagus nerve is identified, and care is taken to avoid injury to this nerve. The TEF is identified and divided, and the esophagus and trachea are each repaired. The proximal esophageal pouch is mobilized and anastomosed to the distal esophagus. Before closure of the chest, a nasogastric tube is passed through the esophagus into the stomach to ensure patency of the esophagus. Postoperatively, feeding through the nasogastric tube is initiated. One week after surgery, a contrast dye is given by mouth to check for any leaks from the esophagus. Subsequently, oral feeding is initiated and the baby is discharged from the hospital.

Discussion

Esophageal atresia occurs in approximately 1 of every 4000 live births. In approximately 85% of such cases, there is an associated TEF in the distal portion of the esophagus (i.e., distal to the atretic segment) that typically communicates with the trachea slightly proximal to the tracheal bifurcation; this type is shown in Figure 6.2C. In the remaining 15% of cases, fistulas may be present in the proximal segment of the esophagus or in both the proximal and distal segments, or there may be no fistula at all.

In up to 30% of cases, there is an association of these esophageal abnormalities with several other congenital abnormalities. This is known as the VACTERL association—an acronym for *Vertebral* anomalies, *Anal* atresia, *Cardiac* defects, *Tracheoesophageal* fistula, *Esophageal* atresia, *Renal* defects, and *Limb* defects. For this reason, careful evaluation of infants with any one of these defects must be done to determine whether any of the other associated defects also exist. In this patient, such other defects were not found. The genetic cause of this grouping of defects is not clear, although it is associated with several trisomies.

Normal Development of the Lower Airway

During the fourth week of development, an endodermal diverticulum evaginates from the ventral midline of the cervical portion of the endodermal gut tube. This is known as the *respiratory diverticulum* (Fig. 6.1). The site of this diverticulum marks the boundary between the future pharynx and the future esophagus. The respiratory diverticulum descends on the ventral side of the gut tube and then bifurcates. The distal ends of each branch of the bifurcation expand to become a lung bud.

The respiratory diverticulum becomes the epithelial lining of the larynx, trachea, and bronchi and the epithelium of the lower airway all the way to the alveolar epithelium. The mesenchyme from the fourth and sixth pharyngeal arches (largely composed of neural crest cells) coalesces around the endoderm to form the laryngeal cartilages. Splanchnic mesoderm coalesces around the remainder of the endodermal diverticulum to form the cartilages of the trachea and bronchi as well as the smooth muscle and connective tissue of the airway.

During the fourth and fifth weeks of development, the airway is separated from the gut tube by the tracheoesophageal folds. If these folds do not fuse properly, a TEF will result. If these folds are improperly positioned, atresia of the esophagus can result.

Polyhydramnios

During fetal life, urine that is produced by the fetus is released into the amniotic cavity and is the major component of amniotic

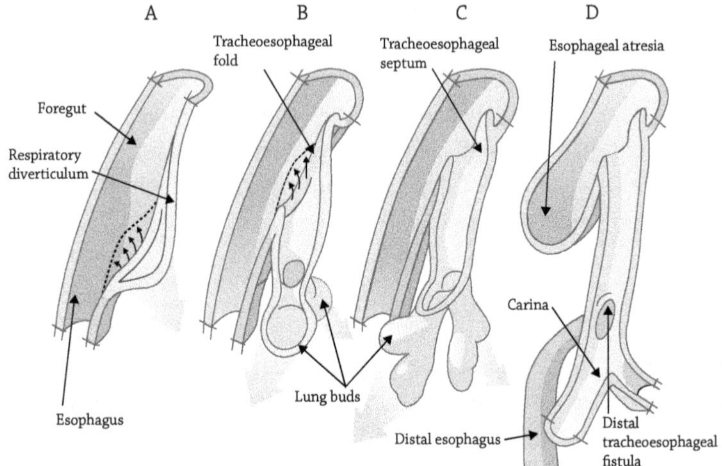

FIGURE 6.1

[1] Development of the respiratory diverticulum. **A,** A ventral midline diverticulum forms during the fourth week of gestation. **B,** The diverticulum descends anterior to the foregut and bifurcates, and the tracheoesophageal folds meet to separate the airway from the gut tube. **C,** The distal ends of the diverticulum branch to become the bronchi of the lungs. **D,** Abnormal communication between the airway and the gut tube forms a tracheoesophageal fistula.

fluid. This amniotic fluid is normally "inhaled" by the fetus and is important for the normal development of the lungs. The fluid is also normally swallowed by the fetus and then absorbed in the digestive tract to eventually be recycled as urine. If there is an obstruction of the gastrointestinal (GI) tract or a neurological defect that interferes with the swallowing reflexes, excess fluid will accumulate in the amniotic cavity. This results in an abnormally large volume of amniotic fluid, known as *polyhydramnios*. The volume of amniotic fluid typically increases during pregnancy to reach a maximum of about 800 mL at 34 weeks of gestation. Usually, the volume then decreases to about 600 mL at 40 weeks of gestation, when a full-term baby is born.

This patient reported that she had a large abdomen during her pregnancy and expected the baby to be bigger. This was caused by polyhydramnios resulting from the esophageal atresia and the resultant obstruction of the GI tract. If the patient had received standard prenatal care, the polyhydramnios would have been noted and confirmed by ultrasonography, and the esophageal atresia may have been diagnosed prenatally.

Tracheoesophageal Fistula

Although esophageal atresia may develop without a TEF, this occurs in only about 10% of cases. In approximately 85% of cases, as in this patient, there is a fistula between the distal segment of the esophagus and the trachea (Fig. 6.2C). In the remaining cases, there is a fistula in the proximal segment or in both the proximal and distal segments (Figs. 6.2A and 6.2B, respectively). Additionally, a TEF sometimes develops without atresia of the esophagus (Fig. 6.2D).

The presence of a fistula can allow passage of air from the trachea into the esophagus or passage of food and liquids from the esophagus into the trachea, depending on the site of the fistula. This patient had a distended abdomen, a result of air in the stomach that had passed from the trachea, through the fistula into the esophagus, and then into the stomach. In contrast, babies who have esophageal atresia without a fistula present with a scaphoid abdomen with the absence of gas.

The most important complication associated with esophageal atresia and TEF is aspiration. Because of the atresia, saliva and other secretions from the mouth and pharynx cannot pass into the stomach. When they fill the proximal segment of the esophagus, they overflow and may be aspirated into the airway. Obviously, attempts to feed the baby further exacerbate this problem. This patient was placed on continuous suction to reduce or prevent aspiration. When there is a fistula between the distal segment of the esophagus and the trachea, as in this patient, an even more serious problem exists. The acidic gastric contents can reflux into the esophagus and then pass through the fistula into the trachea and down into the lungs.

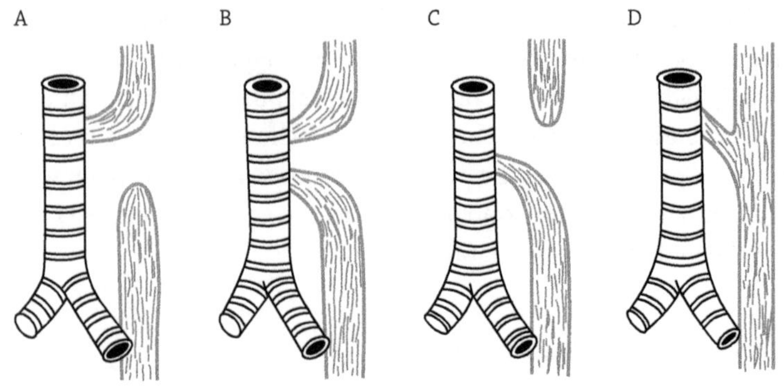

FIGURE 6.2

Types of tracheoesophageal fistulas. **A,** Fistula in the proximal segment of the esophagus. **B,** Fistulas in both the proximal and distal segments of the esophagus. **C,** Fistula in the distal segment of the esophagus. **D,** Fistula without esophageal atresia.

This can result in a very serious pneumonitis, which can significantly compromise the baby's respiration. Because of the risk of pneumonia, antibiotic therapy was initiated in this patient.

Surgical Repair

Because in this patient the atretic segment of the esophagus was short and the proximal and distal segments of the esophagus were fairly close together, primary repair of the esophagus by anastomosis of the two segments was possible at the same time that the fistula was ligated and repaired. If the two segments of the esophagus are too far apart to allow primary repair, the fistula can be closed, and the baby can be maintained on parenteral feeding until a repair of the esophagus becomes possible. Given sufficient time, the growth of the proximal segment provides enough lengthening to allow anastomosis with the distal segment. Sometimes a length of "neo-esophagus" must be created from a segment of a different portion of the GI tract to bridge the gap between the esophageal segments.

Azygos Vein and Vagus Nerve

In the approach to the esophagus from the right side of the chest, the arch of the azygos vein must be ligated and divided. The azygos vein receives venous drainage from the chest wall and the abdominal wall. It is formed by the union of the ascending lumbar vein and the right subcostal vein and receives drainage from right intercostal veins as it ascends along the posterior wall of the thorax on the right side of the vertebral column. It also receives drainage from the hemiazygos vein which, in turn, receives drainage from left intercostal veins. At about the level of the fourth thoracic vertebra, the azygos vein arches forward over the right main bronchus to reach the superior vena cava, into which it drains.

The arch of the azygos lies on the right side of the esophagus and therefore is in the field of surgery. Because of the extensive collateral communications between the ascending lumbar vein and the inferior vena cava, the ligation and division of the arch of the azygos does not prevent the return of the azygos venous drainage to the heart. The blood in the azygos vein travels retrograde to reach the ascending lumbar vein and then the inferior vena cava, returning to the right atrium through that vein rather than the superior vena cava. The right vagus nerve, which passes between the arch of the azygos and the esophagus, must be identified and protected from injury. The vagus nerve in that region is carrying parasympathetic motor innervations to the GI tract and also sensory nerve fibers coming from the GI tract to the brain stem. Because the recurrent laryngeal nerve on the right side branches from the vagus nerve as it passes the right subclavian artery, the motor nerve fibers to the laryngeal muscles on the right are not in the vagus nerve at the level of surgery. In contrast, on the left side, the motor fibers to the laryngeal muscles do not exit from the vagus nerve until it crosses the aortic arch.

7

Fracture of the Mandible

A 23-year-old man is seen in the emergency department shortly after a car accident. His car was struck broadside by another car just after he entered an intersection near his home. He was restrained and the front airbags deployed, but his head impacted the door frame as there was significant intrusion into the driver's compartment. He was awake and alert at the scene, reporting no loss of consciousness, but he could not close his mouth or speak clearly. He also reported difficulty swallowing. The pain in the left side of his jaw is intense, and blood-stained saliva drools from his lips. He has no other complaints. He takes no medications, has no allergies, and is a nonsmoker.

Examination

After a primary survey, an oral examination in the emergency department reveals a malocclusion with a steplike deformity of the mandibular teeth in the left canine area. There is evidence of hemorrhage from a tear in the mucoperiosteum. A hematoma is beginning to form in the floor of the mouth, medial to the tear. Gentle bimanual examination reveals abnormal mobility of the left part of body of the mandible, which is quite painful when even slight pressure is applied. There is circumscribed tenderness in the left mandibular canine region. When the patient attempts to bring his teeth together, the left posterior portion of the mandible is displaced medially and superiorly. There is anesthesia and numbness over the left side of the chin and left lower lip near the midline. He has no cervical spine tenderness to palpation. The remainder of the secondary survey reveals no apparent injuries.

Radiographic examination reveals a break in the continuity of the mandible between the left canine and second premolar teeth posterior to the mental foramen. There is displacement of the fragments as described previously. The first left lower premolar is missing and presumably was avulsed by the blow.

Diagnosis

The diagnosis is left-sided fracture of the body of the mandible with displacement of the fragments.

Therapy and Further Course

The airway is assessed to ensure that there is no upper airway obstruction. Careful evaluation of the cervical spine and the spinal cord is performed, because a force strong enough to fracture the mandible could also injure the cervical spine. Thorough imaging of the mandible is done to determine whether any additional fractures occurred. Because of the horseshoe shape of the mandible and its articulations at both ends, it is common for fractures of the mandible to occur at more than one site. Because the patient is missing a tooth, a chest radiograph is taken to determine whether the missing tooth was aspirated.

Options for repair of the mandible (i.e., open or closed repair) are discussed with the patient. The open repair is accomplished with the patient under general anesthesia. A wide exposure of the fracture site is made, and rigid fixation is accomplished with the use of a titanium plate and screws. The alternative closed repair is agreed to by the patient and the surgeon. This may be done with regional anesthesia by means of an inferior alveolar nerve (mandibular) block. The mandibular block is performed by injecting an anesthetic near the mandibular foramen. This is the method dentists commonly use to anesthetize the mandibular teeth for dental procedures, because it blocks the inferior alveolar nerve before it enters the mandible.

After the anesthesia takes effect, the oral surgeon secures an arch bar by means of interdental wiring. The teeth are placed into proper position of occlusion and held there by additional interdental wiring between the mandibular teeth anterior and posterior to the fracture and also between corresponding maxillary and mandibular teeth. The jaw is immobilized for about 6 weeks to allow osseous callus to develop and unite the fragments. Antibiotics are also prescribed to avoid infection of the bone. Follow-up study shows healing of the fracture in good position and alignment as well as normal function.

Discussion

Sites and Typical Displacement of Fractures

With the exception of the nasal bone, the mandible is fractured more frequently than any other bone in the skull. Motor vehicle accidents and assaults account for approximately 75% of these fractures. Fractures just posterior to the mental foramen, as in this case, are rather common. Other sites that are predisposed to fractures are areas of structural weakness, such as the region of the incisive fossa near the symphysis, the angle of the mandible, and the neck of the mandible. A look at the structure of the mandible as it appears on cross section at various levels is indicated (Fig. 7.1).

The mandible, the heaviest and strongest bone of the head, consists of spongy or cancellous bone surrounded by heavy compact bone on its outer (buccal) and inner (lingual) surfaces and on its lower border, where the compact bone is particularly well developed. The mandibular canal, which transmits the important inferior alveolar nerve and blood vessels of the lower jaw, passes through the spongy inner part with only a thin protective shell of dense bone around it.

As in most cases of fracture of the mandible, the fracture in this patient is compound; it extends through an alveolus (tooth socket) and the mucosa of the oral cavity and, therefore, into a contaminated area, the oral cavity. This is the reason for the administration of antibiotics to the patient. Oral surgeons usually regard the danger of osseous infection from the oral cavity as minimal unless

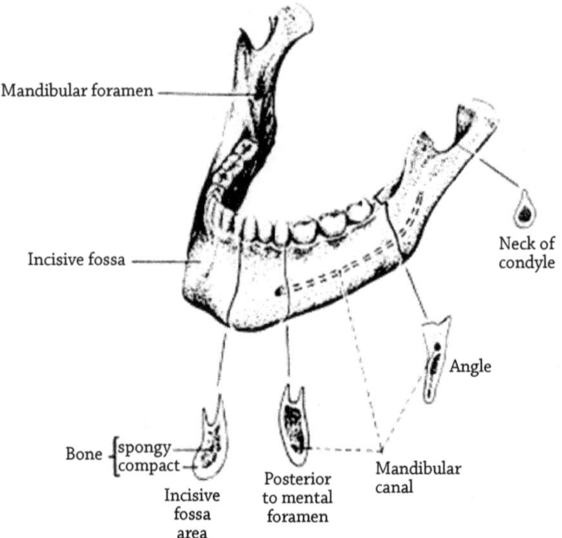

FIGURE 7.1

Drawing of the mandible as it appears on cross section at the incisive fossa, posterior to the mental foramen, at the angle, and at the neck of the condyle.

there are teeth in the line of fracture. In these instances, traumatic disruption of the blood supply to the pulp results in an infarction of the pulpal tissue. The tooth may develop an apical abscess that may be followed by osteomyelitis (inflammation of the bone marrow and adjacent bone).

What determines displacement of the fragments in fractures of the mandible and the consequent malocclusion? Important factors in all fractures are the direction of the initial force, the structure of the bone at the site of the fracture, and, most significantly, the traction of the muscles that attach to the fragments. In this patient, the posterior fragment was displaced upward and medially. The muscles responsible for this misalignment are the masseter, medial pterygoid, and temporalis muscles, all of which are elevators of the mandible, a function that can be deduced from their origins and insertions. The medial pterygoid, which is directed downward and laterally from its origin to its insertion, accounts for the medial displacement. The anterior fragment of the mandible is displaced by the actions of the digastric, the geniohyoid, and, minimally, the mylohyoid muscles. All of these pull the anterior part of the body of the mandible downward toward the hyoid bone when the latter is fixed by the infrahyoid muscles (Fig. 7.2).

Arterial Supply of the Mandible

Because the fracture in this case intersected the mandibular canal, it interrupted the continuity of the inferior alveolar vessels. This was borne out by the presence of a considerable hemorrhage at the site of the fracture and the developing hematoma in the floor of the mouth.

The inferior alveolar artery, a branch of the first part of the maxillary artery, enters the mandible through the mandibular foramen (Fig. 7.3). It traverses the mandibular canal to the mental foramen and divides into its two terminal branches, the larger mental and the smaller incisive arteries. In its course through the mandibular canal, it gives off dental branches to the roots of the lower teeth. These branches enter the pulp cavity as minute vessels through the apices of the roots. Other branches supply the alveolar septa, adjacent bone, and periodontal ligaments and then terminate in the gingiva. The incisive branch anastomoses with the incisive artery of the other side. The mental (from the Latin word, *mentum*, meaning "chin") branch passes through the mental foramen to emerge under the skin and anastomoses with its partner on the other side and also with labial branches on the same side.

The anastomoses of the inferior alveolar artery with branches of the labial, buccal, and submental arteries and their counterparts on the opposite side are rich. This ample blood supply not only discourages infection but also promotes healing of the fracture. For this reason, it is advisable to avoid extensive manipulation of the fragments, which could further traumatize the tissues and blood vessels.

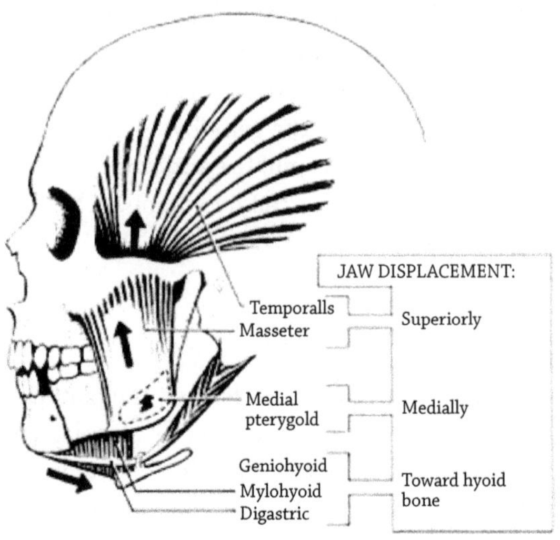

FIGURE 7.2

Displacement of the fractured mandibular body caused by the contraction of attached muscles. The temporalis and masseter pull the mandible superiorly; the medial pterygoid pulls the mandible medially; and the geniohyoid, digastric, and mylohyoid pull it toward the hyoid bone.

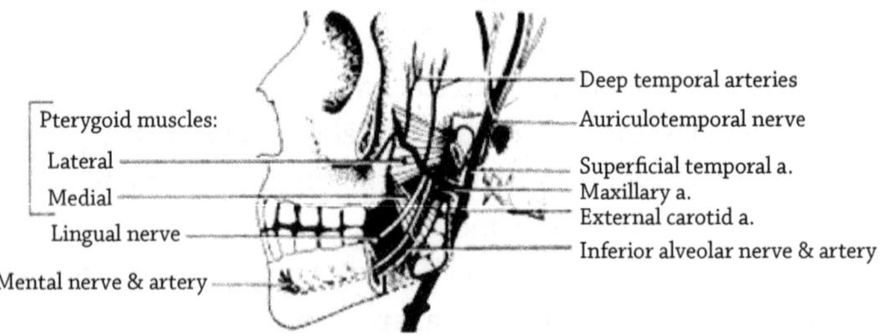

FIGURE 7.3

Lateral view of the arterial and nerve supply of the mandible. Notice the inferior alveolar artery and nerve in the mandibular canal. a., artery.

Healing of the fracture by callus formation is dependent on a sufficient blood supply to the mandible, where the blood vessels have been torn. As the resulting hematoma organizes, blood vessels proliferate and are transformed into small arteries for the supply of the callus, periosteum, cortex, and spongy portion of bone. The callus passes through various stages, from soft connective tissue into spongy and finally dense bone, which is heavily calcified. This healing process usually takes several months, which is the reason for the total immobilization of the jaws in the stage of callus formation.

Sensory Nerve Supply to the Mandible

Interference with the sensory nerve supply has taken place in this case, as indicated by the anesthesia and numbness around the chin and anterior portion of the lower lip. The inferior alveolar nerve from the mandibular division of the trigeminal nerve (V_3) has been interrupted. More important than the anesthesia around the mouth is the deficiency in the nerve supply to the anterior teeth (i.e., the incisors and canine). Loss of sensory nerve supply may result in a devitalized tooth.

The inferior alveolar nerve follows the inferior alveolar artery in its course through the mandibular canal (Fig. 7.3). It provides dental branches that form plexuses in the bone, similar to the corresponding arteries. These supply the molar and premolar teeth by fine fibers that enter the pulp cavity through the apices of the root canals. Interdental branches supply the adjacent alveolar bone, periodontal ligaments, and gingiva. As with the artery, the terminal incisive nerve continues in the direction of the inferior alveolar nerve and supplies the canine and incisor teeth, their alveolar septa, and the labial aspect of the gingiva. The mental nerve continues through the mental foramen to supply the chin and anterior lower lip.

During the healing process, slow regeneration of the nerve within the mandibular canal takes place, starting from the proximal stump of the interrupted nerve; many months may be required for complete regeneration. Other nerves, such as fibers from the gingival portions of the buccal and lingual nerves, contribute to recovery of the sensory innervation, and after some time, no sensory defect can be detected in the supply of teeth, skin, and mucosa.

8

Tracheostomy

A male infant who was born at 34 weeks of gestation with Goldenhar syndrome (oculoauriculovertebral dysplasia) presented at 6 months of age for elective tracheostomy because of upper airway obstruction and developmental anomalies of the lower respiratory tract. His history was significant for concurrent congenital heart defects requiring surgical repair. Since that time, he has experienced frequent bouts of hypoxemia, and his airway is difficult to manage. A recent serious desaturation required intubation, and the patient is currently endotracheally intubated on minimal mechanical support. However, he still has thick secretions that require suctioning and precipitate episodes of cyanosis, dyspnea, tachypnea, and use of accessory muscles of respiration.

Examination

On examination, there is no evidence of cyanosis. The head, eye, ear, nose, and throat (HEENT) examination demonstrates the following findings: the patient's right ear is totally absent, and the right side of his mouth is drawn up. The right mandible is hypoplastic. Examination of the chest reveals scattered coarse rhonchi over both lung fields. The remainder of the examination is within normal limits.

Diagnosis

The diagnosis is persistent upper airway obstruction secondary to Goldenhar syndrome requiring tracheostomy.

Therapy and Further Course

The infant is taken to the operating room and prepared for tracheostomy.

Mild general anesthesia is provided. Local anesthetic is applied to the site of the projected incision. The patient's head is fully extended by placing pillows under his shoulders. The head is stabilized by a ring at the occiput. A 2-cm transverse incision is made 1 fingerbreadth above the jugular (suprasternal) notch about halfway between the cricoid cartilage and the sternal notch. This incision passes through the skin, superficial fascia, platysma, and investing layer of the deep cervical fascia. These structures are widely retracted to give ample access to the area. All superficial veins encountered in the field are ligated and divided. The fascia over the infrahyoid muscles is incised from the thyroid cartilage to the jugular notch of the sternum, and the infrahyoid muscles are retracted laterally. The isthmus of the thyroid gland is pulled superiorly. The pretracheal fascia is incised, and the second, third, and fourth tracheal cartilages are identified (Fig. 8.1).

Nonabsorbable stay sutures are placed through the tracheal rings on either side of the midline and left in place. A vertical incision (*tracheotomy*) is made in the trachea in the midline across two or three rings. The margins of the tracheal incision are spread apart gently by the stay sutures, and the opening in the trachea (*tracheostomy*) is enlarged. The endotracheal tube is identified and gently withdrawn superiorly. A tracheostomy tube of appropriate size is then inserted, and the patency of the tube is checked. The upper and lower ends of the subcutaneous incision are closed by sutures. The tracheostomy tube is held in place by a loose tape around the neck. The margins of the skin wound and the area around the tube are covered with moist gauze dressings.

The infant is placed on mechanical ventilation. The inner tube of the tracheostomy tube is removed and cleaned frequently, and suction of the trachea is employed to aspirate mucus. Over time, the infant is able to be weaned from the ventilator and is discharged to a rehabilitation facility.

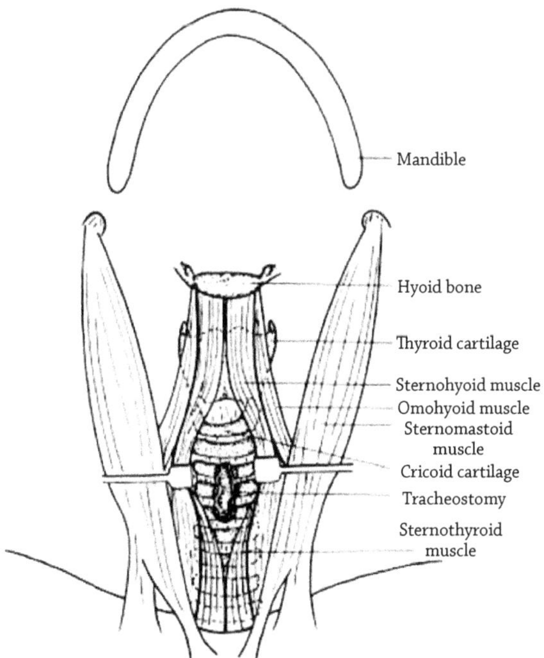

FIGURE 8.1

Site of the tracheostomy in the second, third, and fourth tracheal cartilages. Notice the structures in the midline above the tracheostomy site. Infrahyoid muscles are retracted.

Discussion

This infant has a compromised airway resulting from a rare congenital anomaly. As a consequence, he has had episodes of respiratory distress. The cyanosis observed during these episodes is caused by insufficient oxygenation of blood in the lungs and is most easily detected by inspection of the lips, where a translucent epithelium covers a rich network of blood vessels.

With dyspnea (shortness of breath), accessory muscles of respiration are called into action to add their strength to the normal respiratory muscles. The standard muscles of respiration are the diaphragm and the intercostal muscles. Contraction of the diaphragm increases the superoinferior dimension of the thorax, and contraction of the intercostal muscles can increase the anteroposterior and transverse diameters of the thorax. The accessory muscles of respiration can include any muscle that has an attachment on the chest wall. For example, the scalene muscles attach from the cervical vertebrae to the first and second ribs. Their contraction can elevate these ribs, and by action of the intercostal muscles the other ribs are also elevated, thus expanding the volume of the thorax. The serratus anterior and pectoralis major and minor muscles attach from the scapula and humerus to the chest wall. If the upper limb is fixed by contraction of other muscles, contraction of these muscles will pull on the chest wall, thereby expanding the thoracic volume. Although the thoracic attachment of these muscles is usually thought of as the origin and the upper limb attachment as the insertion, in this use of these muscles, the origin and insertion are reversed.

In forced expiration, maximal contraction of the abdominal muscles is called into play to enhance the action of the normal expulsive forces of the elastic recoil of the ribs.

Tracheostomy is the surgical formation of an artificial opening in the trachea. Tracheostomy is indicated in this case to establish an open airway in the presence of upper airway obstruction.

The patient's neck is placed into full extension in order to lengthen the trachea by pulling it upward from the mediastinum. Additionally, neck extension causes anterior displacement of the trachea into the operative field due to the increased anterior convexity of the cervical portion of the vertebral column. It also tenses the skin and fascia of the anterior neck to facilitate the skin incision. Care is taken to position the neck in a straight line with the superior notch of the thyroid cartilage, trachea, and jugular notch of the sternum in the midline for better identification of the trachea. This is especially important in infants because of the small size of the trachea. Rotation of the head and neck, as may occur under emergency conditions, leads to displacement of the trachea and may induce the operator to miss the trachea entirely and insert the tracheostomy tube into the lax paratracheal connective tissue.

Cervical Fascia Encountered in Tracheostomy

Immediately deep to the skin of the neck is the superficial fascia (subcutaneous layer). In addition to loose connective tissue and some fat, this layer contains the platysma muscle, a skeletal muscle of facial expression. All other fascial layers present in the anterior triangle of the neck are derivatives of the deep fascia of the neck (Fig. 8.2). The first fascial layer that is incised in approaching the trachea, after the skin and superficial fascia have been retracted, is the investing layer of the deep cervical fascia. This layer bridges the anterior triangle, from one sternocleidomastoid muscle to the other, as a sheet with offshoots that surround the infrahyoid muscles. The investing layer of the deep cervical fascia splits inferiorly to attach to both anterior and posterior aspects of the manubrium of the sternum, thus forming a suprasternal space that extends upward for a variable distance. It is, therefore, frequently opened in tracheostomy. Along with fat and possibly some lymph nodes, the suprasternal space contains an important anastomosis between the right and left anterior jugular veins, often called the *jugular arch vein*.

Deep to the investing layer of fascia near the anterior midline are the infrahyoid muscles. The sternohyoid is the more superficial,

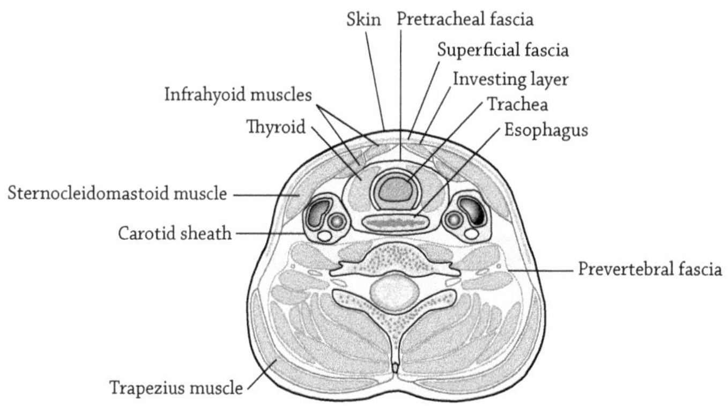

FIGURE 8.2

Fascial layers of the neck.

and the sternothyroid is the deeper. It is the sternothyroid muscles that converge from the thyroid cartilage to the midline at the site of their attachment to the posterior surface of the manubrium and thus make the operative field narrow if a low tracheostomy is undertaken (Fig. 8.1).

The next fascial layer that must be divided is the pretracheal fascia, another part of the deep cervical fascia. It covers the larynx and trachea and forms a sheath for the thyroid gland. It continues inferiorly behind the sternum into the mediastinum.

Landmarks in the Midline

With the cutting of the pretracheal fascia, the level of the trachea has been reached, and it is now time to review the important landmarks in the infrahyoid part of the midline of the neck. Identify these on yourself by palpation, and with the help of a mirror point them out, passing from superior to inferior.

The hyoid bone is a subcutaneous structure that can be easily felt below the mandible and above the larynx. It is somewhat moveable from side to side. Inferior to the hyoid bone and connected to it by the thyrohyoid membrane is the thyroid cartilage, which is characterized by the laryngeal prominence in the midline (the "Adam's apple") and the laminae of the thyroid cartilage on each side of the prominence. These structures form the superior thyroid notch just superior to the prominence. Inferior to the thyroid cartilage, the arch of the cricoid cartilage can be palpated. Connecting these two cartilages in the midline is the strong cricothyroid ligament. Below the cricoid cartilage are the tracheal rings, which give the trachea its corrugated surface. Partly covering the trachea in the midline is the isthmus of the thyroid gland, which covers the second, the third, and sometimes the fourth tracheal ring. The trachea recedes as it descends toward the mediastinum.

In infants, the neck is very short, so the field of operation is quite small. The isthmus of the thyroid gland can be easily dislodged by retracting it upward or downward and snipping through the loose fibrous tissue that attaches it to the trachea. It can also be bisected and the parts retracted after ligation of bleeding vessels.

Larynx, Trachea, and Esophagus

If the correct site of tracheostomy is not properly identified by palpation, tracheostomy may be done too far superiorly. In that case, the cricoid and even the thyroid cartilages may be damaged, and laryngeal stenosis and severe interference with the voice may result.

The approximately 20 rings of hyaline cartilage, which form the supporting framework of the trachea, occupy only two-thirds of the tracheal circumference; they are U-shaped and open posteriorly. The membranous portion of the trachea, consisting of fibrous connective tissue and smooth muscle, closes this gap posteriorly.

Immediately posterior to the membranous posterior wall of the trachea is the esophagus. During tracheostomy, the posterior membranous portion of the trachea may be perforated, particularly in emergency operations, and a tracheoesophageal communication may be established. Such an accident would allow liquids and solid food to be aspirated into the lung through the fistula, causing an aspiration pneumonia. This complication is more apt to occur in infants because of their small tracheas, the diameter of which may be further reduced by protrusion of the anterior esophageal wall into the lumen of the trachea during swallowing and coughing spells. In small children, under emergency conditions, even the anterior surface of the vertebral column located just posterior to the esophagus may be injured by the knife of the surgeon.

In emergency situations in adults, an artificial airway is typically made through the cricothyroid membrane rather than the trachea as a lifesaving operation under adverse and catastrophic conditions. The procedure is termed *cricothyroidotomy*. When this approach is used, there is little risk of perforating the posterior wall of the airway, because the cricoid cartilage, which is located immediately above the trachea, is a complete cartilaginous ring and therefore has a cartilaginous posterior wall that protects the esophagus against perforation. The greater ease of locating and palpating the cricothyroid membrane makes this procedure easier to perform. However, the more superior location of entrance into the airway increases the risk of damage to the larynx and may not bypass the region of obstruction of the airway if the obstruction is below the level of the cricoid cartilage. This procedure is not performed in children because of the risk of damage to the vocal mechanism.

Complications of Tracheostomy

One of the most troublesome and occasionally fatal complications of tracheostomy, particularly when it is performed under emergency conditions, is hemorrhage from veins and arteries. Because one of the prime requirements of an orderly tracheostomy is to stay in the midline, the first question that arises is, Are there blood vessels of any size in the midline that may be endangered?

The following structures are noteworthy (Fig. 8.3):

1. The communication between the anterior jugular veins that crosses the midline within the suprasternal space has been mentioned previously.
2. The left brachiocephalic vein is apt to be located above the jugular notch in infants and children and may cause technical difficulties and severe complications in low tracheostomy.
3. The inferior thyroid vein, instead of being paired, may be unpaired, and the right and left veins may unite to form a single large vein that runs in the midline and usually drains into the left brachiocephalic vein.
4. In 10% of all persons, an additional artery to the thyroid gland arises from either the brachiocephalic trunk, the arch of the aorta, or the right common carotid artery. It is named the lowest thyroid, or *thyroid ima* (lowest) artery, and it can be quite large. It may ascend in the midline in front of the trachea on its way to the thyroid gland and may complicate the operation.
5. Rarely, the brachiocephalic trunk may ascend above the jugular notch and be endangered in the operation.

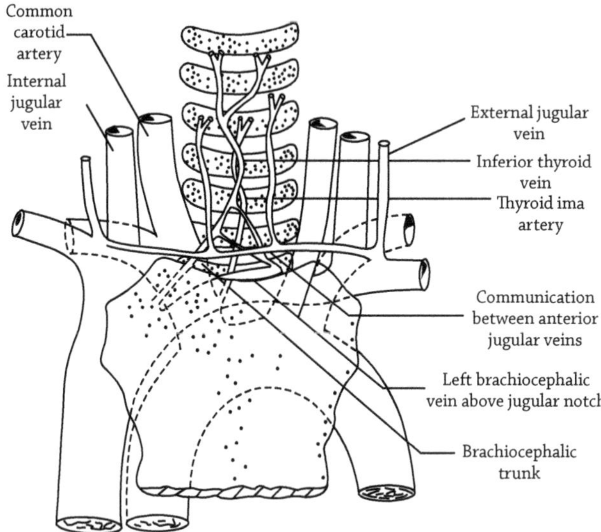

FIGURE 8.3

Potential sites of blood vessel injuries in tracheostomy as listed in text.

6. Although it is difficult to conceive, and only understandable if emergency conditions in a very restless, suffocating child are visualized, the common carotid artery, the internal jugular vein, or the recurrent laryngeal nerve may be injured. Such cases have been reported.

The brachiocephalic veins are cervical structures in infants and occupy a position of considerable danger, especially if they are distended as a result of intrathoracic pathology. The cupola, or dome of the cervical pleura, reaches upward above the clavicle and comes into the surgical field if the surgeon strays laterally from the midline. A resultant pneumothorax should be suspected if respiratory distress occurs after insertion of the tracheostomy tube.

The sternocleidomastoid muscle overlies and protects the carotid sheath and its contents. Under proper operating room conditions, venous hemorrhage and bleeding from an injured thyroid ima artery can be controlled by ligation of the damaged vessel without further consequences to the patient.

In infants, a large thymus may protrude into the neck in front of the trachea and cause some operative difficulties in low tracheostomy. Moreover, the neck in infants is relatively short, and the trachea is softer, more mobile, and quite small (no larger than a pencil), so that the esophagus and adjacent blood vessels are readily endangered by the surgeon's knife.

If the skin is closed too tightly around the tracheostomy tube, expired air may be forced into the tissues of the neck, causing a subcutaneous accumulation of air (emphysema) in the loose tissue of the cervical region. Because the loose connective tissue of the neck continues into the mediastinum, it is anatomically possible for this air to leak gradually downward into the mediastinum and cause circulatory embarrassment by compressing the large vessels of the mediastinum. If the resulting mediastinal emphysema is disregarded and remains untreated, the air may rupture into the pleural cavity and cause filling of the pleural sac (pneumothorax). If this happens on both sides, it can quickly become disastrous. Infection may likewise travel from the site of the tracheostomy down into the mediastinum and cause serious complications.

An emergency tracheostomy can have up to five times as many complications as an elective procedure in the operating room and should be done only in the last resort as a lifesaving measure. Cricothyroidotomy is preferred in adults under such dire conditions. Elective open tracheostomy is done less frequently now; it has been replaced in many cases by a percutaneous approach.

Goldenhar Syndrome

Goldenhar syndrome, also known as oculoauriculovertebral dysplasia, is a genetic syndrome that affects the morphology of many structures of the head and neck. Many of the structural anomalies are related to derivatives of the neural crest component of the first and second pharyngeal arches. These include abnormalities of the mandible, maxilla, palate, external ear, and middle ear as well as multiple other structural abnormalities.

9

Parathyroidectomy

A 37-year-old female presented to her physician's office with a 2-year history of generalized fatigue and depression associated with difficulty concentrating and significant mood swings. She had no significant past medical or family history and took no medications. She was a nonsmoker and denied recreational use of drugs or alcohol. Her physical examination was noncontributory. After the evaluation, the patient was prescribed an antidepressant and scheduled for a follow-up visit in 3 months.

Two months after her initial visit, the patient presents to the emergency department complaining of severe right-sided flank pain. The pain is constant, waxing and waning in intensity, and she rates it 10 out of 10 at its worst. The pain radiates to the right groin.

Physical Examination

On physical examination, the patient is found to be afebrile and tachycardic to 100 bpm. The remaining vital signs are normal. The head, eye, ear, nose and throat (HEENT) examination and lung and heart examinations are all normal. The patient has right costovertebral angle tenderness, in addition to moderate right-sided abdominal tenderness, without peritoneal signs. A urinalysis demonstrates 2+ hematuria. A noncontrast spiral computed tomography scan of the abdomen is performed and demonstrates multiple right intrarenal calculi with associated hydronephrosis (dilatation of the calyces). Laboratory evaluation reveals a serum calcium concentration of 12.8 mg/dL (normal range, 8.5–10.2 mg/dL). Subsequent determination of the serum parathyroid levels reveals a parathyroid hormone (PTH) concentration of 125 pg/mL (normal range, 25–65 pg/mL).

Diagnosis

Primary hyperparathyroidism is diagnosed.

Therapy and Further Course

The need for surgical exploration of her parathyroid glands is discussed with and agreed to by the patient. The patient is placed in the supine position. Under general anesthesia, the patient's neck is extended and the head is placed on a foam donut to ensure stability. The thyroid cartilage and the suprasternal notch, which are landmarks for the incision, are identified and palpated. A transverse incision is made about 2.0 cm above the suprasternal notch between the medial borders of the sternocleidomastoid muscles. The incision is extended through the skin and subcutaneous fat to the platysma muscle, which is then divided by electrocautery. An avascular plane is entered deep to the muscle, allowing the creation of superior and inferior flaps that are retracted to facilitate exposure. The midline is identified, and the fascial plane is divided with the use of electrocautery, exposing the infrahyoid strap muscles. The dissection proceeds until the thyroid isthmus is identified.

Gentle traction is exerted on the left thyroid lobe. A plane is gently developed between the overlying strap muscles and the left lobe of the thyroid, allowing the muscles to be retracted to the left. Once the lateral edge of the left thyroid lobe is reached, the middle thyroid vein is identified, and the carotid sheath is visualized posteriorly. The middle thyroid vein is then divided between sutures. With continued medial rotation of the thyroid, the tissues posterior to the thyroid are identified and inspected. The inferior thyroid artery is identified after blunt dissection of the areolar tissue anterior and medial to the common carotid artery and posteromedial to the thyroid lobe. The recurrent laryngeal nerve is identified next, inferior and lateral to the lower lobe of the thyroid gland. The intersection of the inferior thyroid artery and the recurrent laryngeal nerve is identified. Most parathyroid glands, superior and inferior, are located within 2 cm of this area, with the superior glands found dorsal to the upper two-thirds of the thyroid lobe and posterior to the recurrent laryngeal nerve. The inferior glands, which are more variable in location, can usually be found inferior to the inferior thyroid artery and anterior to the recurrent laryngeal nerve.

No obvious masses are initially identified. However, gentle palpation is performed, and a small mass about the size of an olive is identified off the superior pole of the thyroid. At that time, blood is drawn and the PTH levels are checked and found to be elevated at 110 pg/mL. The mass is then carefully isolated by blunt dissection with a sponge. The inferior pole of the thyroid is examined, and a parathyroid of normal size is identified. Exploration of the right side is then performed. The right superior parathyroid is also identified in its normal position and also appears to be normal. Biopsies of each of the identified glands are taken, and parathyroid tissue is confirmed by frozen section. However, the location of the right inferior gland is not immediately apparent. The superior thyroid vessels are identified and the right carotid sheath is opened, without identification of the fourth gland. The right tracheoesophageal groove is then carefully palpated by entering the groove through the space immediately superior to the inferior thyroid artery. No masses are identified.

At this time, attention is turned to the presumptive adenoma on the left. Care is taken to delineate the adenoma's relationship to the recurrent laryngeal nerve and to preserve this structure uninjured throughout the dissection. After complete mobilization, the adenoma's vascular pedicle is ligated using silk suture. The mass is removed and sent for frozen section. About 10 minutes later, a second blood sample is sent to measure the PTH levels. The PTH remains elevated at 95 pg/mL, suggesting that the patient may be suffering from parathyroid hyperplasia or that a second adenoma is present. At this time, the neck is closed in layers with the plan being to obtain further imaging studies to locate the missing parathyroid gland.

Discussion

Parathyroid Glands

The parathyroid glands are closely associated with, but separate from, the thyroid gland. Most people (84%) have four parathyroid glands (superior and inferior on the right and left); most of the remainder have five or more glands, and a few people (3%) have three glands. PTH is essential for the regulation of calcium. PTH causes the release of calcium from bones to increase serum calcium levels. This patient was diagnosed with primary hyperparathyroidism, meaning that an excessive amount of PTH was being secreted, not caused by some other factor such as hypocalcemia. Primary hyperparathyroidism is the most common cause of hypercalcemia; in this patient, primary hyperparathyroidism was the cause of the renal calculi and possibly of her depressive symptoms as well.

The mnemonic, *Stones, bones, abdominal moans, and psychic groans,* has been used to describe the constellation of symptoms and signs of hypercalcemia. "Stones" refers to nephrolithiasis or nephrocalcinosis; "bones" refers to musculoskeletal complications such as osteoporosis and osteitis fibrosa cystica; "abdominal moans" refers to gastrointestinal complications such as constipation, peptic ulcer disease, and pancreatitis; and "psychic groans" refers to neuropsychiatric complications such as depression, psychosis, and personality changes.

In 90% of cases, primary hyperparathyroidism is caused by an adenoma (a benign tumor) of one of the parathyroid glands. Multiple adenomas are present in a small number of patients (4%), and parathyroid hyperplasia accounts for approximately 6% of cases of primary hyperparathyroidism. Surgical excision of the abnormal gland usually provides a cure. It should be noted that the parathyroid adenoma in this patient was not excised until after other, normal parathyroid tissue was identified. Because of the critical role that PTH plays in calcium regulation, the chance cannot be taken of excising the only source of PTH from the patient.

The parathyroid glands are usually 4 to 6 mm in diameter and 1 to 2 mm thick; they are located on the posterior surface of the lateral lobes of the thyroid gland. However, because of the developmental migration of the parathyroid glands (discussed later), they are sometimes found in abnormal locations.

Infrahyoid Muscles and Cervical Fascia

The thyroid gland lies posterior to the infrahyoid (strap) muscles. The surgical approach to the thyroid gland from the anterior midline requires that these muscles be moved out of the way. The anterior incision passes through the skin and superficial fascia. Contained within the superficial fascia of the anterior neck is the platysma muscle, a skeletal muscle that is innervated by the cervical branch of the facial nerve. Deep to this muscle is found the investing layer of the deep cervical fascia, which crosses from one sternocleidomastoid muscle to the other. Deep to the investing fascia is the infrahyoid fascia, which encloses the infrahyoid muscles. The infrahyoid muscles in this region include the sternohyoid muscle, which is close to the midline and attaches to the sternum below and to the hyoid bone above. Lateral to the sternohyoid muscle is the superior belly of the omohyoid muscle; it ascends from its intermediate tendon, which is tethered to the clavicle, to the hyoid bone. Deep to the sternohyoid muscle is found the sternothyroid muscle, connecting the sternum to the thyroid cartilage, and the thyrohyoid muscle, connecting the thyroid cartilage to the hyoid bone. All of the infrahyoid muscles are innervated by cervical spinal nerves by way of the cervical plexus.

The sternohyoid and sternothyroid muscles, which are close to the midline, lie anterior to the thyroid gland. Incision of the infrahyoid fascia in the midline and mobilization of the fascial plane between the infrahyoid muscles and the pretracheal fascia allows the infrahyoid muscles to be retracted laterally to provide access to the thyroid gland. The pretracheal fascia encircles the visceral compartment of the neck and contains within it the trachea, the thyroid gland, and the parathyroid glands. This is the last layer of cervical fascia that must be incised to reach the thyroid gland (see Fig. 8.2 in Chapter 8 for cervical fascia).

Blood Supply

The parathyroid glands receive their blood supply from branches of the thyroid arteries. There is usually a superior and an inferior thyroid artery on each side (Fig. 9.1). The superior thyroid artery is the first branch of the external carotid artery; it descends toward the upper pole of the lateral lobe of the thyroid gland. The inferior thyroid artery is a branch of the thyrocervical trunk, which arises from the subclavian artery, immediately distal to the origin of the vertebral artery. The inferior thyroid artery approaches the inferior portion of the lateral lobe of the thyroid gland from an inferolateral direction. In approximately 10% of people, there is an additional artery, the thyroid ima artery. This arises from the arch of the aorta or the brachiocephalic trunk and ascends in the midline in front of the trachea to reach the isthmus of the thyroid gland.

There are commonly three thyroid veins on each side. The superior thyroid vein drains into the internal jugular vein and travels parallel with the superior thyroid artery. The middle thyroid vein also drains into the internal jugular vein. It approaches the thyroid gland from the lateral side and is not accompanied by an artery. In this patient, because of the lateral approach of the middle thyroid vein, it was identified, ligated, and divided to allow reflection of the lateral edge of the thyroid gland. The right and left inferior thyroid veins have courses close to the midline; they may each drain into their respective brachiocephalic veins, or they may join to form a common vein that typically drains into the left brachiocephalic vein near the midline.

Laryngeal Nerves

The innervation to the mucosa of the larynx and the muscles of the larynx is by way of the superior laryngeal nerve and the recurrent laryngeal nerve, both of which are branches of the vagus nerve. The

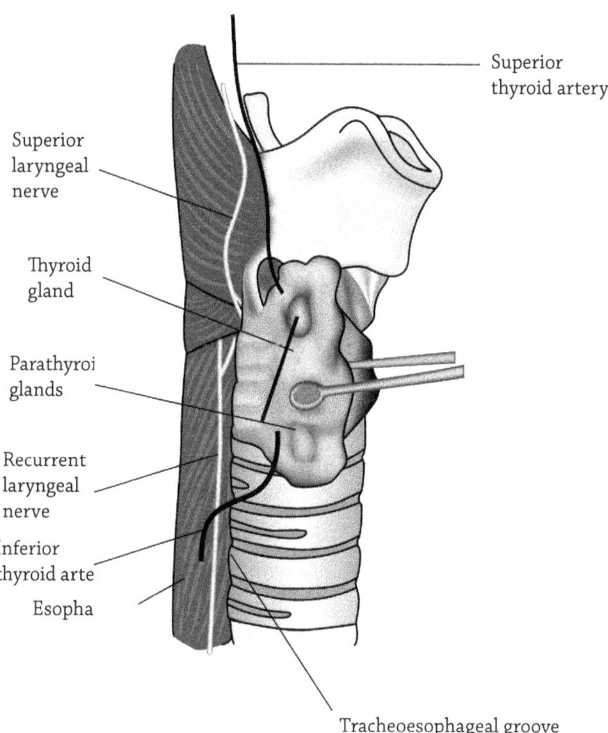

FIGURE 9.1

Thyroid and parathyroid glands and their blood supply.

superior laryngeal nerve divides into an internal and an external branch. The internal branch pierces the thyrohyoid membrane to reach the interior of the larynx and innervates the mucosa above the vocal folds. The external branch continues down to innervate the cricothyroid muscle. This branch parallels the superior thyroid artery in part of its course, and care must be taken to protect this nerve if it is necessary to ligate the superior thyroid artery during thyroid surgery. Inadvertent injury to this nerve will adversely affect vocal quality.

The recurrent laryngeal nerve on the left branches from the left vagus in the thorax as the vagus passes in front of the aortic arch. The left recurrent laryngeal nerve passes under the aortic arch, immediately to the left of the ligamentum arteriosum, and then ascends to the larynx. In its course to the larynx, the nerve passes immediately behind the thyroid gland in close proximity to the inferior thyroid artery. Typically, the nerve and artery cross approximately perpendicular to one another with the nerve either anterior or posterior to the artery. As indicated earlier, the four parathyroid glands are usually found within 2 cm of this intersection, with the superior glands above the intersection and the inferior glands below. This close proximity of nerve, artery, and glands mandates that great care be taken in identifying the recurrent laryngeal nerve when doing thyroid surgery. Injury to this nerve will result in weakness of almost all laryngeal muscles on the injured side and greatly affects vocalization. Injury to the nerve bilaterally results in apposition of both vocal cords, which can emergently compromise the airway.

On the right, the relationship between the inferior thyroid artery and the recurrent laryngeal nerve is similar; however, because the right recurrent laryngeal nerve arises higher than on the left and recurs around the right subclavian artery, its course to the larynx is somewhat less vertical and follows a more horizontal course as it crosses the artery. On both sides, the nerves enter the tracheoesophageal groove after passing behind the thyroid, to continue their ascents to the larynx.

Development of the Parathyroid Glands

The parathyroid glands arise from the endoderm of the third and fourth pharyngeal pouches. Although it is clear that neural crest cells underlying this endoderm play a role in parathyroid development, it is not clear whether neural crest cells actually contribute to the parathyroid or whether they have an inductive relationship with the endoderm that forms the parathyroid.

The superior parathyroid glands are derived from the cells of the fourth pharyngeal pouch. These cells do not have to migrate very far to get to their eventual location, and therefore there is relatively little variability in their location. The inferior parathyroid glands,

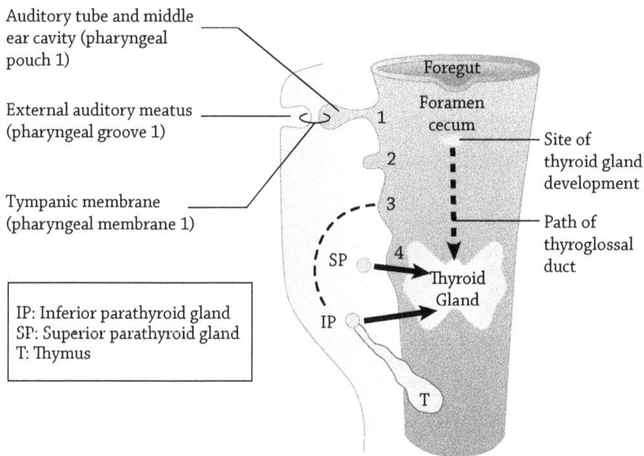

FIGURE 9.2

Development of the parathyroid glands from the third and fourth pharyngeal pouches. IP, inferior parathyroid; SP, superior parathyroid; T, thymus; UB, ultimobranchial body. (Courtesy of Kaplan Medical.)

on the other hand, arise from the third pharyngeal pouch. These cells must migrate further and therefore there is greater variability in their location. Because other cells of the third pharyngeal pouch form the thymus in the thorax, sometimes parathyroid tissue from the third pouch can also be found in the thorax along with the thymus (Fig. 9.2). The fact that an inferior parathyroid gland could not be identified in the neck of this patient necessitates further imaging before proceeding into the chest.

Imaging of the Parathyroid Glands

The patient was referred for imaging studies to locate the additional parathyroid tissue that might be the source of the continued elevated PTH levels. Technetium 99m (Tc^{99m})-sestamibi single-photon emission computed tomography (SPECT) is used to identify parathyroid tissue. Tc^{99m}-sestamibi is an agent used in nuclear medicine imaging. It is injected intravenously and is taken up by the chief cells of the parathyroid tissue. The radioactive decay then allows imaging of the location of the parathyroid tissue.

With preoperative imaging of the parathyroid glands and intraoperative monitoring of PTH levels, minimally invasive parathyroidectomy is now possible with a high degree of success.

Intraoperative Monitoring of Parathyroid Hormone Levels

Intraoperative monitoring of PTH levels was used in this patient to determine whether the source of the excess PTH secretion had been removed. The half-life of PTH is very short (3–5 minutes); if removal of the adenoma had resolved the patient's problem, there would have been a significant reduction in PTH 10 minutes after the adenoma was removed. If the postexcision level of PTH is half or less than half of the preexcision level, the procedure can be considered a success, and it can be anticipated that PTH levels will continue to decline. Because this patient had only a 14% decline in PTH, it is assumed that an additional source of the excess PTH is present that was not identified at the time of surgery. It is hoped that the imaging study will identify the location of this tissue.

Reference

Marcocci C, Cetani F: Clinical practice: Primary hyperthyroidism [erratum appears in *N Engl J Med* 366:2138, 2012]. *N Engl J Med* 365:2389–2397, 2011.

10

Penetrating Injury to the Neck

A 22-year-old man presents to the emergency department after being accidentally shot in the neck with a 0.22-caliber air rifle at a distance of approximately 10 feet. He complains of pain and fullness on the right side of his neck at the site of penetration of the "BB" pellet, accompanied by mild pain with swallowing. He reports no weakness or loss of consciousness. He reports no voice changes or cough. He has had no bloody sputum and is not short of breath. The patient has no significant past medical or surgical history, has no allergies, and is taking no medications. He is a nonsmoker.

Examination

On physical examination, the patient's vital signs are in the normal range, with a blood pressure of 110/65 mm Hg, a heart rate of 76 bpm, and a respiratory rate of 12 breaths/min. Evaluation of the neck reveals an entry wound approximately at the level of the hyoid bone to the right of the midline. There is no exit wound, and the BB is not palpable. A firm, nonpulsatile hematoma, 3 to 4 cm in diameter, is evident deep to the entry wound. No active bleeding is present. Auscultation over the hematoma reveals no bruits. Palpation reveals no subcutaneous emphysema or thrill. The trachea is in the midline, and the thyroid is nonpalpable. Cranial nerves II through XII are intact bilaterally, and the neurological examination demonstrates no deficits. The remainder of the physical examination is within normal limits.

Diagnosis

The diagnosis is penetrating injury to the neck.

Evaluation and Further Course

Cervical spine radiographs demonstrate an airgun pellet embedded in the soft tissues of the right neck and a surrounding mass of 4-cm diameter with a density consistent with hematoma. There is no air in the soft tissue and no deviation of the trachea by the hematoma. A computed tomography scan of the neck reveals a 4 cm by 5 cm hematoma extending from the carotid sheath into the surrounding tissue with the pellet located immediately adjacent. There is no extravasation of intravascular contrast. A marker placed on the entrance wound site reveals the track of the pellet in proximity to the carotid sheath but away from the pharynx. No air is identified in the soft tissues; however, a flexible endoscopic examination is performed to exclude pharyngeal or laryngeal injury. The location of the entrance wound and the underlying hematoma suggest the possibility of injury to a major vessel, and the decision is made to explore the neck in the operating room.

After induction of general anesthesia, the patient is positioned with the head turned toward the left to expose the right sternocleidomastoid (SCM) muscle. An incision is made in the skin parallel to the anterior border of the muscle, extending through the skin and platysma muscle. After incision of the fascia overlying the SCM and retraction of the muscle laterally, the hematoma is encountered and evacuated, revealing an entrance wound in the carotid sheath. On further inspection, there is continuous pulsatile flow of bright red blood from the site. With an arterial injury suspected, proximal and distal control of the carotid artery and its branches is obtained. On entry into the carotid sheath, an injury to the internal carotid artery is evident. Repair of the injury is performed using 6-0 nonabsorbable suture. No patch is required. Examination of the common and external carotid arteries, internal jugular vein, and vagus nerve reveal no evidence of injury. The BB pellet is palpated immediately posterior to the sheath and is removed. The incision is then closed.

The patient is neurologically intact and does well postoperatively. He is discharged home on the second postoperative day.

Discussion

Injuries to the neck can present a management challenge because of the concentration of vital structures in a small anatomic space. Fatality rates for penetrating neck trauma in the civilian population range from 3% to 6%. The most commonly injured structure, in both civilian and combat injuries, is the carotid artery, followed by the trachea and larynx (10%) and the esophagus (6%). Other structural injuries of significance include nerve injuries and injuries to the vertebral artery or the internal jugular vein. Despite its size, injuries to the thyroid are rare.

With civilian trauma, an injury is not considered to have penetrated the neck unless the platysma muscle layer was penetrated. The platysma is a superficial muscle in the neck that lies in the superficial fascia just deep to the skin. It originates in the superficial fascia overlying the pectoralis major and deltoid muscles and inserts onto the inferior border of the mandible. The most anterior fibers of the right and left platysma decussate before attaching to the mandible, and the muscle blends in with other facial muscles in the region. The action of the muscle is either to depress the mandible or to pull up on the skin of the neck and upper chest. When contracting, the platysma creates vertical ridges in the skin of the neck. Like other muscles of facial expression, it is innervated by a branch of the facial nerve. Penetration through this superficial muscle layer indicates real risk to the vital structures below and historically governs the need to perform further workup on the patient, either a neck exploration or a series of noninvasive studies to evaluate the vasculature and aerodigestive tracts.

Regions of the Neck

The neck is classically divided into a number of triangles. The two largest triangles, the anterior triangle and the posterior triangle, are separated by the SCM muscle (Fig. 10.1). The SCM muscle originates from the anterior surface of the sternum and the sternal end of the clavicle, and its insertion is into the mastoid

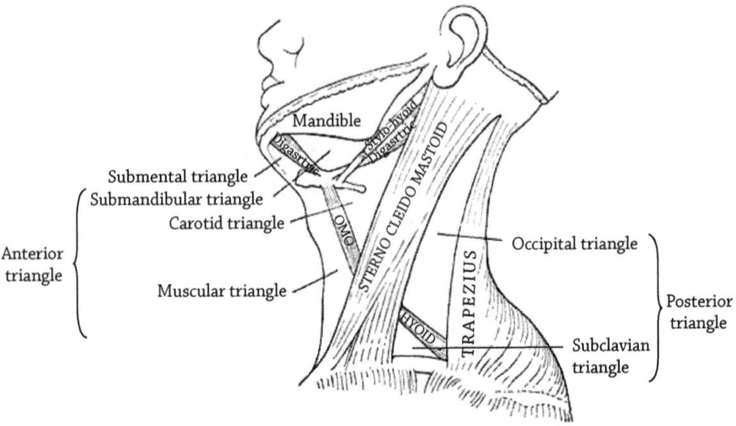

FIGURE 10.1

Regions of the neck.

process and the superior nuchal line. When acting unilaterally, its action is to turn the head obliquely upward and to the opposite side. Acting bilaterally, the muscles function to flex and extend the neck.

The anterior triangle is the region bounded by the SCM, the mandible, and the midline. The posterior triangle is the region bounded by the SCM, the trapezius, and the clavicle. The anterior and posterior triangles are important to the discussion of penetrating trauma because injuries to the area of the neck posterior to the SCM muscle rarely involve the esophagus, the airway, or major vascular structures. Most of these vital structures are located in the anterior or lateral regions. Injury in the posterior triangle may endanger the neurovascular supply to the upper limb.

Classically, the anterior triangle is further subdivided into four smaller triangles. The digastric (or submandibular) triangle is bounded by the two bellies of the digastric muscle and the mandible. The submental triangle is bounded by the anterior belly of the digastric, the mandible and the midline. The carotid triangle is bounded by the posterior belly of the digastric, the superior belly of the omohyoid and the SCM. The muscular triangle is bounded by the superior belly of the omohyoid, the SCM, and the midline.

For trauma evaluations, the anterior region of the neck has classically been divided into three zones, using anatomic landmarks and dividing the neck into horizontal planes. Each zone has a group of vital structures that can be injured and therefore can determine the kind of trauma management. Zone I is the horizontal area between the clavicle and suprasternal notch and the cricoid cartilage, representing the base of the neck and the thoracic outlet structures. The proximal common carotid, vertebral, and subclavian arteries and the trachea, esophagus, thoracic duct, thyroid, parathyroid, and thymus are located in zone I. Injuries in this region historically have the highest mortality because of the risk of major vascular and intrathoracic injury. Zone II is the area between the cricoid cartilage and the angle of the mandible. Because it is the largest region, injuries to this area are most common. Zone II contains the distal common carotid and internal and external carotid arteries, jugular veins, pharynx, larynx, esophagus, and recurrent laryngeal nerves. Zone III is the area that lies between the angle of the mandible and the base of the skull. It contains the distal extracranial carotid and vertebral arteries and the uppermost segments of the jugular veins.

Surgical Exposure

This patient's entrance wound is located in zone II. The presence of the overlying hematoma, in conjunction with imaging studies suggesting that the pellet penetrated the carotid sheath, warrants surgical exploration. Certainly, the patient needs to be evaluated for clinical signs that would indicate significant injury to a major structure. With regard to a major vascular injury, these signs include an expanding hematoma, active external hemorrhage, or decreased carotid pulse. Selecting an operative incision that allows easy access to these important structures is therefore warranted. This can be accomplished by using an incision parallel to the anterior border of the SCM muscle. This incision can be used to expose the carotid sheath, the pharynx, and the cervical esophagus, and it also can be extended both superiorly and inferiorly should additional exposure be warranted.

With the patient in the supine position, the head is turned away from the side of exploration. The entire neck and side of the face and head are prepped and draped. The incision is then made along the anterior border of the SCM muscle and is carried through the dermis and the platysma. After the platysma has been divided in the direction of the incision, the fascia overlying the anterior border of the SCM muscle (the investing layer of fascia) is incised, and the muscle is retracted laterally and posteriorly to expose the carotid sheath.

The tight fascial compartments of neck structures may limit hemorrhage from vascular injuries, minimizing the chance of exsanguination, as was the case in this patient. However, these tight fascial boundaries may increase the risk of airway compromise, because the airway is relatively mobile and compressible by an expanding hematoma. This may be assessed by palpating the position of the trachea at the sternal notch or. alternatively, evaluating its position on cervical radiographs, as was done in this case.

Fascia of the Neck

The deep fascia of the neck is divided into several layers (Fig. 10.2). Immediately deep to the superficial fascia is the outermost layer of deep fascia, which is called the *investing fascia* because it covers all the other layers. The investing fascia splits to enclose each of the SCM muscles and each trapezius muscle. In the posterior midline, it attaches to the spinous processes of the vertebrae.

Deep within the neck, there are two compartments, each surrounded by a layer of fascia. The *prevertebral fascia* surrounds a compartment that contains the vertebral column and the muscles related to the anterior, posterior, and lateral sides of the vertebral column. Included among these muscles are the longus colli anteriorly, the scalene muscles laterally, and the erector spinae, splenius, and semispinalis muscles posteriorly. Anterior to this compartment, the *pretracheal (visceral) fascia* surrounds a compartment that contains

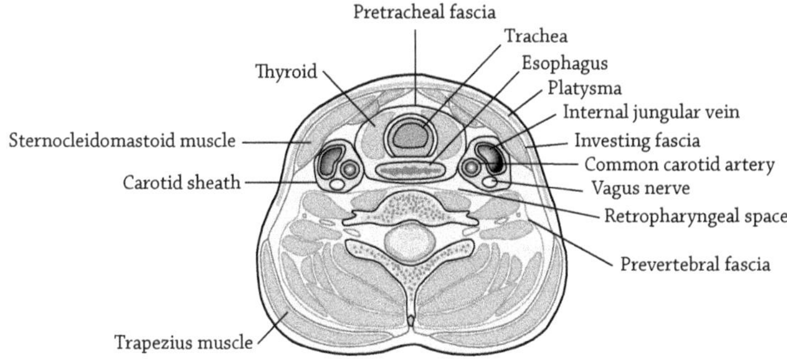

FIGURE 10.2

Fascia of the neck. Notice the carotid sheath containing the common carotid artery, internal jugular vein, and vagus nerve.

the viscera of the neck: the pharynx and esophagus, the larynx and trachea, and the thyroid and parathyroid glands. Between the prevertebral fascia and the pretracheal fascia is a fascial plane called the *retropharyngeal space*. This fascial plane allows for movement of the visceral structures within the pretracheal fascia on the more stable bones and muscles of the neck within the prevertebral fascia. It also provides a pathway for the spread of infection within the neck.

Anterior to the pretracheal fascia is the *infrahyoid fascia*, a thin layer of fascia that encloses the infrahyoid muscles. Located laterally in the neck, deep to the SCM muscle and lateral to the retropharyngeal space, are found the *carotid sheaths*. The carotid sheath is composed of fascia that is continuous with each of the other layers of deep cervical fascia. Within the carotid sheath are found the common carotid artery, the internal carotid artery, the internal jugular vein, and the vagus nerve.

Surgical Approach to the Carotid Arteries

Classic principles of vascular surgery apply. Proximal and distal control should be obtained before exploration of a carotid artery injury. Obtaining proximal control before entering a perivascular hematoma is more important than having distal control; if necessary, distal bleeding can be controlled with digital pressure while the dissection of the injured vessel is completed. For injuries near the carotid bifurcation, it is necessary to control the common, internal, and external carotid arteries as well as the proximal branches of the external carotid artery. This should be done with vessel loops; ligation of vessels should be avoided.

The common carotid artery arises within the thorax from the aortic arch on the left and from the brachiocephalic trunk on the right. The common carotid artery ascends within the carotid sheath and bifurcates at about the level of the fourth cervical vertebra, which corresponds to the upper border of the thyroid cartilage. From this point, the internal carotid artery continues to ascend within the carotid sheath but does not provide any branches within the neck. It enters the carotid canal at the base of the skull to enter the cranial cavity and supply the brain and structures within the orbit.

The external carotid artery provides many branches within the neck. Its first branch is typically the superior thyroid artery, which arises from the anterior side of the external carotid and descends to the thyroid gland. It also provides supply to the larynx. Two other important branches of the external carotid artery in the neck, which also arise from its anterior side, are the lingual and facial arteries. Arising from the posterior side of the external carotid are the occipital and posterior auricular arteries. Arising from its medial side is the ascending pharyngeal artery. The external carotid artery ends at the level of the neck of the mandible by dividing into the maxillary and superficial temporal arteries. Because there is excellent collateral circulation between the left and right superior thyroid arteries, left and right lingual arteries, and left and right facial arteries, during surgery these arteries may be occluded without concern about depriving their target organs of adequate blood supply. It is because of these extensive collateral channels that distal control of the external carotid artery is necessary in our patient.

During dissection of the carotid sheath and retraction of the jugular vein, care must be taken to avoid injuring the vagus nerve, which is within the carotid sheath posterolateral to the artery.

Division of the facial vein, which is superficial to the carotid bifurcation, facilitates jugular vein retraction.

Exposure of the proximal common carotid artery at the base of the neck may require division of the omohyoid muscle at the point where its superior and inferior bellies are joined. For proximal control of the common carotid artery, it may be necessary to enter the chest via a median sternotomy. If exposure of the distal internal carotid artery is needed, a number of important structures must be identified and protected. Of particular note is the hypoglossal nerve. Injury to the hypoglossal nerve results in impaired motor function of the tongue and can lead to dysarthria and dysphagia. Although the ansa cervicalis lies on the carotid sheath and is subject to injury during surgical procedures involving that sheath, such injury causes little or no morbidity. The ansa cervicalis provides motor innervations to several of the infrahyoid muscles.

11

Flexion-Extension Injury of the Neck

A 52-year-old female banker comes to her physician's office complaining of headaches, neck pain, and stiffness in the neck. These symptoms started 4 days ago after an automobile accident. Her car had stopped at a traffic light and was struck from the rear by another car. She states that at the time of the accident she was badly shaken and noticed immediate pain in her neck that radiated into both shoulders. However, the pain gradually resolved over the next 30 minutes, and she refused transport to the hospital for evaluation. The following day, she noticed an aching in her neck that gradually increased in severity over the next 2 days. She states that the pain is currently constant and aching, and she rates it as 9 out of 10 in severity (with 10 being most severe). The pain does not radiate to her shoulders or arms. Slight flexion, extension, or rotation of her neck increases the pain. She has taken acetaminophen and ibuprofen with no relief. She has no prior history of neck or back injury. She denies any weakness, numbness, or tingling in her extremities.

Examination

On examination, the patient's head is held rather rigid. Flexion, extension, and lateral rotation of head and neck cause pain and are resisted by the patient. There is some local tenderness on palpation, particularly over the area of the transverse processes of the fourth and fifth cervical vertebrae. A screening neurological examination, including evaluation of deep tendon reflexes and plantar responses, reveals normal findings. A thorough radiographic examination shows disappearance of the normal cervical lordosis. There are slight degenerative changes at the middle cervical vertebrae, with some bony spurs, particularly around the intervertebral foramina between C4 and C5, but the radiologist states that these alterations could be in keeping with the patient's age. The most important radiographic finding is the absence of any signs of fracture of the cervical vertebrae. Subsequent magnetic resonance imaging does not detect any evidence of disc herniation, ligamentous disruption, or muscle hematoma.

Diagnosis

The patient has a cervical spine sprain/strain injury due to hyperextension-hyperflexion (whiplash) injury caused by a rear-end traffic collision.

Therapy and Further Course

The patient is given a sponge rubberneck collar and told to wear it intermittently. She is told to apply ice packs for 5 to 10 minutes every 1 to 2 hours. Local application of ice or a cold compress is effective at reducing muscle spasm. After at least 24-hours of cryotherapy, the patient is instructed to begin gentle, active range-of-motion exercises. She is also given a prescription for physical therapy. Nonsteroidal antiinflammatory medication is prescribed, as well as a muscle relaxant, if needed. She is cautioned not to drive her car, in order to avoid sudden twisting motions of her head and neck. Under this treatment, the symptoms gradually improve.

Discussion

The term *whiplash injury* refers to the mechanism of the trauma, not to the underlying lesion. "Whiplash" describes the rapid change in motion, from hyperextension to hyperflexion of the head and the upper part of the neck in rear-end collisions and from extreme flexion to maximal extension in head-on collisions.

The term *flexion-extension syndrome due to rear-end or head-on collision* is now preferred by most clinicians instead of "whiplash injury of the neck." The broad spectrum of injuries to various tissues, with possible involvement of muscles, ligaments, cartilage, bone, spinal cord, peripheral nerve structures, and blood vessels, requires familiarity with the underlying anatomy.

In descending order of frequency, the potential tissue damage in the neck includes the following:

1. Muscle strain or sprain of the cervical ligaments
2. Rupture of the ligaments and the intervertebral disks
3. Fractures of the vertebrae
4. Injury to the cervical spinal cord and emerging cervical nerves
5. Damage to the vertebral artery with resulting interference with cerebral circulation

Underlying Anatomy of the Condition

Muscular Injuries

Muscle strains in flexion-extension injuries of the neck involve the flexors of the head, such as the sternocleidomastoid, and perhaps the rectus capitis anterior and longus capitis. These muscles lie along the anterior and anterolateral surfaces of the cervical vertebrae. The damage ranges in severity from minor tears of a few muscle fibers to partial or total avulsion (traumatic separation) of the muscular attachments to the cervical vertebrae.

Ligamentous Injuries

Ligamentous sprains are the mildest form of neck injuries. A sprain denotes a ligamentous injury with stretching of some of the fibers and tearing of others but with preservation of the continuity of the ligament. Ligaments that resist extension of the vertebral column would most likely be sprained in a forceful hyperextension of the neck; those that resist flexion would most likely be sprained with forceful hyperflexion.

The thick anterior longitudinal ligament is a broad band that extends along the anterior surface of the vertebral column from the atlas to the front of the sacrum. Its more superficial fibers bridge several vertebrae, and its deeper portions extend from one vertebral body to the next. It is particularly these deeper portions of the ligament that may be stretched or torn in hyperextension injuries (Fig. 11.1).

Hyperflexion injuries may expose the posterior longitudinal ligament to undue traction. The posterior longitudinal ligament likewise extends over all vertebrae from the neck to the sacrum, with its superficial fibers crossing several vertebrae and its deeper portions connecting adjacent vertebrae. The posterior longitudinal ligament attaches to the posterior aspect of the vertebral bodies anterior to the spinal cord and checks extreme flexion. In this function, it is

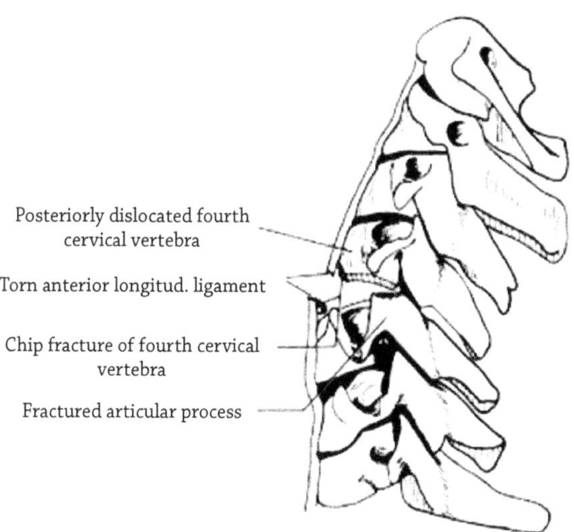

FIGURE 11.1

Depiction of extensive hyperextension injury with tearing of the anterior longitudinal ligament, posterior dislocation of the fourth cervical vertebra with chip fracture of its body, and fracture of the articular process of the fifth cervical vertebra.

assisted by the ligamenta flava, which connect the laminae of the vertebrae, and the interspinous and supraspinous ligaments. The supraspinous ligaments are particularly well developed in the neck as the ligamentum nuchae (ligament of the nape of the neck), which forms a fibrous, intermuscular septum in the midline by attaching to the bifid spinous processes. The posterior longitudinal ligament and the ligamenta flava may be stretched or torn in hyperflexion.

Intervertebral Disk Injuries

Injury to the cervical disks in rear-end collisions is considered likely by many neurologists, although these disks are "preradiographic," generally appearing normal for some time. It is also likely that these flexion-extension injuries accelerate degenerative disk disease, which does not become apparent until new bone formation and calcification are seen years after repair of the injury.

The intervertebral disk has two portions, an outer portion and an inner portion. The outer ring, or *anulus fibrosus*, consists of concentric layers of collagenous fiber bundles, which by their lamellar arrangement are able to withstand multidirectional strains. The centrally located *nucleus pulposus* consists of a soft, highly elastic, compressible, semigelatinous mass with a high water content. It acts as a shock absorber.

The cervical disks are thicker anteriorly than posteriorly and thus are responsible for the lordotic curvature of the cervical vertebral column. Degenerative changes resulting from chronic trauma and age predispose the anulus fibrosus to rupture under severe compression and the nucleus pulposus to prolapse or herniate. This is particularly apt to occur in the neck at the level of the disks between C5 and C6 and between C6 and C7.

Spinal Nerve and Cord Involvement

Because the intervertebral disk forms part of the anterior boundary of the intervertebral foramen, when the nucleus pulposus herniates in a posterolateral direction, it may compress a cervical spinal nerve passing through this foramen. Such a nerve compression explains the occurrence of nerve root symptoms such as shoulder pain and paresthesias (burning and tingling) in the affected dermatomes, which can be perceived as far distally as the fingers if there is involvement of C6 and C7. The commonly observed reflex spasm of the neck muscles with straightening of the normal curvature of the spine is another effect of nerve or nerve root irritation. Most serious is a protrusion of the disk in, or close to, the midline, which leads to cervical spinal cord compression.

Vertebral Injuries and Dislocations

There is a gradual transition in severity from the relatively harmless, common stretching of the anterior longitudinal ligament to its rupture, wrenching, displacement of the disks, and chip fracture of the anteroinferior corners of the vertebral bodies (Fig. 11.1). If the trauma is more destructive, the articular processes of the vertebrae may also fracture, and the upper part of the cervical vertebral column may be dislocated posteriorly, with pressure on and damage to the spinal cord. In these cases, open reduction by surgical means is often required to remove pressure on the cord.

The Intervertebral Foramina and Synovial Joints

The intervertebral foramina in the cervical region are short canals that contain the ventral and dorsal roots and spinal ganglia within a meningeal sleeve, the recurrent meningeal nerves, the spinal arteries, and venous plexuses—all embedded in fat and connective tissue. The venous plexuses connecting the internal and external spinal veins allow blood to be expelled in movements of the cervical column, thus cushioning and protecting the nerve structures against pressure. The same holds true for the fat, which is semifluid at body temperature.

Immediately posterior to the intervertebral foramina are the superior and inferior articular processes of adjacent vertebrae; they form the synovial (facet) joints, which are surrounded by joint capsules (Fig. 11.2). Synovial joints are subject to many inflammatory

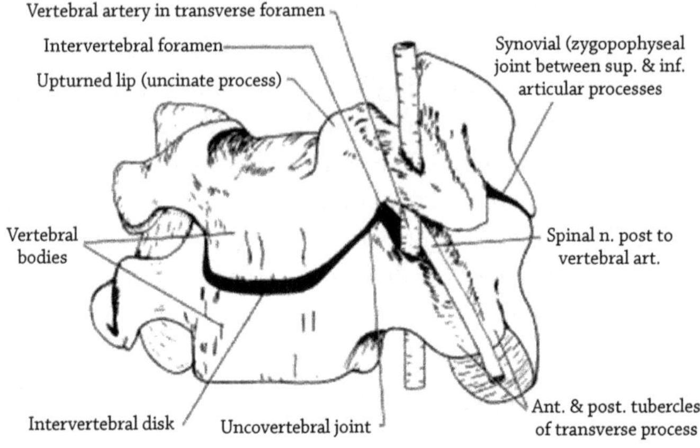

FIGURE 11.2

Oblique view of two articulated cervical vertebrae showing (1) anterior to the intervertebral foramen, the cartilaginous joint between vertebral bodies with the intervertebral disk and also the uncovertebral joint; and (2) posterior to the intervertebral foramen, the synovial joint between articular processes. Notice that the vertebral artery passes through the transverse foramen, in front of the cervical nerve which emerges from the intervertebral foramen. ant., anterior; art., artery; inf., inferior; post., posterior; spinal n., spinal nerve; sup., superior.

arthritic and degenerative diseases that frequently lead to changes in joint configuration by narrowing the articulations, thickening the joint capsules, and causing bony spur formation. These changes result in alterations in spatial relationships and encroachment on the intervertebral foramina; in hyperextension trauma, the nerve structures within the foramina are exposed to stretching over preexisting abnormal bone formation. The presence of bony spurs adjacent to the intervertebral foramina between C4 and C5 was mentioned in this case and could partly explain the patient's symptoms.

Occasionally, a nerve root or parts of a nerve root may be caught, pincer-like, between deformed articular facets. It was mentioned previously that the intervertebral disks make up the immediate anterior boundary of the intervertebral foramina and that protrusion of these disks as a result of trauma may explain the signs and symptoms of nerve involvement in disk degeneration (Fig. 11.2).

Uncovertebral Joints

The uncovertebral joint (lateral interbody joint, joint of Luschka) is an anatomical feature that is found only in the cervical vertebral column. These joints have been the subject of extensive discussion in the clinical literature, although they are often ignored in anatomical texts. Although they are not true synovial joints, but apparently the result of degenerative processes starting in the cervical disks in childhood and adolescence, they give the appearance of joints. They are formed by the upward, liplike projections on the superolateral surfaces of the cervical vertebral bodies (uncinate processes) and corresponding beveled grooves on the inferolateral surfaces of the overlying vertebrae. These bony areas are covered with cartilage and surrounded by synovial-like capsules. The presence of these joints predisposes to arthritic changes with bone proliferation. They form part of the anterior boundary of the intervertebral foramina and lie in close relationship to their nerve root contents (Fig. 11.2). As with other degenerative and proliferative joint changes, superimposed trauma on these joints leads to or aggravates the clinical condition of nerve root compression.

In summary, the nerve structures within the intervertebral foramina are bounded anteriorly by the cartilaginous joints between vertebral bodies (intervertebral disks), anterolaterally by the uncovertebral joints, and posteriorly by the intervertebral synovial (facet) joints. All these articulations alter their configuration during flexion, extension, and torsion of the cervical spine and thereby encroach on the intervertebral foramina and their contents. This is particularly true in hyperextension and more so if the joints are already deformed by degenerative or proliferative bone changes. It is easily realized that the emergence of spinal nerves from the spinal canal through foramina that are bounded anteriorly and posteriorly by movable joints is conducive to injury of these nerves.

Vertebral Artery Injury

An unusual and sometimes quite serious complication of hyperextension injury is compression of the vertebral artery as it runs through the neck. The vertebral artery, the first branch of the subclavian artery, ascends through the transverse foramina of the cervical vertebrae, starting with C6, and exits through the transverse foramen of the atlas to enter the cranial cavity through the foramen magnum. It joins with its partner from the opposite side to form the basilar artery, which supplies the cerebellum, the posterior portion of the cerebrum, and much of the brain stem. As the vertebral artery passes through the transverse foramina, it lies anterior to the emerging nerve roots. Hyperextension injury may occasionally traumatize the intima of the artery, particularly if its walls have become atherosclerotic and rigid, and this may lead to vascular insufficiency of the posterior portions of the brain caused by a dissecting aneurysm and secondary thromboembolism. Bizarre clinical pictures, such as vertigo, ataxia (loss of muscular coordination), disturbances of vision and bearing, and temporary loss of consciousness, may result.

The symptoms in this patient were transitory. They can probably be explained by a ligamentous sprain with resulting muscle spasm and some temporary injury to the cervical nerves, which may have been stretched over existing bone proliferations at levels C4 and C5.

For more information on the vertebral artery and its collateral circulation in case of atherosclerotic obstruction, see Chapter 41, Subclavian Steal Syndrome.

12

Central Venous Catheterization

A 45-year-old man is brought to the emergency department. He reports a 36-hour history of midepigastric pain that has gradually increased in severity so that it is now 10 out of 10 with 10 being maximal pain. The pain is constant and radiates to his back. There are no exacerbating features, but the pain is slightly relieved by lying still. He has never had pain like this before. He denies fever or chills but has had several episodes of bilious vomiting. There has been no change in his bowel habits. The patient reports no alcohol use and is a nonsmoker.

Examination

His temperature is 38.5° C, blood pressure is 70/40 mm Hg, heart rate is 135 bpm, and respiratory rate is 24 breaths/min. The patient appears pale and is mildly agitated. His extremities are cool, his sclera are anicteric (no evidence of jaundice), and his mucous membranes are dry. His lungs are clear, and his heart sounds are normal except for the tachycardia. Abdominal examination reveals distention, an absence of bowel sounds (paralysis of the intestine), and epigastric tenderness with guarding on palpation. No ecchymoses (bruising), referred to as Cullen's sign in the umbilical region or Grey-Turner's sign in the flank, are evident.

A plain radiograph of the abdomen shows multiple air-fluid levels within dilated loops of the small intestine overlying the splenic flexure. The patient's hemoglobin is low (12 g/dL), and his white cell count is high (22,000 cells/mm^3). Laboratory tests show markedly elevated amylase (1110 IU) and lipase (850 IU); normal values are 35 to 85 IU for amylase and 100 to 500 IU for lipase.

Diagnosis

The patient's condition is diagnosed as acute pancreatitis. The two most common causes of acute pancreatitis in adults are alcohol abuse and gallstones. The patient denies alcohol use, so his symptoms could have resulted from transient blockage of the main pancreatic duct by a gallstone. This may occur where the pancreatic duct joins the common bile duct to form the hepatopancreatic ampulla, which then enters the medial wall of the descending part of the duodenum. Clinicians commonly call the hepatopancreatic ampulla by its eponym, ampulla of Vater.

Therapy and Further Course

The principal treatment for acute pancreatitis is supportive care to ensure adequate oxygenation and maintenance of intravascular volume. The emergency department physician rapidly administers intravenous fluid through a catheter placed in the right internal jugular vein (IJV), which is effective in combating the patient's hypovolemia (abnormal reduction in circulating blood volume). Central venous catheterization is chosen because the blood volume depletion had collapsed the peripheral veins. The IJVs and the subclavian veins are equally satisfactory for the infusion of fluids. The choice is usually based on the physician's previous experience, and placement can be aided by ultrasonographic imaging.

During the first hour, the patient receives 3 L of crystalloid. He also is given analgesics to control his pain and is placed on supplemental oxygen. A nurse inserts a bladder catheter, and urine output is soon adequate at 0.5 mL/kg per hour. The vital signs improve: blood pressure rises to 110/70 mm Hg, heart rate falls to 90 bpm, and respiratory rate diminishes to 18 breaths/min. Frequent assessment of his vital signs ensures that the patient is receiving adequate volume resuscitation.

Cultures of blood and urine are taken. A nasogastric tube is placed, and slow suction is started. Contrast-enhanced computed tomography (CT) of the abdomen demonstrates a large edematous pancreas with mild dilatation of the extrahepatic and intrahepatic biliary ducts. There is no evidence of decreased pancreatic perfusion or peripancreatic fluid collections. A sonogram of the right upper quadrant of the abdomen corroborates the CT findings and also shows numerous small gallstones in the gallbladder. The patient is admitted to the hospital for observation and supportive care.

His condition improves the next day, but he is still experiencing epigastric pain and bloating. His nausea is largely resolved, however, and the nasogastric tube is replaced with a feeding tube that is positioned, using fluoroscopic guidance, through the pylorus into the duodenum. Bowel sounds remain hypoactive, and his amylase and lipase levels continue to be elevated. Because his course of therapy may be protracted, enteral nutrition is initiated via the feeding tube. To minimize the chance of infection, the central venous catheter is removed and peripheral intravenous access is achieved.

The patient's health improves during the next week of hospitalization. On the fourth day, his pain is largely resolved and bowel sounds have returned (resumption of motility). His feeding tube is removed. The patient tolerates liquids administered orally and remains asymptomatic. By the end of the week, he is able to eat solid food. He is then discharged and told that a cholecystectomy will be necessary in the next 2 to 4 weeks to avoid passage of another gallstone and recurrent pancreatitis.

Discussion

The patient underwent successful treatment for hypovolemia by infusion of fluid. The pancreatitis resolved spontaneously after the presumed passage of the gallstone into the duodenum. Enteral feeding and supplemental oxygen also aided the patient's recovery.

The elevated amylase and lipase levels in the blood represented responses to autolytic injury in the exocrine portion of the pancreas caused by transient blockage of the main pancreatic duct. In this case, the blockage took place where the main pancreatic duct empties into the hepatopancreatic ampulla.

What caused the paralysis of the small intestine, which was revealed by the lack of bowel sounds and the multiple air-fluid levels on the abdominal films? The best explanation is that inflammatory agents from the pancreas crossed the peritoneum covering the pancreas to enter the peritoneal cavity and affect the motility of the small intestine, producing a localized ileus. The radiographic finding of multiple loops of the small intestine with air-fluid levels is indicative of stasis of the intestinal content.

Central venous catheterization allows invasive hemodynamic monitoring, temporary cardiac pacing, and safe delivery of a wide variety of drugs and hypertonic solutions that irritate peripheral veins. Central venous catheters are also vital in providing intravenous fluids, drugs, and total parenteral nutrition to patients with diminished peripheral venous access sites, as in this case.

Anatomy of Central Venous Catheterization

Subclavian Vein

Those learning or reviewing IJV or subclavian central venous catheterization may consult a standard anatomy atlas to review the venous anatomy of the axilla and root of the neck. The osteology of the upper chest and clavicle is especially relevant to these procedures because it provides important topographical landmarks for guiding the catheter accurately. In reviewing the clavicle, one should pay particular attention to its S-shaped form, which divides it into thirds, known as the medial, middle, and lateral components. The junction between the medial and middle thirds (commonly referred to as the *break* of the clavicle) is emphasized because it serves as the landmark for subclavian vein cannulation. The sternoclavicular joint should be located, because the brachiocephalic vein, which is formed by the union of the IJV and the subclavian vein, lies directly behind it.

The subclavian vein travels medially from the axilla toward the brachiocephalic vein in the narrow space between the clavicle and the first rib. It passes over the first rib just in front of the insertion of the anterior scalene muscle, behind the medial part of the clavicle. After crossing the inner border of the first rib, it lies on the cupula of the pleura. The adventitia of the subclavian vein is directly attached to the periosteum of the posterior surface of the medial third of the clavicle, the costoclavicular ligament, and the fasciae of the subclavius and anterior scalene muscles. The tethering of the subclavian vein to surrounding structures by connective tissue has great clinical importance because it prevents the subclavian vein from completely collapsing, even in the case of hypovolemia.

When the operator is ready to perform the procedure, the first step is to place the patient in the Trendelenburg position (feet up; head down) to increase venous pressure. The operator then selects the skin entry site for subclavian venipuncture. This site is located 1 cm inferior and 1 cm lateral to the convex bend (the break) between the medial and middle thirds of the clavicle. An 18-gauge "finder" needle, 2.5 inches long, is inserted into the skin at the entry site and aimed toward the tip of the index finger of the opposite hand, which is placed deeply in the patient's suprasternal notch. This trajectory aligns the needle with the longitudinal axis of the subclavian vein as it courses posterior to the medial third of the clavicle (Fig. 12.1). The operator should be aware that this positioning keeps the needle directed horizontally in a coronal plane, thereby minimizing the risk of puncturing either the lung or the subclavian artery. In some patients, the shoulders jut so far forward that it is difficult to direct the needle horizontally. In these cases, it may be necessary to move the shoulders posteriorly by placing a rolled towel between the shoulder blades.

During needle advancement, the operator should apply slight back-pressure on the plunger of the syringe to provide continuous negative pressure. Confirmation of needle entry into the vein is made when dark-colored venous blood is aspirated into the syringe. The syringe is removed, and the needle is covered to prevent entry of air. A guidewire is inserted through the bore of the needle into the vein. The needle is removed, leaving the guidewire in place. A small incision is made in the skin along the wire. Next, the operator feeds a dilator down the wire to expand the tissue to the size of the catheter. The dilator is removed, and the catheter is inserted into the vein, sutured in place, and covered with a sterile dressing.

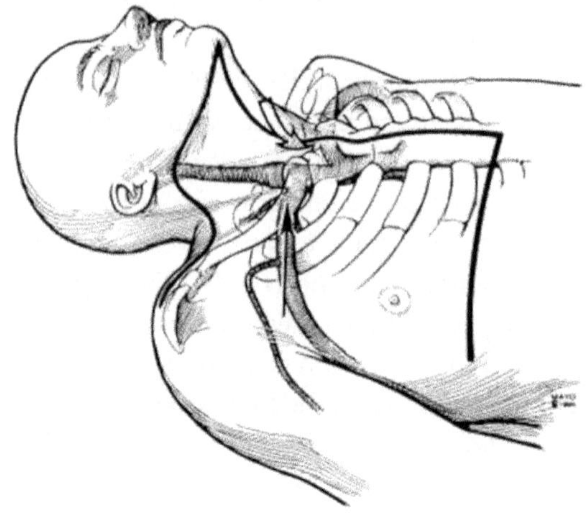

FIGURE 12.1

Diagrammatic representation of a catheter (*straight arrow*) within the subclavian vein directed toward the suprasternal notch (*curved arrow*). The catheter enters the vein deep to the medial third of the clavicle in the direction indicated by the straight arrow.

Different points of resistance are usually encountered with the finder needle in seeking the subclavian vein. The points of resistance vary according to the laterality of the entry site. When the entry site is more medially placed, the points of resistance are (1) the skin and superficial fascia, (2) the subclavius muscle, (3) the costoclavicular ligament, and (4) the posterolateral surface of the bulky medial end of the clavicle if the needle pass is too shallow. When the entry site is more laterally placed, the subclavius muscle and the costoclavicular ligament may not be encountered.

Internal Jugular Vein

The surface anatomy used to locate the skin entry site for successful catheterization of the IJV can be reviewed by examining the lower part of the sternocleidomastoid muscle, either on a volunteer or on oneself while looking in a mirror. To examine the right sternocleidomastoid, the head should be rotated downward toward the left shoulder and vice versa for the left sternocleidomastoid. This action brings the sternocleidomastoid muscle into relief, so that the cord-like form of the sternal head contrasts with the less-defined, thinner, flat clavicular head. In practice, the operator will ask the patient to lift his or her head off the table to define further the two heads of the sternocleidomastoid. The legs of the triangle, brought into relief by this action, are formed by the superior aspect of the medial third of the clavicle, the lateral border of the sternal head, and the medial border of the clavicular head of the sternocleidomastoid.

The apex of this triangle, located about 5 cm above the clavicle, serves as the skin entry site for the approach to IJV catheterization. The IJV (within the carotid sheath) lies against the deep surface of the sternocleidomastoid, requiring a penetration depth by the finder needle of only 10 to 15 mm from the skin surface before it enters into the vein. The IJV is a superficial structure. The structures that separate the IJV from the surface of the neck are the skin (2 mm thick), the superficial fascia containing the thin platysma muscle (3–6 mm thick), and the sternocleidomastoid muscle (5–6 mm thick).

Three other anatomical points help to ensure safe central venous catheterization via the IJV. First, the IJV lies on the anterior surface of the cupula covering the apex of the lung. This relationship makes the lung vulnerable to accidental puncture when the needle is pushed through the vein. Second, the easy collapsibility of the vein may complicate entry into the lumen (interior of the vessel). When the needle encounters the anterior wall of the vein, the external pressure from the advancing needle may exceed the distending pressure of the vein, which is low in patients with hypovolemia. In such cases, the needle may press the anterior wall of the vein against its posterior wall. Then, as the needle advances, it may pass through both walls without entering a patent (open) lumen. If no blood rushes into the syringe at a depth of about 2 to 2.5 cm, the needle should be slowly withdrawn while back-pressure is maintained on the syringe. This action is intended to draw the anterior wall of the vein away from the posterior wall and to create a lumen, allowing blood to enter the needle. Third, the trajectory for catheterization of the IJV is critical to the success of the procedure. The method described here is to enter the skin at the apex of the triangle of the sternocleidomastoid and clavicle while aiming the needle at a downward angle of 45 degrees to the horizontal plane, directing the needle toward the ipsilateral nipple.

Complications of Central Venous Catheterization

The juxtaposition of the apex of the lung to the subclavian and IJVs poses a risk for lung puncture by misdirected needles, and this can lead to pneumothorax (collapsed lung). The cupula is at the level of the first rib posteriorly, but the first rib slopes downward and forward. Therefore, the cupula and apex of the lung extend above the level of the anterior part of the first rib and above the thoracic inlet into the root of the neck. They lie behind the sternocleidomastoid muscle, 3 cm above the level of the medial third of the clavicle. The important anterior relationships of the cupula are with (1) the subclavian artery and its branches, anterior to which are the anterior scalene muscle and the phrenic nerve lying on the anterior surface of that muscle, and (2) the IJV and the subclavian vein, which pass anterior to the insertion of the anterior scalene muscle on the first rib.

Complications during the insertion of central venous catheters include pneumothorax, arterial puncture, and hematoma. The incidence of pneumothorax is reported to be between 1.5% and 3.1% for subclavian vein catheterization but considerably lower for the IJV (<0.2%). Because an estimated 5 million central venous catheter procedures are performed annually in the United States, a great number of people suffer complications of these procedures. The use of ultrasound guidance reduces the incidence of mechanical complications of central venous catheterization.

Pneumothorax is caused by the creation of an opening between the lung and the pleural cavity. The injury to the visceral pleura and lung from the penetrating catheter allows atmospheric air within the lung to enter the pleural space. This breaks the suction effect (surface tension) between the parietal and visceral pleurae, allowing the natural tendency of the chest wall, lined with parietal pleura, to expand outward, and of the lung, covered by visceral pleura, to retract inward upon itself. In essence, the normal negative pressure in the pleural space, which keeps the lungs inflated against the parietal pleura, is lost. The lung retracts on itself toward the lung root because of the pull of its elastic tissues and smooth muscle; thus, it becomes ineffective in respiration. Less threatening, but still of concern, is accidental puncture of the arteries that travel alongside the veins: the subclavian artery located just behind the subclavian vein and the common carotid artery lying medial to the IJV. IJV catheterization has a higher incidence of arterial puncture (6.3–9.4%) than does subclavian catheterization (3.1–4.9%).

Unit I

Review Questions

The number in parentheses is a reference to the page on which information about the question may be found.

1. In what part of the temporal bone does the facial nerve course, and through what opening does it emerge onto the face?
The facial nerve passes through the facial canal within the petrous portion of the temporal bone and then emerges through the stylomastoid foramen onto the face. (6)

2. Why does the face appear asymmetrical when there is a facial nerve lesion?
The muscles of facial expression on the normal side are unopposed by the paralyzed muscles on the side of the lesion. (7)

3. Why is vision at risk when a patient has a facial palsy?
Because the orbicularis oculi is paralyzed, the patient loses the blink reflex on the side of the lesion; therefore, the cornea is at risk for desiccation and ulceration. (6–7)

4. Why does food and saliva leak from the mouth of a patient with facial palsy?
The orbicularis oris and the buccinator muscles are responsible for keeping food in the mouth and against the teeth while chewing. When these muscles are paralyzed, food and saliva will leak from the mouth. (7)

5. Why might a patient with facial palsy experience hyperacusis?
The facial nerve innervates the stapedius. This muscle in the middle ear is responsible for attenuating sound. Paralysis of the stapedius eliminates this attenuation and causes sounds to be perceived as louder. (9)

6. In addition to the innervation of skeletal muscle, what other functions are served by the facial nerve?
The facial nerve carries taste sensation from the palate and the anterior two-thirds of the tongue. It is also responsible for general sensation from the skin behind the ear. It is responsible for secretion from the lacrimal gland, the submandibular gland, and the sublingual gland. (8–9)

7. What are the three divisions of the trigeminal nerve, and what regions of skin do they innervate?
The three divisions are the ophthalmic, maxillary, and mandibular divisions. The ophthalmic division innervates the skin from the lateral angle of the eye up to the interauricular line. The maxillary division innervates the skin from the lateral angle of the eye to the lateral angle of the mouth. The mandibular division innervates the skin from the angle of the mouth to the margin of the mandible and the skin anterior to the ear. (16)

8. Where are the sensory cell bodies of the nerve fibers in the trigeminal nerve found?
The sensory cell bodies are in the trigeminal ganglion, which is on the anterior face of the petrous bone in the middle cranial fossa. (16)

9. What are emissary veins, and what role do they play in the transmission of infection?
Emissary veins are veins that communicate between superficial regions of the face and scalp and the dural venous sinuses. Because these veins do not contain valves, blood can flow in either direction. Infections of the skin of the face and scalp can travel into the dural venous sinuses. (23–24)

10. Why might a patient with cavernous sinus thrombosis have swelling of the eyelid and conjunctiva?
The ophthalmic veins, which drain the eyelids and conjunctiva, communicate with the cavernous sinus. Thrombosis in the sinus impedes venous drainage from these regions. (25)

11. Which cranial nerves pass through the cavernous sinus and could be affected by a cavernous sinus thrombosis?
The oculomotor nerve, the trochlear nerve, the abducens nerve, and the ophthalmic and maxillary divisions of the trigeminal nerve all pass through the cavernous sinus in their course to the superior orbital fissure and the orbit. (25)

12. What are the venous connections of the cavernous sinus through which infection could spread?
The cavernous sinus communicates with the superior ophthalmic vein anteriorly, the superior and inferior petrosal sinuses posteriorly, the anterior and posterior intercavernous sinus medially, and the cerebral and meningeal veins. (24)

13. Why might a cavernous sinus thrombosis cause loss of all eye movement and dilatation of the pupil?
All of the extraocular muscles that cause eye movement are innervated by nerves that pass through the cavernous sinus. The oculomotor nerve innervates the superior rectus, medial rectus, inferior rectus, and inferior oblique. The trochlear nerve innervates the superior oblique, and the abducens nerve innervates the lateral rectus. Additionally, the oculomotor nerve carries the preganglionic parasympathetic nerves, which are responsible for the constriction of the pupil. (26)

14. What are the bony openings in the back of the orbit, and what passes through them?
The openings in the back of the orbit are the optic canal, the superior orbital fissure, and the inferior orbital fissure. The optic nerve and the ophthalmic artery pass through the optic canal. The oculomotor nerve,

the trochlear nerve, the abducens nerve, and the ophthalmic division of the trigeminal nerve, along with the superior ophthalmic vein, pass through the superior orbital fissure. The infraorbital nerve and artery, the zygomatic nerve, and the inferior ophthalmic vein pass through the inferior orbital fissure. (30)

15. Which two extraocular muscles, when contracted together, cause elevation of the eyeball?
When the superior rectus and the inferior oblique muscles contract together, they cause elevation of the eyeball. The superior rectus causes elevation and adduction; the inferior oblique causes elevation and abduction. When they contract together, the abduction and adduction actions cancel, and pure elevation results. (32)

16. Why can damage to the floor of the orbit cause sensory disturbance to the upper teeth?
The infraorbital nerve travels along the floor of the orbit. This nerve gives rise to branches that descend through the floor of the orbit and pass through the wall of the maxillary sinus to reach the roots of the maxillary teeth and provide sensory innervation. If the infraorbital nerve is damaged in the floor of the orbit, disruption of the sensory pathway from the maxillary teeth may occur. (32–33)

17. What muscles are responsible for movements at the temporomandibular joint (TMJ)?
Movement at the TMJ is provided by the four muscles of mastication (masseter, temporalis, medial pterygoid, and lateral pterygoid) as well as the anterior digastric and mylohyoid muscles. (40)

18. Which muscles are responsible for closing the jaw?
The masseter, temporalis, and medial pterygoid are responsible for closing the jaw. (40)

19. Why might dislocation of the mandible occur during extreme opening of the jaw but not during closing of the jaw?
When the jaw is opened, the condyle of the mandible and the intraarticular disk move forward; this may cause the condyle to pass over the articular tubercle and thus dislocate from the joint. Closing of the jaw moves the condyle posteriorly, where it is well seated in the joint. (41)

20. At what location is an inferior alveolar nerve block done?
The inferior alveolar nerve enters the mandible at the mandibular foramen, on the medial side of the ramus of the mandible. The nerve can be blocked at this location. (52)

21. In addition to the mandibular teeth and gums, what region of skin receives sensory innervation from the inferior alveolar nerve?
The terminal branch of the inferior alveolar nerve is the mental nerve. This nerve emerges from the mandibular canal through the mental foramen and innervates the skin overlying the anterior portion of the mandible. (57)

22. What are accessory muscles of respiration?
The primary muscles of respiration are the diaphragm and the intercostal muscles. Accessory muscles of respiration are any muscles that have an attachment to the chest wall and can cause expansion of the chest if the other attachment of the muscle is stabilized. For example, upper limb muscles such as the pectoralis major, pectoralis minor, and serratus anterior can expand the chest if the upper limb is stabilized. Similarly, the scalene can elevate the ribs, thus expanding the thorax, when the cervical spine is stabilized. (62)

23. What are the major layers of the deep cervical fascia?
The outermost layer of deep cervical fascia is the investing layer, which covers the trapezius and sternocleidomastoid muscles and encircles all the layers of cervical fascia. The pretracheal fascia encloses the visceral compartment, and the prevertebral fascia encloses the vertebral column and the paravertebral muscles. The carotid sheath encloses the internal jugular vein, the common and internal carotid arteries, and the vagus nerve. (63–64)

24. What structure lies immediately posterior to the trachea and could be perforated if a tracheostomy tube is inserted too far?
The esophagus is located immediately posterior to the trachea. Because the cartilages of the trachea are incomplete posteriorly, the membranous posterior wall of the trachea can be penetrated. (65)

25. Why does cricothyroidostomy avoid the possibility of injury to the esophagus?
The cricoid cartilage is a complete ring with a wide posterior lamina that prevents penetration of the esophagus. However, cricothyroidotomy presents the possibility of injury to the vocal mechanism. (65)

26. What are the bony and cartilaginous structures that can be palpated in the anterior midline of the neck?
From superior to inferior, the palpable midline structures are the hyoid bone, the thyroid cartilage with the superior thyroid notch in the midline, the cricoid cartilage, the tracheal rings, and the suprasternal notch of the manubrium. (64)

27. Which infrahyoid muscles that are close to the midline must be retracted to gain access to the thyroid gland?
The sternohyoid and sternothyroid muscles are close to the midline and lie anterior to the thyroid gland. These muscles are retracted to gain access to the thyroid. (73)

28. What nerve crosses the inferior thyroid artery posterior to the thyroid gland, and what would be the result of injury to this nerve?
The recurrent laryngeal nerve, a branch of the vagus nerve, crosses the inferior thyroid artery. This nerve innervates all of the intrinsic laryngeal muscles except for the cricothyroid. Injury to the nerve results in hoarseness. (76)

29. What is the embryonic origin of the parathyroid glands, and how does this relate to the greater variability of the location of the inferior parathyroid gland?
The parathyroid glands are derived from the endoderm of the third and fourth pharyngeal pouches. The superior parathyroid comes from the fourth pouch, and the inferior parathyroid comes from the third pouch. The longer migration path of the cells forming the inferior parathyroid leads to greater variability in location. (76–77)

30. The carotid pulse can be palpated at the anterior border of the sternocleidomastoid muscle. What are the boundaries of the carotid triangle in which this pulse is felt?
The carotid triangle is a subdivision of the anterior triangle. It is bounded by the posterior belly of the digastric, the superior belly of the omohyoid, and the sternocleidomastoid muscle. (82–83)

31. What is the retropharyngeal space, and what is the relationship of the carotid sheath to this space?
The retropharyngeal space is the fascial plane between the prevertebral fascia, which surrounds the vertebral column and paravertebral muscles, and the pretracheal fascia, which surrounds the visceral compartment of the neck. The right and left carotid sheaths close off the right and left sides of this space. (85)

32. What structures are in the carotid sheath, and what are their relationships to one another?
Within the carotid sheath are found the common carotid artery, the internal jugular vein, and the vagus nerve. The vein is anterolateral, the artery is anteromedial, and the nerve is posterior and between the two vessels. When the common carotid artery bifurcates, the internal carotid remains in the sheath, and the external carotid exits the sheath. (85)

33. Through what pathways do the right and left external carotid arteries anastomose with one another?
Branches of the external carotid artery include the superior thyroid artery, the lingual artery, and the facial artery. Each of these branches anastomoses with its counterpart from the contralateral side. (86)

34. What ligament resists hyperextension of the neck and may be sprained with a hyperextension injury?
The anterior longitudinal ligament is the primary ligament that resists hyperextension of the neck. (90–91)

35. What ligaments resist hyperflexion of the neck and may be injured with a hyperflexion injury?
The ligaments that resist flexion of the neck include the posterior longitudinal ligament, the supraspinous ligament, the interspinous ligament, and the ligamentum flavum. (91–92)

36. What are the characteristics of the two parts of an intervertebral disk?
The outer part of the disk is the anulus fibrosus. This is composed of concentric rings of fibrous tissue and fibrocartilage. The inner portion of the disk is the nucleus pulposus. This is a semigelatinous material with high water content. (92)

37. What is the relationship between the vertebral artery and the cervical vertebrae?
The vertebral artery enters the transverse foramen of the sixth cervical vertebra and then ascends through the transverse foramina of all vertebrae above that level. After exiting from the foramen in the first cervical vertebra, the artery passes through the foramen magnum to enter the cranial cavity. While passing through the transverse foramina, the vertebral artery is subject to injury in neck trauma. (96)

38. Describe the position of the subclavian vein where it may be accessed for central venous catheterization.
The subclavian vein passes under the medial third of the clavicle and over the first rib. It passes anterior to the anterior scalene muscle and then lies on the surface of the cervical pleura. Injury to the pleura at this location can cause a pneumothorax. (100)

39. What surface landmark is used to locate the internal jugular vein for central venous catheterization?
The triangular gap between the sternal head and the clavicular head of the sternocleidomastoid identifies the location of the internal jugular vein. A needle is passed through the apex of this triangle about 5 cm above the clavicle. (102–103)

UNIT II

Back

13

Prolapse of an Intervertebral Disk

A 63-year-old college professor presents to the office with a 2-day history of lower back and right lower limb pain. The patient states that he tried to push his car, which was caught in a snowdrift, and immediately suffered sudden and severe pain in the lower back. He felt as if something had "snapped" in the lower part of his spine. He lay down to rest, applying an ice pack. He also took ibuprofen, a non-steroidal antiinflammatory drug (NSAID), with no relief. Later, his pain extended down the posterior aspect of his right thigh and leg. He also noticed some numbness and tingling over the lateral part of his right leg, foot, and little toe. Currently the pain is 7 on a scale of 10 in severity and is worse with both prolonged sitting and standing. The radiation of the pain down the right leg is worsened with straining or coughing. He reports that for several years he has had episodes of "bad back," particularly after lifting heavy objects from a stooping position. He reports having difficulty urinating and feels as if he is not emptying his bladder; however, he reports no incontinence. He has no history of unexplained weight loss or diagnosis of cancer.

Examination

There is a diminution in the spinal lumbar curve and a tilt of the trunk to the left side. Because of his pain, he has marked limitation of movement in the lumbar vertebral column. Supine straight-leg testing is performed and elicits radiating pain at 50 degrees of hip flexion. On further examination, tenderness to palpation along the course of the sciatic nerve in the right thigh is noted, and there is some weakness in plantar flexion of his right foot as well as some loss of sensory perception over the lateral heel and fifth toe. The Achilles tendon reflex is absent.

Because of the patient's reported urinary symptoms, there is concern about possible involvement of the autonomic innervation to the pelvic organs, and an magnetic resonance imaging study is ordered.

Diagnosis

This patient has a rupture of the intervertebral disk between the fifth lumbar and first sacral vertebrae (L5/S1) with herniation of the nucleus pulposus and nerve root involvement of the first sacral nerve (slipped disk) (Fig. 13.1).

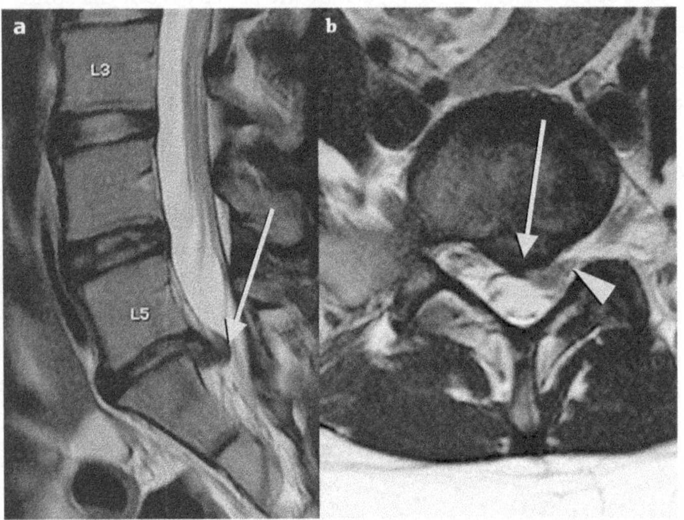

FIGURE 13.1

A, A sagittal magnetic resonance image of the vertebral column from the level of the third lumbar vertebra (L3) downward through the second sacral vertebra (S2) shows the herniated L5/S1 disk (*arrow*) as it protrudes posteriorly into the vertebral canal, where it impinges on the nerve roots of the first sacral nerve. **B,** An axial magnetic resonance image at the level of the L5/S1 disk shows a herniated nucleus pulposus (arrow) in the vertebral canal where it impinges on a spinal nerve (arrow head).

Therapy and Further Course

Under conservative treatment and bed rest for 2 days, the patient improves sufficiently to start a set of exercises recommended to strengthen the flexor and extensors of the vertebral column.

Discussion

The combination of low back pain and pain along the course of the sciatic nerve aggravated by straining is typical of a disk lesion. The intervertebral disks act as shock absorbers; each consists of an outer firm fibrocartilaginous ring, the anulus fibrosus, and an inner softer, more pliable, gelatinous center, the nucleus pulposus. Chronic trauma, particularly in middle-aged or older patients with degenerative changes in their intervertebral disks, may lead to a posterior tear in the anulus fibrosus at the site of greatest mechanical stress. A later consequence, particularly in conjunction with further acute or chronic trauma, is protrusion or herniation of the nucleus pulposus into the vertebral canal. Usually the herniation takes place to one side or the other of the midline because of the ligamentous reinforcement in the midline provided by the posterior longitudinal ligament. The posterior longitudinal ligament attaches to the occiput above and extends all the way down the vertebral column along the posterior surfaces of the vertebral bodies into the sacral canal. It narrows behind each vertebral body but broadens as it passes over each disk. This ligament resists flexion of the vertebral column.

The "snap" that the patient felt may have been caused by the anular tear, with partial expulsion of the nucleus pulposus. The lower lumbar disks are among the most flexible areas of the vertebral column and are the most common sites of herniation. The disappearance of the normal lumbar concavity, or lordosis, results from contraction of flexors of the spine. The chief flexors of the lumbar vertebral column are the rectus abdominis and the external and internal abdominal oblique muscles.

Cauda Equina and Subarachnoid Space

The spinal cord is not subject to injury from disk herniations at this vertebral level because the spinal cord in the average adult ends inferiorly at the L2 vertebra or the disk between L1 and L2. The subarachnoid space ends at the S2 level. Within the subarachnoid space (thecal, meningeal sac) below the level of the spinal cord are the cauda equina and the filum terminale within the cerebrospinal fluid. The cauda equina consists of dorsal and ventral nerve roots that extend downward in the vertebral canal within the subarachnoid space from the spinal cord to the level of emergence from their respective intervertebral foramina. At these levels, as the nerve roots exit from the subarachnoid space, they are covered by meningeal sleeves as far as the spinal ganglia, where the meningeal membranes become continuous with the epineurium.

Posterolateral herniation of the nucleus pulposus may readily impinge on the nerve roots within the vertebral canal as they course diagonally downward toward their exit (Fig. 13.2). The prolapse is particularly apt to compress the roots of the next lower spinal nerve. Therefore, herniation of the disk between L5 and S1 involves most commonly the roots of the first sacral nerve, as in this case (Figs. 13.2 and 13.3). The fifth lumbar nerve leaves the vertebral canal above the fifth lumbar disk, and the first sacral nerve crosses this disk in its course to the first sacral foramina (anterior and posterior).

Straining and coughing increase intravenous pressure, which also increases the pressure of the cerebrospinal fluid, adding to the pressure on the involved nerve roots. Tilting of the trunk away from the compressed roots decreases the pressure on them and lessens the pain.

Sciatic Nerve and Its Roots

The roots of the first spinal sacral nerve represent one of the important components of the sciatic nerve. The sciatic nerve takes origin from the L4, L5, and the first three sacral nerves. Raising the

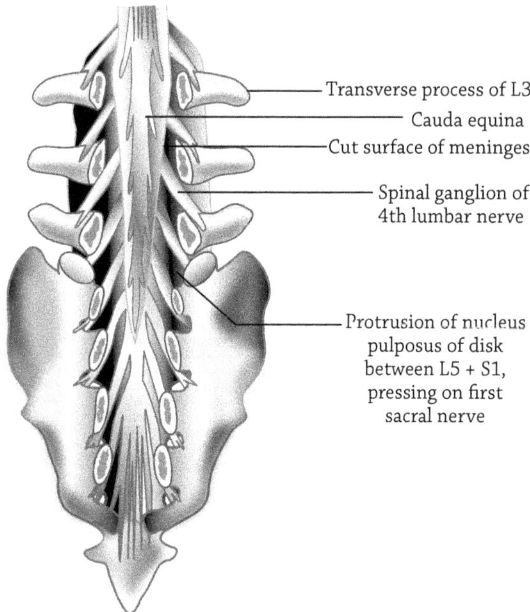

FIGURE 13.2

Vertebral arches have been removed and the spinal canal has been exposed. The dura and arachnoid have been cut and reflected. The oblique course of spinal nerves is shown. The prolapsed nucleus pulposus is pressing on the first sacral nerve and ganglion. L3, third lumbar vertebra; L5, fifth lumbar vertebrae; S1, first sacral vertebra.

extended leg of a patient in the recumbent position stretches the sciatic nerve and is painful in cases of sciatic nerve root compression, as is direct pressure on the sciatic nerve itself in its course along the thigh. The nerve runs almost vertically down the thigh, passing midway between the greater trochanter and the ischial tuberosity.

Weakness of plantar flexion of the right foot in this patient is a sign of involvement of the motor root of the first sacral nerve. The branch of the tibial nerve that innervates the main plantar flexor, the gastrocnemius muscle, contains mainly fibers from the first and second sacral nerves. The sensory area of the skin (dermatome) supplied by the first sacral nerve varies somewhat. The most typical

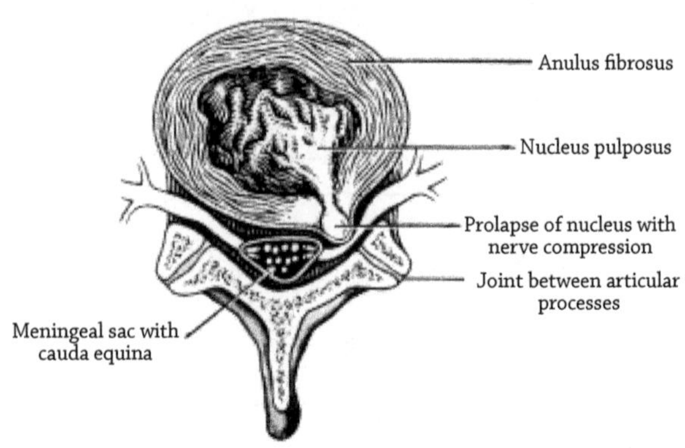

FIGURE 13.3

Cross section of intervertebral disk and spinal canal. Notice the ruptured anulus fibrosus with posterior protrusion of nucleus pulposus and compression of the spinal nerve on the right.

TABLE 13.1 Motor and Sensory Findings with Disk Herniations at Levels L2 through S1

Herniated Ditsk	*Spinal Nerve Affected*	*Motor Findings*	*Area of Sensory Disturbance*
L1/L2	L2	Weakness of hip flexors	Groin and anterior thigh
L2/L3	L3	Weakness of knee extensors	Anteromedial thigh
L3/L4	L4	Weakness of ankle dorsiflexors	Anterior leg and medial foot
L4/L5	L5	Weakness of big toe extensor	Dorsum of foot
L5/S1	S1	Weakness of ankle plantar flexors	Lateral foot

area of disturbed sensation in involvement of the first sacral nerve comprises the lateral aspect of the leg below the knee and the lateral side of the foot (Table 13.1). These are the areas involved in this patient.

Conservative treatment will usually suffice, but if objective signs (e.g., atrophy of the calf muscles, reflex anomalies with sensory deficiencies) and pain do not resolve with conservative therapy, surgical treatment may be indicated.

14

Lumbar Puncture

A 15-year-old boy is referred to the hospital by his family physician. He had presented to the physician's office with a 2-day history of fever, severe headache, nuchal rigidity (neck stiffness), and photophobia (sensitivity to light). He reports no recent upper respiratory tract infection and has no significant past medical history. He has never been hospitalized, has no allergies, and takes no medication. Of note, he recently returned from a 1-week hiking trip and reports that he had a tick bite during that time.

Examination

On physical examination, the boy appears ill and restless. His temperature is 103.5° F, and his pulse rate is accelerated. He complains of severe headache, which extends into the neck and is symmetrical on both sides of the head. On forward bending of the head and neck (flexion), the neck appears rather stiff. This movement is painful and is actively resisted by the patient. Additionally, he responds to flexion of his neck by flexing his hips and knees; this is a positive Brudzinski sign, suggesting the presence of meningitis.

Neurological examination does not reveal any specific defect in the central nervous system. Functions of the cranial and spinal nerves are intact. Examination of the fundus of the eye (eye grounds) with the ophthalmoscope shows the interior of the eye to be normal. There is no swelling of the optic disc, the site of entrance of the optic nerve into the eyeball; significantly increased intracranial pressure is therefore less likely. Examination of the heart and lungs is within normal limits. However, on the posterior aspect of his trunk, there is a large circular lesion, approximately 8 cm in diameter, that is erythematous with central clearing. A diagnosis of Lyme disease is suspected. Blood is drawn for a complete blood count (CBC) and differential and for a Lyme titer. To confirm or exclude the diagnosis of Lyme meningitis, a lumbar puncture (LP) is done. The cerebrospinal fluid (CSF) pressure is somewhat elevated at 28 mm Hg, but the fluid itself is clear and colorless. Microscopic examination of the CSF reveals the white blood cell count to be mildly elevated (15 cells/mL^3).

Diagnosis

The diagnosis is Lyme disease and presumed Lyme meningitis.

Therapy and Further Course

Intravenous antibiotics are started, and the patient is admitted overnight for observation. Acetaminophen and ibuprofen are prescribed for the fever, headache, and general discomfort. His fever is further reduced by frequent sponging with tap water.

By the next day, the patient's headache has considerably lessened and he is afebrile. The patient is discharged home on 4 weeks of antibiotic therapy. Follow-up shows that he has completely recovered.

Discussion

What is Lumbar Puncture?

In an LP, the subarachnoid space in the lumbar region is tapped for the removal of CSF or for the introduction of drugs such as antibiotics or anesthetics. The LP was introduced into the diagnostic and therapeutic armamentarium more than 100 years ago and has proved to be of unforeseen value as a sensitive diagnostic procedure and therapeutic tool.

Why should edema (papilledema) of the optic papilla, a sign of increased intracranial pressure, be excluded before an LP is undertaken? Sudden pressure reduction in the subarachnoid space caused by LP in the presence of elevated intracranial pressure can lead to herniation of the tonsils of the cerebellum through the foramen magnum into the spinal canal or to prolapse of portions of the temporal lobe through the tentorial notch. The result in either case may be a serious or fatal compression of vital portions of the brain.

Site of Lumbar Puncture

The optimal site of LP is in the lower part of the lumbar spinal column between vertebrae L3 and L4 or between L4 and L5. A landmark available for identifying the proper site of entrance of the LP needle is a horizontal line connecting the highest points of the iliac crests, as seen from the posterior aspect. This line crosses the midline at about the level of the spinous process of L4. The adjacent interspinous spaces above or below are then chosen as the site of LP. In the lumbar area, there is a wide space between adjacent, horizontally directed spinous processes; this space allows easy access to the spinal canal (Fig. 14.1). Entrance into the canal between thoracic spinous processes is impossible because they are directed inferiorly at a sharp angle and overlap each other so much that there is very little area in the midline that is free of bone.

Flexion of the lumbar vertebral column widens the space between adjacent spinous processes and is therefore used in positioning of the patient for LP. Maximal flexion of the vertebral column is applied either in the sitting position or in the lateral decubitus (horizontal) position with the patient's knees drawn as close to the chin as possible.

Lowest Extent of the Spinal Cord

Obviously, needle puncture of the spinal cord with resulting injury to the central nervous system must be avoided. The problem then focuses on the question of what the lowest extent of the spinal cord is in terms of vertebral landmarks. In the average adult, the lowest point of the cord is the tip of the conus medullaris, which is located at the lower border of L1 or at the level of the body of L2. In some individuals, it is a bit higher or a bit lower.

In the young fetus, the spinal cord extends through the entire length of the spinal canal down to the coccyx. As development

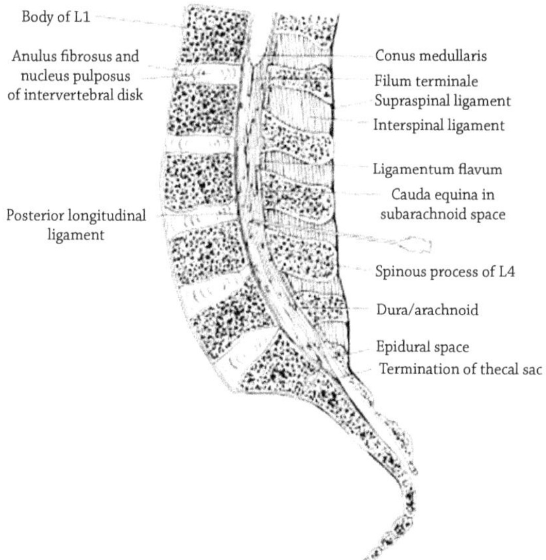

FIGURE 14.1

Midsagittal section through the lumbar spinal column with spinal puncture needle in place between the spinous processes of lumbar vertebrae L3 and L4. Notice the slightly ascending direction of the needle. The needle has pierced three ligaments and the dura/arachnoid and is in the subarachnoid space.

progresses, the growth of the spinal cord does not keep pace with the longitudinal growth of the vertebral column (differential growth). Already at birth, considerable discrepancy exists between the length of the cord and that of the column, with the cord ending, on average, at the inferior border of L3. Ultimately, the disproportion in length becomes even greater, so that in adults the end of the cord is usually two vertebrae higher (i.e., at the lower border of L1).

Subarachnoid Space and Cauda Equina

The CSF fills the subarachnoid space between arachnoid and the pia mater. The lowest extent of the subarachnoid space is at the level of S2. The fused sacral vertebrae form a solid bony mass as the posterior boundary of the sacral canal and prevent entrance into that part of the subarachnoid space. Within the subarachnoid space below the spinal cord is found the cauda equina ("horse's tail"), a collection of spinal nerve roots (sensory and motor) that descend from the lumbar and sacral segments of the cord to their exits as spinal nerves through the lumbar intervertebral and sacral foramina. The filum terminale, a strand of pia mater that descends from the conus medullaris, is considered one of the strands of the cauda equina.

If one of the nerve roots of the cauda equina is touched by the needle, it usually escapes injury, because it is easily displaced in the fluid medium of the CSF; however, contact with a sensory root may cause the patient to perceive a shooting pain in the lower extremity on that side, and the needle should be withdrawn slightly. It may be helpful to think of the spinal cord and cauda equina as analogous to a straw broom and its bristles: It would be easy to stick a needle into the handle of a broom (spinal cord) but almost impossible to stick it into one of the bristles (dorsal or ventral root).

Ligaments of the Spine

In the typical midline LP, three ligaments must be traversed by the needle: the supraspinous ligament, the interspinous ligament, and the ligamentum flavum (Fig. 14.1). Although the ligamenta flava are frequently described as not being continuous across the midline, they often are, and because the needle often strays from the theoretical midline, they must be considered structures encountered by the needle. After the needle has pierced the skin and superficial fascia, these ligaments are encountered in the order given.

The length of the needle is adjusted to the amount of fat in the subcutaneous tissue and to the size of the patient. The supraspinous ligaments connect the tips of the spinous processes; the interspinous ligaments join the superior and inferior borders of adjacent spinous processes and are fairly well developed in the lumbar area. The ligamenta flava are strong plate-like membranes, composed of yellow elastic fibers, that in the lumbar area may reach a thickness of 1 cm. They offer a noticeable resistance to the entering needle, and their penetration is felt as a "snap" or "click." They connect adjacent laminae and run from the anterior-inferior border of the lamina of the higher vertebra to the posterior-superior aspect of the lamina of the adjacent lower vertebra. Thus, they cover the interlaminar space between two vertebrae, which on inspection of the skeleton and on radiographs appears to be quite large in this area. The ligamenta flava fuse laterally with the capsules of the joints formed by the articular processes and blend posteriorly with the interspinous ligaments in the midline. The function of the ligamenta flava is to assist the erector spinae muscle in maintaining the upright position by resisting flexion of the vertebral column. They are put on stretch in flexion, and their elastic pull helps to restore the upright (extended) posture. Because flexion is the position assumed by the patient undergoing LP, the ligaments are stretched and easily traversed by the needle.

Epidural Space and Epidural Anesthesia

After the needle has penetrated the ligamentum flavum, thus traversing the interlaminar space, it enters the epidural (extradural) space, which extends from the foramen magnum to the sacral hiatus and communicates through the intervertebral foramina with the space outside the vertebral column. The epidural space surrounds the spinal meninges and separates the dura mater from the wall of the vertebral canal (Fig. 14.1). Its contents are the ventral and dorsal nerve roots, which are enveloped by their meningeal sleeves; a substantial amount of fat; and an elaborate plexus of veins called the *internal vertebral venous plexus*. The practical importance of the epidural space and its contents for LP lies in the possibility of inadvertently puncture of the venous plexus, which results in a bloody tap. Striking the roots of a spinal nerve is another mishap that may lead to long-lasting paresthesias.

The epidural space is commonly used as the site of anesthesia of the spinal nerves. This procedure should not be confused with spinal anesthesia, in which the anesthetizing fluid is injected into the subarachnoid space. Epidural anesthesia can be induced through LP or through the caudal approach. In caudal anesthesia, the needle is inserted through the sacral hiatus into the inferior part of the sacral canal without penetration of the dural sac, which ends at S2. It is a useful method of obtaining analgesia of the perineum in obstetrics.

Subdural and Subarachnoid Spaces

The next step in LP, after the ligamentum flavum has been penetrated and the epidural space passed, is the piercing of the dura and arachnoid, which again may be perceived as a "snap." The needle is then in the subarachnoid space, and under normal conditions, CSF will appear at the hub of the needle (Figs. 14.1 and 14.2). The pressure of the CSF should be determined and its clearness, color, and cell and protein count investigated. Fluid for bacterial cultures also should be collected.

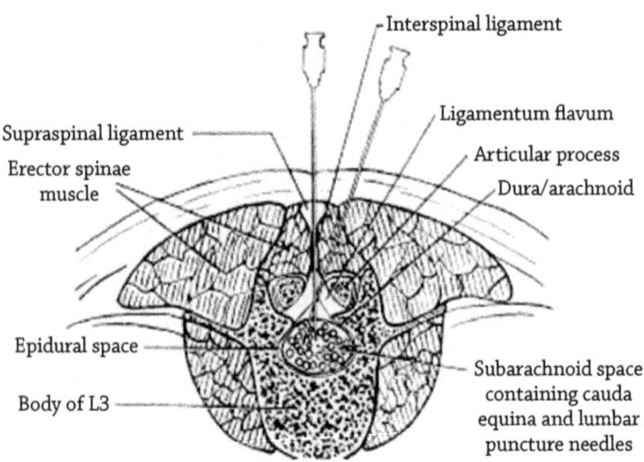

FIGURE 14.2

Horizontal section through the body of lumbar vertebrae L3. Notice that there are two puncture needles in the subarachnoid space. The median one is in the midline, corresponding to the position in Figure 14.1. The lateral one exemplifies the lateral approach, which avoids the occasionally calcified supraspinal ligament. Notice that the lateral needle pierces the intrinsic musculature of the back and only one ligament, the ligamentum flavum.

The subdural space is a potential space. An actual space does not normally exist, because the arachnoid is directly in contact with the dura and held tightly against it by the CSF pressure. However, because the arachnoid and dura are not fused together, they can be separated, for example when blood or other fluid enters this space and separates the layers.

Posterolateral Approach

In older people or and in patients with metabolic disease, the supraspinous ligament may be ossified or calcified, and perforation by the puncture needle may be difficult. Such a calcified ligament may also deflect the needle from its intended course so that it strikes the bony lamina above or below the puncture site. In such cases, a slightly lateral approach to one side of the midline may be chosen (Fig. 14.2). The needle is directed slightly superiorly to miss the lamina of the lower vertebra and slightly medially to compensate for the lateral point of entrance. In this approach, the needle passes through skin, a variable amount of superficial fascia and fat, the dense posterior layer of the thoracolumbar fascia, and the erector spinae muscles. The needle must now penetrate only the ligamentum flavum (i.e., the supraspinous and interspinous ligaments have been bypassed), the epidural space, and the dura-arachnoid before CSF escapes.

Side Effects and Complications

One of the side effects of LP has already been mentioned: a bloody tap resulting from puncture of the epidural venous plexus. Acute root pain or longer-lasting neuralgia of a spinal nerve may be caused by contact with the needle if it is misdirected in the lateral approach. A serious, often fatal, complication is herniation of the temporal lobe or cerebellum with compression of the vital centers of the brain stem in patients who have increased intracranial pressure as a result of sudden release of the pressure (see earlier discussion). If the needle passes through an infected area or if a faulty, nonsterile technique is employed, septic meningitis may result. Other incidents include puncture of the posterior longitudinal ligament and the anulus fibrosus, resulting in prolapse of the nucleus pulposus of the intervertebral disk.

Post-puncture Headache

The most common side effect of LP is post-puncture headache, which is slow in starting, and takes 2 to 3 days to reach its peak. The pain is caused by leakage of CSF at the site of puncture of the dura; this causes decreased hydrostatic pressure in the subarachnoid space, which leads to slight dislodgment of the brain and traction on pain-sensitive blood vessels and intracranial dura. The surface of the brain does not contain pain fibers. The headache is increased when the patient is in the erect position and is temporarily relieved by a second LP with injection of saline solution. Placing the patient in a horizontal position, with the head flat and unsupported by pillows, alleviates the pain. The headache typically lasts only a few days. It is obvious that use of small-gauge puncture needles and avoidance of multiple punctures will reduce the frequency of many of the side effects of LP.

Unit II

Review Questions

The number in parentheses is a reference to the page on which information about the question may be found.

1. Why are herniations of the nucleus pulposus usually in a posterolateral direction?
The anulus fibrosus is thinner posteriorly than anteriorly, so it is easier to herniate through the posterior portion of the disk. However, the posterior longitudinal ligament reinforces the disk in the posterior midline. Therefore, the posterolateral direction is most common for herniation. (121)

2. What is the vertebral level of the most inferior portion of the spinal cord?
The inferior tip of the spinal cord (the conus medullaris) is at the level of the L1/L2 intervertebral disk in the average adult. However, the location varies from person to person. (122)

3. What is the inferior limit of the subarachnoid space?
The subarachnoid space extends down to the S2 vertebral level in the average adult. Again, there is variability from person to person. (122)

4. What is the cauda equina?
The cauda equina is the collection of dorsal and ventral roots from lumbar and sacral levels that extend below the bottom of the spinal cord. The cauda equina is in the subarachnoid space surrounded by cerebrospinal fluid. (122)

5. If there is a herniation of the L4/L5 disk, which spinal nerve is most likely to be affected?
If the L4/L5 disk herniates, the spinal nerve most likely to be involved is the L5 spinal nerve. Because of the downward slope of the spinal roots forming the lumbosacral nerves, the nerve exiting though the intervertebral foramen below the herniated disk is the one most likely to be compressed. (122)

6. What is the optimal site for performing a lumbar puncture?
Lumbar puncture is performed most frequently at the L3/L4 interspace or the L4/L5 interspace. This is done to ensure that the puncture will be below the bottom of the spinal cord but above the bottom of the subarachnoid space. (128)

7. What landmark is used to identify the proper level for performing a lumbar puncture?
The iliac crest is a palpable landmark. A horizontal line connecting the highest points of the iliac crests is used to identify the L4 level. The spinous process is palpated at this level, and the interspaces immediately above and below it are the L3/L4 and the L4/L5 interspace, respectively. (128)

8. What ligaments of the spine must be traversed when inserting a lumbar puncture needle?
The ligaments traverses are the supraspinous ligament, the interspinous ligament, and the ligamentum flavum. (130)

9. Why is a lumbar puncture done with the spine in a flexed position?
Flexing the spine widens the interspinous and interlaminar spaces and thereby provides more space for the introduction of the needle. It also puts the ligaments on stretch, making it easier to penetrate them. (128)

10. What is the internal vertebral venous plexus, and what is its significance when performing a lumbar puncture?
The internal vertebral venous plexus is an elaborate plexus of veins in the epidural space. When the lumbar puncture needle traverses the epidural space, a vein may be punctured, and blood may enter the needle, giving rise to blood in the cerebrospinal fluid that is withdrawn. (131)

UNIT III

Thorax

15

Cancer of the Breast

A 51-year-old woman presents to the office with a 1-month history of a lump in her right breast which she discovered during breast self-examination. The lump is not tender and has not changed in size since she first noticed it. She reports no skin changes or nipple discharge. She has always been in good health and has no significant medical history. She had her first menstrual period at age 13 and has had three full-term pregnancies, the first at age 22. She reached menopause 3 years ago. She has no family history of breast or ovarian cancer and has never had a mammogram. Her last gynecological examination was 1 year ago and was normal. She takes no medications or hormonal supplements. Her past medical and surgical histories are noncontributory.

Examination

The patient has been in good health. On inspection with the patient seated, the breasts are symmetrical and there are no skin changes, dimpling, or erythema. The nipples are both everted. The breasts are then examined with the patient in a supine position. In the upper outer quadrant of the right breast there is a pea-sized nodule in the 10 o'clock position, 3 cm from the areolar border. The nodule is 1 cm by 1 cm in size, firm, and nontender. The borders are well circumscribed, and it is mobile. There are no palpable masses in the left breast. There is no cervical, supraclavicular, or axillary adenopathy. The remainder of the examination is within normal limits.

Diagnosis

The diagnosis is right breast mass.

Therapy and Further Course

To complete the examination of both breasts, a mammogram is ordered. Bilateral mammography is performed and confirms the location of the mass in the upper outer quadrant of the right breast. The borders are well circumscribed. There are no associated calcifications. The remainder of the right breast examination and the examination of the left breast are normal. The patient is referred directly for ultrasound examination to determine whether the mass is solid or fluid-filled (a cyst). Ultrasonography demonstrates a solid mass.

Sonographic guidance is used to perform a core biopsy of the mass, which confirms a diagnosis of infiltrating ductal carcinoma of the right breast. After lengthy discussion regarding her treatment options, the patient elects to have a sentinel lymph node biopsy (SLNB) followed by a lumpectomy (localized excision of the mass). The SLNB result is positive, and the patient undergoes complete axillary lymph node dissection as an outpatient procedure. She is referred for follow-up care to both radiation and medical oncologists.

Discussion

For patients who are newly diagnosed with invasive breast cancer, the status of the axillary lymph nodes is an important prognostic indicator. Staging depends not only on the size of the metastatic deposits but also on the total number of lymph nodes involved. If the lymph nodes in the axilla are clinically negative (i.e. not palpable), what is the best way to determine whether the breast cancer has spread to this lymph node basin?

Historically, the gold standard procedure for staging breast cancer was a complete axillary lymph node dissection (ALND) with histopathological study of the axillary specimen. However, the low (<3%) rate of axillary recurrence in patients undergoing level I or II ALND (discussed later) is achieved at the cost of significant morbidity, with an acute complication rate of 20% to 30% and a significant chronic lymphedema rate. Therefore, for those women with small

(<2 cm) tumors and favorable pathological features who have a low risk of axillary metastasis or for those who would receive adjuvant therapy regardless of axillary involvement, clinicians have sought alternative methods for managing the axilla.

Recent introduction of intraoperative lymphatic mapping and sentinel lymphadenectomy (SLNB) for primary breast cancer allows directed and accurate assessment of axillary involvement with minimal morbidity. More recent data have suggested that the long-term survival of patients found to have metastatic disease in the axillary nodes is equivalent whether the patient had SLNB alone or complete ALND. Therefore, the practice of traditional axillary staging for breast cancer may become increasingly rare.

The Axilla

The axilla is a pyramid-shaped space between the upper limb and the chest wall (Fig. 15.1). It has an anterior wall composed of the pectoralis major and pectoralis minor muscles. It has a posterior

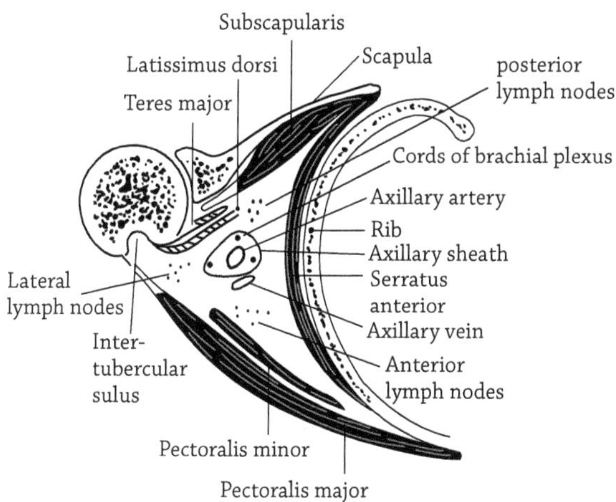

FIGURE 15.1

Horizontal section through the axilla.

wall composed of the subscapularis, teres major, and latissimus dorsi muscles. It has a medial wall composed of the serratus anterior muscle covering the ribs. Its small lateral wall is composed of the intertubercular sulcus of the humerus, between the humeral attachments of the pectoralis major and the teres major. The base of the pyramid is composed of skin and fascia. The apex of the pyramid is the space between the clavicle and the first rib. Much of the axillary space is filled with fat.

Passing through the axilla is the neurovascular supply to the upper limb, including the axillary artery and vein and elements of the brachial plexus. A large collection of lymph nodes is found in the axilla. These lymph nodes receive lymphatic drainage from the anterior chest wall (including the breast), the posterior chest wall, the scapular region, and the upper limb. The lymph from these nodes enters the subclavian lymph trunk, which then joins the thoracic duct on the left side or the right lymphatic duct on the right side to return the lymph to the venous system.

Axillary Lymph Nodes

There are five groups of axillary lymph nodes, the first three of which can be regarded as peripheral outposts. These are the anterior nodes, which receive drainage from the anterior chest wall and breast; posterior nodes, which receive drainage from the posterior chest wall; and the lateral nodes, which receive drainage from the upper limb. These three groups of nodes drain to the other two groups, the central and apical nodes. The efferent drainage from the apical nodes forms the subclavian trunk (Fig. 15.2).

Because of this anatomy, the anterior, central, and apical axillary lymph nodes are interposed in the pathway of cancerous emboli from the breast before they reach the venous bloodstream. Supraclavicular nodes in the low neck may also receive some of this drainage. Because shortcuts that bypass one, two, or even three of the more peripheral lymphatic stations may occur, direct drainage from the breast into the central or apical or even the supraclavicular set can take place. The goal of an ALND is to remove all nodal

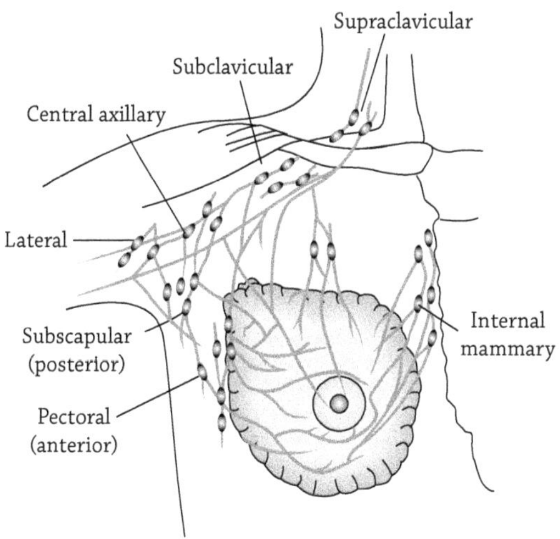

FIGURE 15.2

Lymph nodes associated with drainage from the breast.

tissue in the space defined by the axillary vein superiorly, the latissimus dorsi muscle inferolaterally, the medial border of the pectoralis minor muscle medially, and the subscapularis muscle posteriorly.

Clinically, the axilla is divided into levels using the pectoralis minor muscle as a reference. Level I lymph nodes are found in the space inferolateral to the pectoralis minor muscle; level II nodes are those found posterior to the pectoralis minor; level III nodes are those found superomedial to the pectoralis minor. The ALND focuses specifically on level I and level II nodes only and can usually yield from 7 to 15 nodes. Level III nodes are typically not removed unless clinically suspicious.

Accessory Lymphatic Channels

Additional lymph vessels connect the breast, particularly its medial half, with the parasternal nodes. These vessels traverse the pectoralis major and intercostal muscles and follow the anterior intercostal branches of the internal thoracic vessels. They terminate in parasternal nodes (internal mammary nodes) located in the upper intercostal spaces near the internal thoracic vessels, close to the lateral margin of the sternum (Fig. 15.2). Their efferents go to the supraclavicular nodes and lymph trunks in the neck. Direct lymphatic connections between the right and left parasternal nodes provide a pathway for direct metastasis to the contralateral breast.

In this discussion on lymphatic drainage of the breast and lymphatic spread of cancer, it must be realized that obstruction of the normal lymph flow by metastatic growth in the lymph nodes may lead to reversal of the lymph flow and to involvement of lymph nodes in atypical locations, such as the inguinal region.

Vulnerable Nerves in Axillary Lymph Node Dissection

There are three nerves in the operative field during ALND that are susceptible to injury and deserve special note in this discussion. The long thoracic nerve arises in the neck from branches of the anterior rami of cervical vertebrae C5, C6, and C7 and innervates the important serratus anterior muscle. This nerve lies on the medial wall of the axilla and may be injured during the procedure. Injury to this nerve may paralyze the serratus anterior. Because this muscle helps to hold the scapula against the posterior chest wall and to upwardly rotate the scapula, paralysis results in "winged scapula" and a severely compromised ability to rotate the scapula upward. Patients suffering winged scapula have difficulty in raising their hand as in brushing their hair or reaching to retrieve items from an overhead shelf.

The thoracodorsal nerve arises from the posterior cord of the brachial plexus, passes through the axilla, and descends on the posterior wall to innervate the latissimus dorsi muscle. Because the latissimus dorsi is an important extensor, adductor, and medial rotator of the arm at the shoulder, injury to this nerve results in difficulty with these movements.

The intercostobrachial nerve arises as a branch of the second intercostal nerve. It crosses the axilla to reach the medial side of the arm, where it provides cutaneous sensory innervations. Injury to this nerve during ALND can result in chronic postoperative pain in this region or numbness of the region.

Anatomy of Edema

The lymphatic system is the primary pathway for drainage of extracellular or interstitial fluid. Because all of the lymphatic drainage from the upper limb flows to the axillary lymph nodes, removal of these nodes may significantly interfere with lymphatic drainage of the limb with resultant accumulation of fluid, known as *lymphedema*. A substantial percentage of patients who have ALND experience some amount of lymphedema of the upper limb. They experience swelling of the limb and may have a feeling of fullness, tightness, or pain. Keeping the limb elevated above the level of the heart, exercise, and the use of a compression sleeve may be effective in reducing the edema. The use of SLNB rather than complete ALND reduces the incidence of lymphedema in the limb.

Historical Comments on Breast Cancer Surgery

In 1882, William Halsted introduced the radical mastectomy. In this procedure, the breast, the pectoral muscles, and the axillary lymph nodes are removed. The rationale for this procedure was the desire to excise all possible metastatic cells. Because lymphatic channels from the breast penetrate the pectoral muscles to reach the axilla, it was believed that removal of these muscles would remove such metastatic cells. This disfiguring and disabling procedure was widely used through most of the twentieth century. In 1971, a large controlled study demonstrated that radical mastectomy produced no higher cure rates than a less aggressive modified radical mastectomy in which the chest wall muscles are spared along with the uninvolved axillary lymph nodes. This began a period of pursuing less extensive surgery with adjuvant chemotherapy and radiation therapy.

It is currently common to do a lumpectomy, removing only the tumor and some surrounding tissue. This procedure is frequently followed by ALND for staging or therapy or both. As indicated earlier, even this procedure is now being reduced in scope with the use of SLNB, in which a colored dye and a radioactive dye are injected into the region of the tumor and then the very few lymph nodes to which the dye drains are removed. The rationale for this approach is that the dye identifies the axillary lymph node or nodes to which the region of the tumor drains, and the removal of those nodes for biopsy is sufficient to determine whether the tumor has metastasized and to prevent metastasis.

16

Aspiration Pneumonia

A 77-year-old woman who is recovering from a recent cerebrovascular accident (CVA) that resulted in mild right-sided weakness and difficulty swallowing (dysphagia) presents with fever and increased respiratory rate. She had been well until 2 days earlier, when she began experiencing cough productive of greenish sputum. She notes that the cough has gotten progressively worse and kept her awake the previous night. She has had no blood in her sputum. She has felt warm over the previous 12 hours and reports that she had fever to 101.8° F accompanied by chills. She has had no upper respiratory tract symptoms, sore throat, or runny nose. She reports no chest pain. Of note, she was previously evaluated for swallowing difficulty as a residual deficit from her stroke and is receiving occupational therapy for management. She has no history of pulmonary disease, is a nonsmoker, and is negative on purified protein derivative (PPD) skin testing for tuberculosis. She currently takes only a baby aspirin daily and has no medication allergies. She is residing at a rehabilitation facility.

Examination

The patient is an ill-appearing female and is slightly tachypneic (rapid respiratory rate). Her temperature is 102.3° F, respiratory rate is 22 breaths/min, heart rate is 95 bpm, and blood pressure is 140/80 mm Hg. There is no evidence of cyanosis. She is found to have 92% oxygen saturation on room air by pulse oximetry. Her conjunctivae are clear. There is no nasal discharge or polyps. She is edentulous. The oropharynx is normal, without erythema or exudate. However, she has a diminished cough reflex. She has no cervical or supraclavicular adenopathy. Cranial nerves II through XII are intact, although there is mild facial droop. Examination of the chest reveals diminished breath sounds over the right upper lobe posteriorly, with dullness to percussion. There is increased tactile fremitus and diffuse rales over the upper right lung field. The remainder of the physical examination is noncontributory. Anteroposterior and lateral chest radiographs are obtained and demonstrate an infiltrate in the posterior segment of the right upper lobe.

Diagnosis

The diagnosis is pneumonia, possibly due to aspiration.

Therapy and Further Course

A sputum sample is obtained from the patient and sent for Gram staining and culture. She is admitted to the hospital and begun on intravenous, broad-spectrum antibiotics designed to cover both gram-negative and gram-positive bacteria. She is also given supplemental oxygen through a nasal cannula. A respiratory therapist visits to encourage coughing and to provide chest percussion to help the patient clear secretions. This is aided by the provision of a mucolytic to thin her secretions. A swallowing evaluation is performed, and aspiration precautions are instituted. The patient steadily improves and is discharged to the rehabilitation facility for additional recovery.

Discussion

The presumptive diagnosis in this patient is aspiration pneumonia, yet she presents no history of aspiration, nor was there a witnessed event. Clearly, this diagnosis may not be an easy one to make. There are several factors that support the consideration of aspiration as the etiology for pneumonia in this patient. First, although the overall incidence of aspiration is relatively low, this patient has several risk factors that increase both the likelihood of aspiration and the probability that the aspiration will lead to pneumonia. These include increased age, debilitation, recent stroke, dysphagia, diminished cough reflex, and residence at a long-term care facility. Whereas some aspiration of oropharyngeal contents normally occurs during sleep in adults, the amount of aspirate and the virulence of the typical oropharyngeal bacteria are usually low enough that normal clearance mechanisms prevent pneumonia from developing. The presence of both dysphagia and a poor cough reflex (as in this patient) increases the chance that the volume aspirated will lead to aspiration pneumonia. Her edentulous condition is also associated with an increased bacterial burden. Finally, her residence in a rehabilitation facility increases the risk that she is colonized with bacteria that have enhanced virulence and are therefore more likely to cause a problem should aspiration occur.

The second factor that contributes to the diagnosis is the location of the pneumonia as determined by the physical examination and radiography. Her physical examination findings of diminished breath sounds, rales, dullness to percussion, and increased tactile fremitus all support a diagnosis of pneumonia. This assessment is supported by the chest radiograph. The location of the pneumonia in the posterior segment of the right upper lobe is strongly associated with an etiology of aspiration.

Anatomy of the Airway

The upper pharynx (nasopharynx and oropharynx) serves as an aerodigestive pathway. The pathway bifurcates at about the level of the fourth cervical vertebra (C4) into the more anterior airway (the larynx) and the more posterior digestive tract (the laryngopharynx). At the level of C6, the downward continuation of the laryngopharynx is the esophagus and the downward continuation of the larynx is the trachea. The trachea continues down into the thorax, and at the level of T4 it bifurcates into the right and left main bronchi. This bifurcation is not symmetrical. The right main bronchus takes a more vertical course than the left (i.e., closer to the long axis of the trachea) and is wider than the left. The left main bronchus diverges more from the long axis of the trachea (i.e., is more oblique) and is

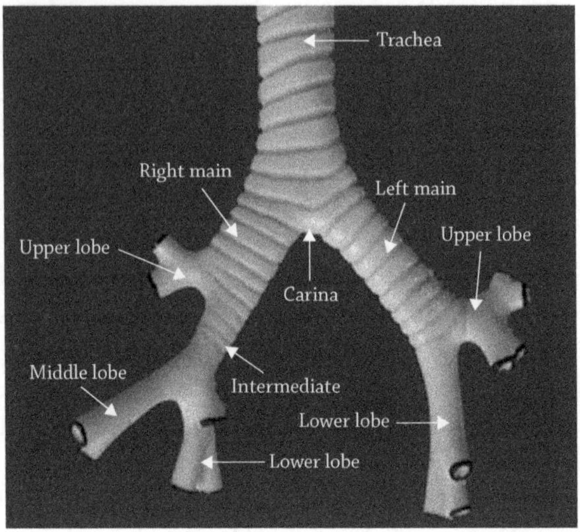

FIGURE 16.1

Bifurcation of the trachea.

narrower than the right main bronchus (Fig. 16.1). For these reasons, any aspirated material is more likely to enter the right bronchus than the left. Similarly, if an endotracheal tube is placed too far into the trachea, it is more likely to enter the right bronchus than the left. In this patient, the presumptive aspiration pneumonia is in the right lung.

The main bronchus enters the hilum of the lung and divides into lobar bronchi, three on the right and two on the left. Each lobar bronchus is the airway to one lobe of the lung. On the right side, the upper lobar bronchus arises just before the main bronchus enters the hilum, and the remainder of the main bronchus continues more distally into the lung to divide into the middle and lower lobar bronchi. On the left side, the main bronchus enters the hilum and then divides into upper and lower bronchi (Fig. 16.1). Each of the lobar bronchi divides into segmental bronchi. There are a total of 10 segmental bronchi in each lung. Each segmental bronchus is the airway to a bronchopulmonary segment.

Because each bronchopulmonary segment is supplied by its own segmental bronchus and its own segmental branch of the pulmonary artery, the bronchopulmonary segment can be viewed as the structural and functional unit of the lung. Bronchopulmonary segments tend to be separated from their neighboring segments by connective tissue septa. Disease processes may be limited to one segment or may extend beyond the segment to involve the whole lobe or even the whole lung. The anatomical separation of segments makes surgical resection of a bronchopulmonary segment possible. Branches of the pulmonary veins are located in the intersegmental planes and serve as landmarks for the surgeon during a segmental resection. For detailed description of the bronchopulmonary segments, the reader should refer to a standard anatomy text.

As indicated earlier, aspiration is more likely to occur on the right side. The specific segmental bronchus into which aspiration is most likely to occur depends on the position of the patient. If the patient is supine at the time of aspiration, as was likely the case in this patient, then the posterior segment of the right upper lobe is the most likely segment to be affected. This is because the upper lobar bronchus takes a slightly posteriorward direction when it arises from the main bronchus, and the posterior segmental bronchus arises from the posterior wall of the upper lobar bronchus. Therefore, with the patient supine, the effect of gravity directs the aspirate to the posterior segmental bronchus of the upper lobe. In this patient, the pneumonia is localized in the posterior segment of the upper lobe. This location is strongly associated with aspiration as the etiology of the pneumonia. If the patient were standing or sitting up at the time of aspiration, the effect of gravity would tend to direct the aspirated material toward the right lower lobe and then into either the posterior basal or the medial basal segment, because these are the segmental bronchi with the most vertical courses.

The Swallowing Mechanism

This patient was at risk for aspiration in part because her swallowing mechanism was compromised due to her stroke. The clinician needs to understand the anatomical mechanisms involved with swallowing. The objective of the swallowing reflexes is to get food from the oral cavity to the esophagus and to avoid having the food pass to other regions, especially the airway. The bolus of food is moved posteriorly from the oral cavity to the oropharynx by action of the tongue. As the food approaches the pharynx, the pharynx is elevated by action of the stylopharyngeus, palatopharyngeus, and salpingopharyngeus muscles. This elevation of the pharynx causes the oropharynx to widen, facilitating the entry of the bolus.

Once the food is in the oropharynx, it is propelled by contraction of the pharyngeal constrictors. However, it is necessary to ensure that there is only one pathway for the bolus to follow when the pharynx constricts. To accomplish this, the palatoglossus muscle contracts to approximate the tongue to the soft palate, thereby preventing the food from returning back to the oral cavity. The soft palate is elevated by contraction of the levator palati and tensor palati muscles, thus approximating the soft palate to the posterior wall of the pharynx. This separates the nasopharynx from the oropharynx and prevents the bolus from entering the nasopharynx and thence the nasal cavity. With these two pathways closed, contraction of the constrictors causes the bolus to move downward toward the larynx and the laryngopharynx.

Because the epiglottis is positioned behind the tongue and above the laryngeal aditus, the bolus tends to pass around the epiglottis and into the right and left piriform recesses of the laryngopharynx. From these recesses, the food returns toward the midline and enters the esophagus, having bypassed the larynx. However, the epiglottis does not form a tight seal over the aditus of the larynx, so another mechanism is needed to protect the airway if any food enters the larynx. During swallowing, the glottis is closed by reflex adduction of the vocal folds. This is accomplished by contraction of the lateral cricoarytenoid muscles and the interarytenoid muscles. With closure of the glottis, the airway is protected: Neither air nor liquid can pass. It is for this reason that we normally cannot breathe and swallow at the same time. If we attempt to override this reflex, for example by talking while swallowing, we increase the risk that food will enter the airway.

All of the muscles involved in swallowing are innervated by cranial nerves (Table 16.1), and the stroke suffered by our patient presumably compromised or weakened these mechanisms, which increased the risk of aspiration.

TABLE 16.1 The Swallowing Mechanism

Action	*Muscles Involved*	*Innervation*
Movement of food bolus from mouth to oropharynx by the tongue	Palatoglossus Hyoglossus Styloglossus	Vagus Hypoglossal Hypoglossal
Elevation of the pharynx	Palatopharyngeus Salpingopharyngeus Stylopharyngeus	Vagus Vagus Glossopharyngeal
Occlusion of the nasopharynx by the soft palate	Levator palati Tensor palati	Vagus Trigeminal (mandibular division)
Occlusion of the oral cavity by the tongue	Palatoglossus	Vagus
Constriction of the pharynx	Superior, middle, and inferior constrictors	Vagus
Obstruction of the laryngeal aditus by the epiglottis	Aryepiglotticus	Vagus (recurrent laryngeal branch)
Closure of the glottis by the vocal folds	Lateral cricoarytenoid and interarytenoid	Vagus (recurrent laryngeal branch)

The Cough Reflex

Because it is possible for food or other foreign material to enter the aditus of the larynx, it is necessary to have a mechanism to prevent this material from descending through the airway. The interior of the larynx is divided into three regions: the vestibule, from the aditus to the vestibular folds; the ventricle, from the vestibular folds to the vocal folds; and the infraglottic space, below the vocal folds. The glottis comprises the vocal folds and the space between them.

If a foreign body contacts the mucosa of the vestibule, it stimulates the sensory nerve innervating this region, which is the internal branch of the superior laryngeal nerve, a branch of the vagus nerve. This serves as the sensory limb of the cough reflex. In response to this stimulus, the glottis closes tightly, preventing passage of the foreign body or air through the glottis. With the glottis closed, the abdominal wall muscles are contracted and the diaphragm is relaxed, causing an increase in the intrathoracic pressure. As the intrathoracic pressure increases, a pressure gradient is established between the infraglottic space and the vestibule. When the pressure gradient has become high enough, the glottis is rapidly opened by action of the posterior cricoarytenoid muscles, and a high-velocity blast of air moves through the glottis, clearing the retained foreign body from the vestibule. The fact that this patient has a diminished cough reflex as a result of the stroke contributes to her risk for aspiration.

17

Tetralogy of Fallot

A 3-year-old boy is brought to the emergency department by his mother. He is crying and appears cyanotic. The mother reports that the boy fell while running outside, scraped his knee, and began to cry. She reports that as he continued to cry, his lips became blue, followed by his fingers. He has had no recent upper respiratory infections and has no history of asthma. No one in the family is a smoker. The mother reports that her son was delivered by normal vaginal delivery but she received very little prenatal or postnatal care. She reports that the boy has reached his developmental milestones but has had difficulty keeping up with his friends and seems to tire more easily than they do.

On further questioning, the mother reports that she has noticed that when the boy has been very active, he assumes a squatting position while he rests. She further states that at other times his lips have become blue when he cried, but this soon passed after he stopped crying. Because of the more prolonged crying during the current episode and the more noticeable blueness, she brought him to the emergency department. To her knowledge, her son has not received routine vaccinations. He has had no prior hospitalizations. He is taking no medications and has no known allergies. She reports that the family immigrated to this country 2 years ago from Central America.

Examination

The boy is small in stature and is at the 10th percentile for his age in height and weight. He continues to cry during the examination. His pulse and respiratory rates are mildly elevated, whereas his blood pressure is within normal limits. His oxygen saturation is 89% on

4 L of oxygen delivered through a nasal cannula. His lips and nail beds are mildly cyanotic. His head, ears, eyes, nose, and throat examinations are normal. The chest is symmetrical with good excursions. The lungs are clear with no wheezes or rales. Palpation of the chest reveals a systolic thrill present along the left sternal border. Auscultation of the heart reveals a harsh systolic ejection murmur that is most prominent at the upper left sternal margin, in the second intercostal space. There is a normal S_1 heart sound and a single S_2 heart sound; the pulmonic valve closure is not heard. Mild clubbing of the fingers and toes is noted. The remainder of the physical examination is normal.

An electrocardiogram displays a right axis deviation. The patient is sent for chest radiography, which reveals an enlarged heart shadow with a boot-like appearance. Blood tests reveal an elevated hemoglobin concentration and an elevated red blood cell count. Transthoracic cross-sectional echocardiography reveals a large ventricular septal defect with an overriding aorta and right ventricular hypertrophy with outflow tract obstruction, confirming the diagnosis of tetralogy of Fallot (TOF).

Diagnosis

A diagnosis of TOF, confirmed by echocardiography, can be made based on the patient's clinical signs and symptoms. These include the appearance of cyanosis on exertion, a heart murmur indicative of pulmonary stenosis, a smaller than average stature for age, a tendency to tire more easily than his peer group, and findings on electrocardiography and chest radiography that are indicative of right ventricular hypertrophy. TOF consists of a group of four defects: ventricular septal defect, pulmonary stenosis, overriding aorta, and right ventricular hypertrophy (Fig. 17.1).

Therapy and Further Course

A pediatric cardiologist and pediatric cardiac surgeon are consulted for repair of the defect, and the patient is admitted to the hospital.

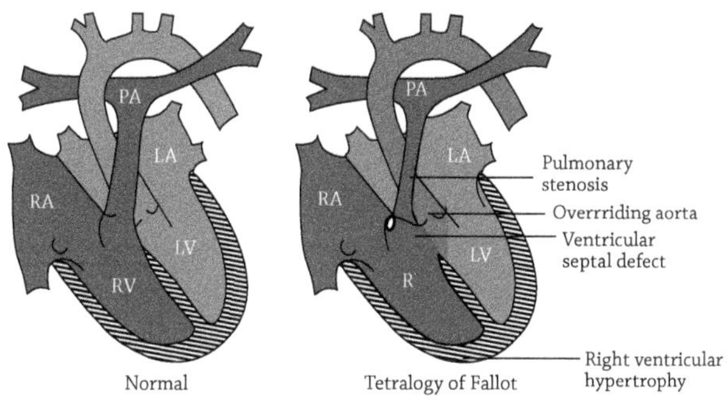

FIGURE 17.1

Schematic diagram of a normal heart and tetralogy of Fallot.

A cardiac catheterization is performed to determine the size of the pulmonary artery and the aorta and to determine the pressure gradient across the obstructed pulmonary outflow tract is determined. At surgery, the ventricular septal defect is repaired with a pericardial patch. This repair also addresses the overriding aorta. The pulmonary outflow tract is enlarged by resecting some of the obstructing muscle and enlarging the pulmonary trunk with a second patch. A few days after surgery, right ventricular function has improved markedly and peripheral arterial oxygen saturation has improved. The patient is discharged from the hospital after 7 days.

Discussion

TOF accounts for approximately 10% of congenital heart disease. Its incidence is about 5 in 10,000 live births and is higher in males than in females. It is often associated with other cardiac defects, including a right-sided aortic arch (25% of patients) and atrial septal defects (10% of patients). It was described in 1888 by Etienne Fallot as consisting of pulmonary stenosis, ventricular septal defect, displacement of the origin of the aorta toward the right, and hypertrophy of the right ventricular wall (Fig. 17.1). There is wide variability in the structural manifestation of this abnormality. The degree of obstruction of the pulmonary outflow tract accounts for the variability in the degree of cyanosis observed in patients.

The cause of TOF is not known, but it is almost certainly multifactorial. Factors that seem to be associated with TOF include hereditary factors and environmental factors such as rubella or other viral infection of the mother during pregnancy, alcohol use by the mother, maternal diabetes, and maternal age older than 40 years. TOF is seen in association with some genetic syndromes such as DeGeorge syndrome, which is characterized by a microdeletion in chromosome 22 (22q11). This region contains the T-box 1 (*TBX1*) gene, a transcription factor that plays a critical role in the developmental patterning of the cardiac outflow tract. TOF is also associated with trisomy 21 (Down syndrome).

Normal Development of the Heart

During the fourth week of development, the embryonic heart tube is a midline structure in the ventral portion of the thorax. The outflow from the embryonic ventricle is through the truncus arteriosus. During the fifth and sixth weeks of development, the embryonic ventricle is divided into right and left ventricles by the formation of the ventricular septum, and the truncus arteriosus is divided into the ascending aorta and the pulmonary trunk by the formation of the aorticopulmonary septum. In normal development, the aorticopulmonary septum forms in the center of the truncus arteriosus and divides the truncus arteriosus into two equal halves. Thus, the diameters of the ascending aorta and the pulmonary trunk are equal (Fig. 17.2).

Tetralogy of Fallot

The error in development that results in TOF is referred to as dextropositioning of the aorticopulmonary septum—that is, the septum is abnormally displaced toward the right side (pulmonary side) of the outflow tract. As a result, the truncus arteriosus is divided into two channels of unequal size. The pulmonary trunk is narrower

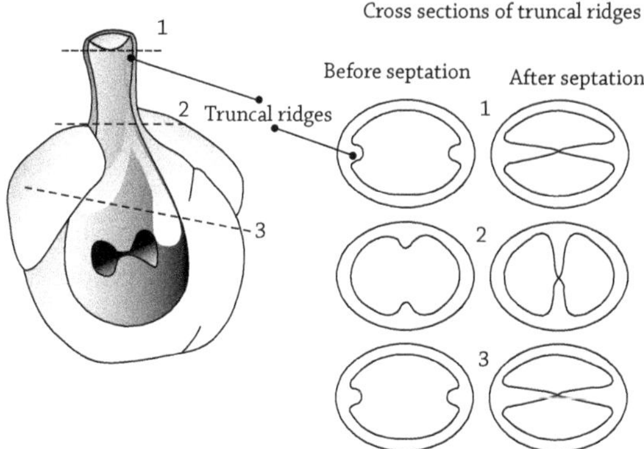

FIGURE 17.2

Formation of the aorticopulmonary septum from the truncal ridges. Notice the spiral shape of the septum.

than normal (pulmonary stenosis), and the ascending aorta is wider than normal and receives outflow from both the left and right ventricles (overriding aorta).

The definitive interventricular septum normally is formed by fusion of the embryonic interventricular septum (which forms the muscular portion of the interventricular septum) and caudal extension of the aorticopulmonary septum (which forms the membranous portion of the interventricular septum). For this to be accomplished, the aorticopulmonary septum must be in its normal position in the center of the truncus arteriosus so that it is aligned with the embryonic ventricular septum and the two septa can meet and fuse. When there is dextropositioning of the aorticopulmonary septum, it is not aligned with the embryonic interventricular septum, and the two cannot meet and fuse, resulting in a ventricular septal defect.

Because of the pulmonary stenosis that results from the dextropositioned septum, the right ventricular myocardium has to pump blood through a narrowed opening. This increased workload causes the right ventricular myocardium to hypertrophy. Accordingly, the right ventricular hypertrophy seen in TOF is not really part of the developmental defect but rather the physiological response of the right ventricle to the defect.

Blood Flow in Tetralogy of Fallot

The pulmonary stenosis results in increased right ventricular pressure. This leads to a right-to-left shunting of blood through the ventricular septal defect and into the overriding aorta. Thus, deoxygenated blood from the right ventricle enters the systemic circulation, leading to cyanosis. The degree of shunting of blood determines the extent to which the child will be cyanotic. Not uncommonly, as in this case, the child is not cyanotic at birth but becomes cyanotic as he gets older and becomes more active. Periods of strenuous activity or periods of crying and agitation may bring on cyanosis. Children learn that squatting during such periods can relieve the distress caused by the cyanosis. It is believed that the squatting increases peripheral arterial resistance, thereby increasing the pressure in the left ventricle. This increased pressure reduces the pressure gradient between the two ventricles, thus reducing the right-to-left shunting of blood and resulting cyanosis.

The elevated hemoglobin value and red blood cell count seen in this patient represent the body's response to the reduced level of oxygen in the peripheral circulation. This is the body's attempt to bring more oxygen to the tissues of the body.

Repair of Tetralogy of Fallot

Most children with untreated TOF die before the age of 10 years, and they rarely live beyond 40 years. Total surgical repair of this defect has been possible for the past few decades, and patients generally do well after repair. Before the availability of open heart surgery, a palliative operative procedure (Blalock-Taussig shunt) was available to improve oxygenation of the peripheral systemic circulation. This procedure was first performed in 1944 on a 15-month-old child with TOF. It did not repair any of the structural defects in the heart but rather addressed the functional issue of not having sufficient oxygenated blood in the systemic circulation. The Blalock-Taussig procedure creates a shunt from the subclavian artery to the pulmonary artery. This takes systemic arterial blood, which is deficient in oxygen, and sends it to the lungs for oxygenation. Thus it provides two pathways for blood to get to the lungs, one from the right ventricle through the stenotic pulmonary outflow and a second from the left ventricle through the subclavian artery. Although this does not correct the underlying structural defect, it does provide an improved quality of life and extended life span.

It is now common for TOF to be diagnosed prenatally by ultrasound imaging or to be diagnosed very soon after birth. The surgical repair is typically done while the child is an infant. In this case, the minimal prenatal and postnatal care presumably accounts for the failure to diagnose this disorder sooner. Variations on the Blalock-Taussig shunt are still used for palliation in patients with a variety of cyanotic congenital heart diseases, often as a temporary measure while awaiting definitive surgical repair. This may be the prudent course to follow if the patient is not a good surgical risk at the time of diagnosis. The procedure provides relief of symptoms while allowing the child's condition to improve so that definitive open heart surgery can be done.

18

Lung Cancer

The patient is a 69-year-old man with a 40 pack-year smoking history who presents with a longstanding history of chronic cough and recent onset of inspiratory stridor (high-pitched breathing sound) and increasing shortness of breath. The patient states that over the past year, he has experienced a progressively worsening cough. Over the past month, he has been awakened from sleep each night with one or two episodes of coughing. The cough is productive of one to two teaspoons of gray sputum, but he denies noticing any blood. He presents now because of the onset of a high-pitched sound on inspiration. He also reports that his exercise tolerance has diminished significantly so that he gets short of breath after walking one block. He denies chest pain or palpitations. He has had no recent weight loss but has felt a generalized fatigue over the past month that he attributed to poor sleeping. He has no history of hypertension, diabetes, or myocardial infarction. He has no surgical history. He denies any medications or allergies.

Examination

On physical examination, there is no evidence of cyanosis. The patient's respiratory rate is slightly elevated at 18 breaths/min. He is afebrile, his pulse is 89 bpm, and his blood pressure is 157/78 mm Hg. Examinations of the head, eyes, ears, nose, and throat (HEENT) are all within normal limits. There is no cervical or supraclavicular adenopathy. The heart examination reveals no jugular venous distention. The S_1 and S_2 heart sounds are normal. There are no gallops, rubs, or murmurs. Examination of the lungs reveals diminished excursion of the left chest. There are diminished breath sounds on the left, with audible inspiratory stridor. On percussion, the left

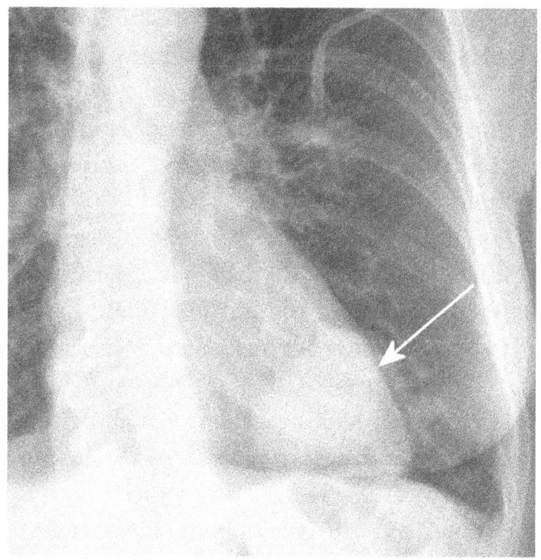

FIGURE 18.1

Chest radiograph shows mass in left lung (*arrow*). The mass is seen as a double density through the heart.

chest has decreased resonance when compared with the right. In addition, diminished vocal and tactile fremitus is noted. Palpation of the trachea reveals a slight shift to the left. The remainder of the physical examination is normal. A chest radiograph is obtained and reveals a large, centrally located mass in the parenchyma of the left lung (Fig. 18.1) with atelectasis of the left lung. There also appears to be hilar lymph node enlargement.

Diagnosis

The diagnosis is lung mass, possibly secondary to malignancy.

Therapy and Further Course

A computed axial tomograph of the chest and abdomen confirms a centrally located mass in the left chest that involves the left main stem bronchus and is closely adjacent to other hilar structures. The mass does not involve the carina. There is minimal left hilar adenopathy. The right lung field and hilum and the abdomen are free of disease. A bronchoscopy is performed and identifies an endobronchial mass in the left main stem bronchus. Biopsy confirms the diagnosis of non–small cell carcinoma of the left lung.

Surgery is recommended, and pulmonary function tests are performed. They demonstrate that the patient can tolerate a left pneumonectomy (removal of the left lung), and he is scheduled for surgery to attempt curative resection. A posterolateral thoracotomy via the fifth intercostal space is used to access the left chest. This procedure provides excellent visualization and access to both the anterior and posterior sides of the hilum. Once the chest is entered, a careful assessment is performed to confirm the extent of the tumor, and the necessity for the pneumonectomy is established.

After retraction of the lung, the pulmonary ligament is identified and divided. The inferior pulmonary vein is then isolated with vessel loops. The superior pulmonary vein is found anterior to the left main bronchus and is similarly dissected and isolated. The inferior and superior pulmonary veins are then divided. The remainder of the hilum is then dissected to expose the main pulmonary artery and the main stem bronchus. After identification of the left recurrent laryngeal nerve, which is free of tumor, the pericardium is opened to allow access to the left pulmonary artery at its origin. The artery is isolated and ligated with suture. The left main stem bronchus is divided 3 mm from the carina, and the specimen is removed. The subcarinal, pulmonary ligament, paraesophageal, and aortopulmonary nodes are dissected and removed for biopsy; they do not appear grossly positive. A small chest tube is left in place to drain any remaining air, and the incision is closed in layers. The chest tube is left for drainage without negative pressure suction, to allow gradual repositioning of the mediastinum in the postoperative period, after which it is removed. The patient's postoperative course is uneventful, and he is discharged home on postoperative day 6.

Discussion

The lung is surrounded by the pleural cavity and is able to move freely within this cavity because of the low friction of the serous surfaces of the visceral and parietal pleurae. The only site of attachment of the lung to other structures is at the root of the lung, which passes through the hilum. Therefore, the removal of a lung (pneumonectomy) is accomplished by the division of all structures in the root of the lung.

Hilum of the Lung

The hilum of the lung is the region bounded by the reflection of pleurae that serves as the entryway into the lung. At the hilum, the visceral pleura, which is fused to the surface of the lung, becomes continuous with the mediastinal parietal pleura, which is fused to the fibrous pericardium. The hilum contains the structures that form the root of the lung. These include the bronchus, the pulmonary artery, the pulmonary veins, the bronchial arteries, the bronchial veins, and lymphatic channels. At the inferior end of the hilum, the anterior pleural reflection and posterior pleural reflection fuse to form the pulmonary ligament (Fig. 18.2).

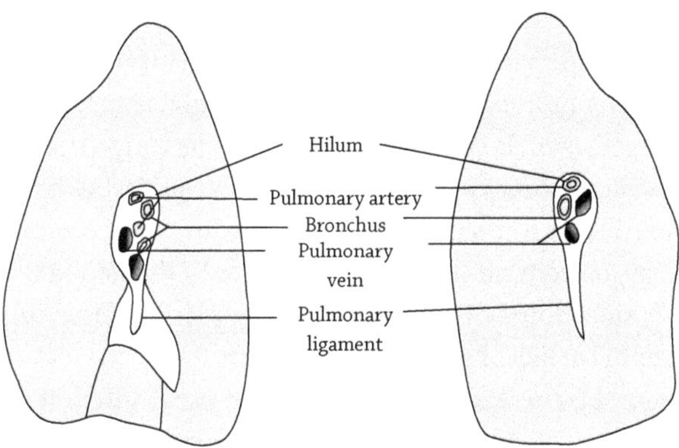

FIGURE 18.2

Hilum of the lung containing the structures of the root of the lung

Root of the Lung

The inferior pulmonary vein is the most inferior structure in the root of the lung. It sometimes extends down into the pulmonary ligament. When the root of the lung is approached from the inferior side of the hilum, the inferior pulmonary vein is the first structure that is encountered. The superior pulmonary vein is the most anterior structure in the root of the lung. The most posterior structure in the root of the lung is the bronchus. The position of the pulmonary artery in the root of the lung is slightly different on the two sides. In the right lung, the pulmonary artery is anterior to the bronchus and posterior to the superior pulmonary vein (i.e., it is the central structure in the root of the lung). In the root of the left lung, the pulmonary artery is anterosuperior to the bronchus and is the most superior structure in the root of the lung (Fig. 18.2).

In the right lung, the upper lobar bronchus branches from the main bronchus before it enters the lung and passes superior to the pulmonary artery to enter the upper lobe. This upper lobar bronchus is sometimes called the *eparterial bronchus* because of its position above the artery. There are one or more bronchial arteries in the root of the lung in variable positions. The bronchial artery on the left is usually a branch of the descending aorta, although it may arise from the aortic arch or from an intercostal artery. The bronchial artery on the right side typically arises from an intercostal artery. In contrast to the pulmonary artery, the bronchial artery carries oxygenated blood, which supplies the cells of the lung. The bronchial veins, which carry deoxygenated blood from the tissues of the lung, exit at variable positions in the root of the lung and typically drain into the azygos vein on the right side and into the hemiazygos vein on the left side. Some of the venous drainage in the bronchial veins drains into branches of the pulmonary vein.

The root of the lung also contains visceral efferent and visceral afferent nerve fibers. The visceral efferent fibers include both parasympathetic and sympathetic nerves. Sympathetic fibers innervate glandular cells in the lung and vascular smooth muscle. Parasympathetic fibers innervate bronchial and bronchiolar smooth muscle. The visceral afferent nerve fibers are branches of the vagus nerve; they carry impulses from stretch receptors and sensation of visceral pain.

Lymphatics of the Lung

The lung has extensive lymphatic drainage, which provides the primary route for spread of bronchogenic carcinoma. Lymphatic channels drain from the visceral pleura, the lung parenchyma, the connective tissue septa in the lung, and the walls of the bronchi. All lymphatic drainage is toward the hilum of the lung (Fig. 18.3). There are pulmonary lymph nodes within the substance of the lung along the course of these lymphatic channels. The efferent drainage

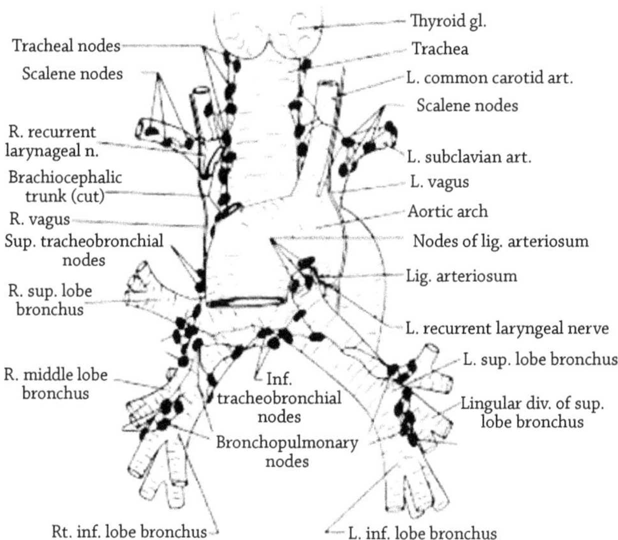

FIGURE 18.3

Diagram of the tracheobronchial tree shows lymph nodes that are particularly apt to be involved in the spread of bronchogenic malignancies. art., artery; div., division; gl., gland; inf., inferior; L., left; lig., ligamentum; n., nerve; R., right; sup., superior.

from these nodes is to the bronchopulmonary lymph nodes (also called *hilar nodes*), which are found at the hilum of the lung. These nodes drain to the tracheobronchial lymph nodes, which are found in the region of the tracheal bifurcation. This group of nodes continues upward along the trachea as the paratracheal lymph nodes. The efferent channels from these nodes coalesce to form the bronchomediastinal lymph trunk. On the left side, this lymph trunk drains into the thoracic duct. On the right side, it may drain directly into the venous system in the region of the junction of the right subclavian vein and the right internal jugular vein, or it may drain into the right lymphatic trunk, which drains into the venous system. Although most of the lymphatic drainage from each lung is to the ipsilateral lymphatic channels, many of the lymphatics from the left lower lobe drain to the right tracheobronchial nodes and then continue along the lymphatic pathway on the right.

Pericardial Cavity

As described earlier, the pericardium was opened to gain access to the proximal portion of the pulmonary artery. Remember that the pulmonary trunk arises from the right ventricle within the pericardial cavity. The full length of the pulmonary trunk is within the pericardial cavity, and it ends by bifurcating into the two pulmonary arteries. Both pulmonary arteries arise within the pericardium and then exit from the pericardium to approach the hila of the lungs. Opening the pericardium allows an increased length of the pulmonary artery to be visualized, which ensures safe ligation.

19

Pneumothorax

A 59-year-old male factory worker comes to the outpatient department because of chest pain and shortness of breath. The patient states that he was well until approximately 2 hours earlier, when he experienced the abrupt onset of sharp, stabbing pain on the right side of his chest. He rates the pain as 8 out of 10 in severity; it is nonradiating and is constant. The pain is worse when he takes a deep breath or when he coughs. He has never experienced anything like this before. The pain is accompanied by a difficulty in breathing that has progressively worsened. He currently is unable to walk more than a few steps before becoming short of breath. The patient has a history of chronic bronchitis with an accompanying chronic cough. However, he reports that this current episode of dyspnea is much worse than any he has experienced in the past. He reports that he used his inhaler but it did not provide any relief of his symptoms. He denies fever or chills or recent sputum production. He reports a history of having smoked about two packs of cigarettes per day for 35 years but was able to quit smoking after chronic obstructive pulmonary disease (COPD) was diagnosed about 4 years ago.

Examination

On examination, the patient is in mild distress and is tachypneic. His pulse is 92 bpm, his respiratory rate is 28 breaths/min, and his blood pressure of 136/92 mm Hg. His temperature is 98.8° F. Pulse oximetry reveals that his oxygen saturation is 89% on room air. Examination of his neck reveals that the trachea is midline and there is no jugular venous distention. His chest excursion is greater on the left than on the right. Auscultation of his chest reveals an absence of breath sounds on the right side and significant wheezing on the

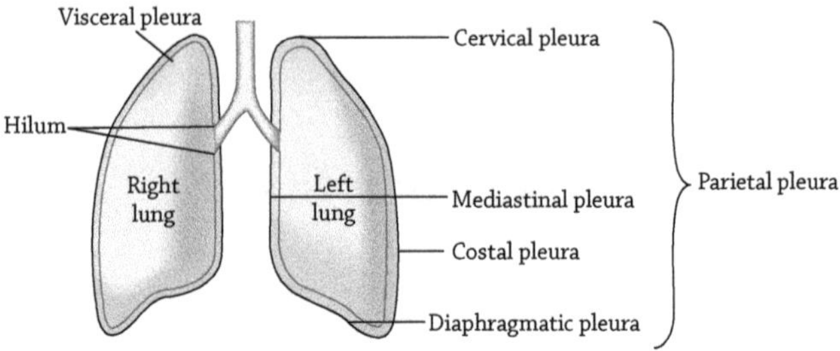

FIGURE 19.1

Schematic diagram through the lung and pleural cavity demonstrates the relationship between the parietal and the visceral pleurae and the pleural reflection at the hilum of the lung.

left side. There is no palpable crepitus (air in the soft tissue) over the chest. He coughs repeatedly during the examination. Radiographic examination of the chest reveals an air-filled right hemithorax with no vascular markings. There is a density in the region of the right lung hilum (Fig. 19.1).

Diagnosis

The diagnosis is right-sided spontaneous pneumothorax, most likely caused by his underlying lung disease.

Therapy and Further Course

The patient is given supplemental oxygen and prepared for the insertion of a small-bore catheter to drain the pleural space. A local anesthetic is administered in the region of the right fourth intercostal space, in the midaxillary line at the inferior border of the fourth rib (the location of the fourth intercostal nerve). A tube is inserted into the right pleural cavity and connected to a low suction through a sterile water seal. The patient remains in the hospital for 3 days with the tube inserted. Chest radiographs are taken daily to confirm that the lung remains expanded. The tube is removed on the third day, and the patient is discharged from the hospital and instructed to avoid any rapid changes in altitude, such as air travel.

Discussion

Each lung is surrounded by a pleural cavity (Fig. 19.1). The pleural cavity is a potential space between two layers of pleura. The inner layer of pleura, called the *visceral pleura*, is fused to the surface of the lung. The outer layer, called the *parietal pleura*, is attached to the walls of the hemithorax. The parietal pleura is given different names in different regions of the chest. The parietal pleural adherent to the chest wall is *costal pleura*. The parietal pleura adherent to the superior surface of the diaphragm is *diaphragmatic pleura*. The lateral surface of the mediastinum is covered by *mediastinal pleura*, and the parietal pleura that extends above the first rib into the neck is *cervical pleura*. Between the two layers of pleura is a potential space containing a thin film of fluid to facilitate smooth sliding of one layer on the other during respiration.

The parietal pleura is continuous with the visceral pleura at the hilum of the lung, where one layer of pleura reflects to become the other layer. This pleural reflection surrounds the root of the lung, which contains the bronchi, the pulmonary artery and veins, the bronchial arteries and veins, and the lymphatic drainage and nerve supply for the lung. Thus, the structures of the root of the lung are able to enter or leave the lung without traversing the pleural cavity.

Functional Relationship of the Pleural Cavity to the Lung

There is a negative pressure within the pleural cavity. The lungs have a considerable amount of elastic tissue. This elastic tissue is continuously attempting to cause the lung to collapse and recoil toward the hilum. The negative pressure in the pleural cavity resists this elastic recoil and maintains the lung in an expanded state. During the respiratory cycle, the intrapleural pressure varies, decreasing as the chest wall expands during inspiration and increasing with recoil of the chest wall during expiration. This causes expansion of the lungs during inspiration and decreased lung volume during expiration.

Causes of Pneumothorax

If there is a breach in either the chest wall or the lung, air will pass from the higher-pressure ambient environment into the lower-pressure pleural cavity, raising the intrapleural pressure. The increase in pressure in the pleural cavity reduces the pressure gradient between the alveolar air space of the lung and the pleural cavity. This allows the elastic fibers of the lung to begin to recoil, resulting in a collapse of the lung. What had been only a potential space is now an air-filled space. This is called a *pneumothorax*. The portion of the lung that is collapsed is no longer functional in respiration. If it is a large pneumothorax, as in this patient, the entire lung is collapsed and the patient is able to respire with only the contralateral lung (Fig. 19.2). The result is reduced oxygen exchange and shortness of breath.

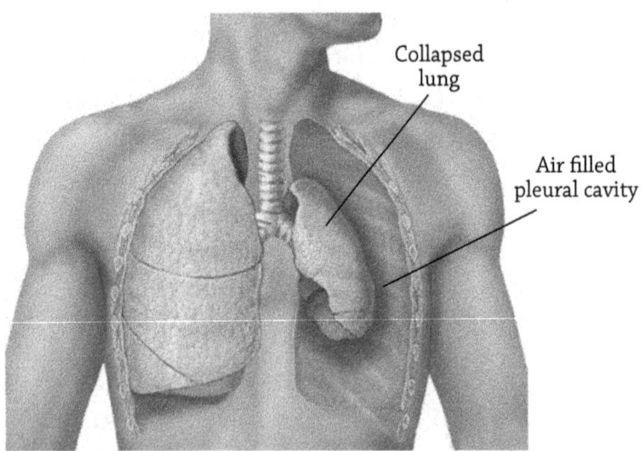

FIGURE 19.2

A collapsed lung caused by a large pneumothorax. The pleural cavity is filled with air.

Types of Pneumothorax

Traumatic pneumothorax occurs when there is trauma to the chest wall (e.g., bullet wound, knife wound) or trauma to the lung (e.g., puncture from fractured rib, transbronchial biopsy of the lung) that allows air to enter the pleural cavity. In the absence of apparent trauma, a spontaneous pneumothorax may occur in which one or more bullae or blebs on the lung rupture, permitting air to enter the pleural cavity. A spontaneous pneumothorax may be primary (i.e., occurring in the absence of any known lung disease) or secondary (i.e., resulting from a preexisting lung disease, such as COPD, as in this patient).

A pneumothorax may be an open pneumothorax or a tension pneumothorax. In an open pneumothorax, there is an open communication between the pleural cavity and atmospheric air, resulting in an equilibration in which the intrapleural pressure rises to atmospheric pressure. This allows the lung on that side to collapse but has no significant effect on the lung on the other side. In a tension pneumothorax, a flap of tissue, either on the chest wall or on the lung, creates a one-way valve that allows air to enter the pleural cavity but not to leave it. This causes the pressure in the pleural cavity to increase with each inspiration, to a point that the intrapleural pressure is higher than atmospheric pressure and therefore higher than the pressure in the other lung. The resulting pressure gradient across the mediastinum causes the mediastinum to deviate toward the opposite lung (Fig. 19.3). Therefore, not only is the lung on the side of the pneumothorax collapsed and unable to participate in respiration, but the other lung can also be compromised because of the compression from the mediastinum. In addition, the deviation of the mediastinum interferes with venous return to the heart through kinking of the venae cavae and compression of the thin-walled right atrium. This diminishes diastolic filling and thereby reduces cardiac output. The compromise of respiration in both lungs, along with the compromise of cardiovascular function, makes tension pneumothorax a life-threatening condition.

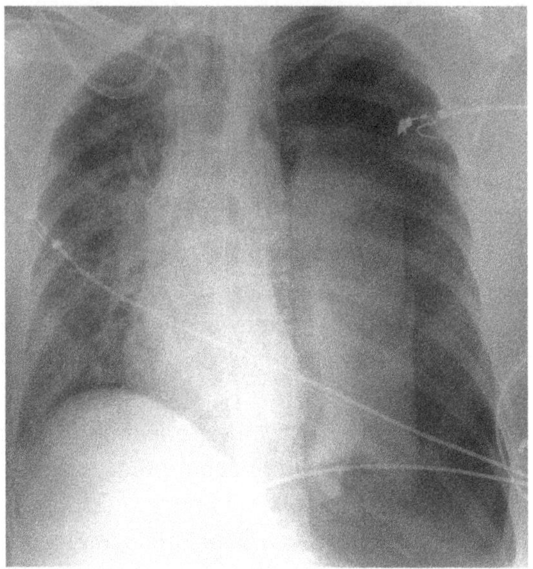

FIGURE 19.3

Chest radiograph of a left tension pneumothorax. Notice the shift of mediastinal structures to the right.

Prognosis

In most cases, pneumothorax has a good prognosis. In fact, it is believed that many cases of small primary spontaneous pneumothorax go unrecognized and resolve on their own when the defect that allowed the entry of air into the pleural space heals and the air in the pleural cavity is absorbed. A pneumothorax that is larger and compromises pulmonary function often requires intervention, such as withdrawal of the air by needle aspiration or insertion of a chest tube, as in this patient. More severe cases may require surgery to repair the lung. However, tension pneumothorax, if not immediately recognized and relieved, may lead to death.

20

Angina Pectoris

A 59-year-old physician who is 30 pounds overweight enters the hospital with a history of attacks of shoulder pain that started 2 years earlier. The pain is located in the left shoulder and is described as a "squeezing pain or heaviness." The pain is almost always accompanied by a burning in his chest that the patient attributes to "heartburn." These attacks of pain usually last from 1 to 5 minutes and had been occurring at most weekly. However, in the preceding 2 weeks, the patient has noted increased frequency of pain that is usually associated with exertion such as walking or climbing stairs, forcing him to stop work. The pain is not severe and is always relieved by rest. The pain does not change with inspiration or with change in position. His left arm feels tired, especially after an attack of pain. He reports no nausea, diaphoresis, or shortness of breath associated with the pain. He has no recent history of injury to that shoulder, and he is right-hand dominant. His past medical history is significant for hypertension and hyperlipidemia. He is a nonsmoker.

Examination

The patient is an overweight male, in no distress at this time. His vital signs demonstrate that he is afebrile. His heart rate is 85 bpm and regular. His blood pressure is 165/90 mm Hg, and respirations are 12 beats/min. His skin is warm and dry. Examination of the head and neck reveals no jugular venous distention and no carotid bruits. The carotid upstrokes are normal. His chest excursion is symmetrical, and the breath sounds are equal and clear to auscultation bilaterally. There are no rales or wheezes. The left chest is nontender to palpation, particularly over the pectoralis major muscle. On cardiac examination, the point of maximum impulse is shifted to the left, indicating that the heart is slightly enlarged. The heart sounds are otherwise normal, and there are no murmurs or gallops. Examination of the shoulder reveals full range of motion with no tenderness elicited. With abduction and lateral rotation of the arm, the patient is also pain-free. The remainder of the examination is unremarkable.

A stress test is performed that demonstrates electrocardiographic changes associated with myocardial ischemia as his treadmill activity increases. Subsequent angiography confirms the preliminary diagnosis of coronary artery disease. The right coronary artery is 85% blocked, and the anterior interventricular artery (left anterior descending, or LAD) is 70% blocked.

Diagnosis

Pain of the type described in a man aged 59 years suggests angina pectoris, which is confirmed in this case by the results of stress testing and angiography.

Therapy and Further Course

The patient's pain is relieved by the administration of nitrates, which dilate the coronary arteries. Coronary angioplasty with placement of stents is suggested to the patient, and he is referred to a cardiologist for further care.

Two weeks later, percutaneous transluminal coronary angioplasty with stent placement is done, and after a 1-day hospital stay the patient is discharged for further recovery at home. He is referred to a dietician and an exercise physiologist. He is put on aspirin and clopidogrel (Plavix) to reduce the likelihood of clot formation at the site of the stent, a low-fat diet, and a program of regular exercise.

Discussion

Angina pectoris is characterized by attacks of moderate to severe chest pain originating in the heart. The attacks are usually precipitated by exertion, excitement, or a heavy meal and are relieved or diminished by rest. The pain is felt behind the sternum and radiates most commonly to the neck, left shoulder, or arm. The pain is customarily explained on the basis of *ischemia*, an insufficient supply of oxygen to the heart muscle as a result of arteriosclerotic narrowing of the coronary arteries, particularly when the heart is required to perform an increased amount of work.

Although the history strongly suggests that this patient's pain is of cardiac origin, involvement of the joints, muscles, periosteum, and peripheral nerves must be considered. Myalgia, an aching condition of the skeletal muscles, is also included in the differential diagnosis, particularly in this age group, whenever unusual physical exercise precedes the attack of pain. The pectoralis major, which is located in the painful area, could cause a similar distribution of pain. In order to stretch this muscle and thereby elicit pain if this muscle is the source of the patient's pain, the examiner abducts and laterally rotates the arm at the shoulder. An absence of pain in performing these motions rules out inflammation of this muscle.

An inflammatory lesion in the richly innervated periosteum over the ribs (costochondritis) can be excluded by the absence of tenderness. Neuralgia of the intercostal nerves can be ruled out by the absence of pressure pain along the course of the intercostal nerves. In a case of neuralgia of one or more intercostal nerves, there would be localized tenderness on pressure along the costal groove and inferior margin of the corresponding ribs.

Pain Pathways in Angina Pectoris

An understanding of the sensory pathway for the perception of pain from the heart is essential for understanding angina pectoris. The sensory nerve fibers that convey pain have a course that is roughly parallel to the pathway for sympathetic innervations to the heart. The pain stimuli are received by free nerve endings in the cardiac connective tissue and the adventitia of the cardiac blood vessels. From there, they travel in visceral sensory fibers through the cardiac plexus and through the middle and inferior cervical cardiac and thoracic cardiac nerves to the sympathetic chain ganglia of the neck and upper thorax. From the middle and inferior cervical chain ganglia, these fibers descend without synapse in the chain to upper thoracic ganglia, where other pain pathways arrive directly via thoracic cardiac nerves.

From the upper four or five thoracic chain ganglia, the fibers continue, again without synapse, via white rami communicantes, to spinal nerves T1 through T5 and their corresponding dorsal roots and dorsal root ganglia. The cell bodies of these sensory nerve fibers are located in the dorsal root ganglia. The central processes of the neurons in these dorsal root ganglia go to the upper thoracic spinal cord segments (Fig. 20.1).

Although there are also sensory nerve fibers that travel from the heart to the brain stem in the vagus nerve, these do not transmit any pain impulses from the heart. Rather, they participate in reflex actions (typical of parasympathetic sensory fibers) related to control of heart rate, control of blood pressure, and similar visceral functions.

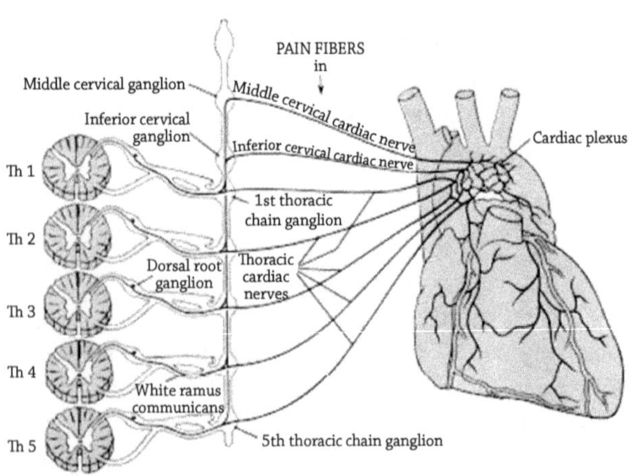

FIGURE 20.1

Schematic diagram of sensory pain pathways from the heart to the first five thoracic spinal cord segments (T 1 through T 5).

The details of referred pain remain incompletely understood; however, cardiac pain is referred to areas of the body surface that send sensory impulses to the same segments of the spinal cord that receive cardiac sensory impulses, that is, mainly C8 through T5. The dermatomes for segments C8 through T5 are represented on the medial side of the upper limb and on the chest wall (Fig. 20.2). Because these regions send their sensory nerve fibers to the same levels of the spinal cord as does the heart, the brain "misinterprets" the source of the pain, and the patient perceives the referred pain as coming from these regions of the body wall. A preponderance of the pain occurs on the left side. In addition to the common sensation of retrosternal pressure and constriction, cardiac pain may atypically be referred to the side of the neck, ear, lower jaw, or back of the

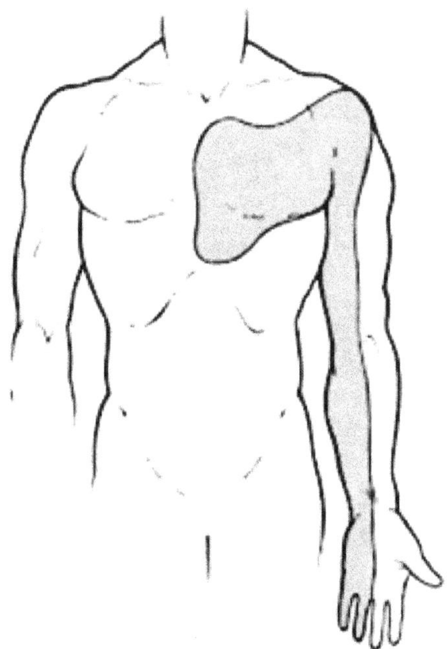

FIGURE 20.2

Typical area of pain referral in angina pectoris.

chest, particularly the interscapular area. This type of pain referral is hard to explain on an anatomical basis.

Access to the Coronary Arteries for Angioplasty

The femoral artery is commonly used as the access point for entry into the arterial system and passage of a catheter to arteries in many parts of the body. The large diameter of this artery, its relatively superficial location, and its ease of identification make it a good candidate for this purpose. The femoral artery is the direct continuation of the external iliac artery; the name simply changes as the artery passes deep to the midpoint of the inguinal ligament. The midpoint of the ligament can be identified by palpating the bony attachments of the ligament at its two ends. The inguinal ligament attaches to the anterior superior iliac spine laterally and to the pubic tubercle medially. Palpation of these two bony landmarks and finding the midpoint between them identifies the midpoint of the inguinal ligament. The pulse of the femoral artery can be palpated immediately inferior to this point.

A small incision is made at this site, and a guidewire is passed into the femoral artery. The guidewire can be advanced under fluoroscopic observation retrograde through the external iliac artery, to the common iliac artery, and then into the abdominal aorta. The wire can then be advanced up the abdominal aorta, into the thoracic aorta, and through the aortic arch into the ascending aorta. A catheter is then passed over the guidewire, and the injection of radiopaque dye allows identification of the coronary arteries.

A balloon catheter is advanced into the coronary artery to the site of the partial occlusion caused by the atherosclerotic plaque (Fig. 20.3). The balloon at the tip of the catheter is then expanded to push the plaque against the wall of the artery and thereby expand the lumen of the artery. If a wire mesh stent is to be placed to maintain the patency of the lumen, the stent surrounds the balloon at the end of the catheter and is expanded by expansion of the balloon. The balloon is then deflated and the catheter is removed,

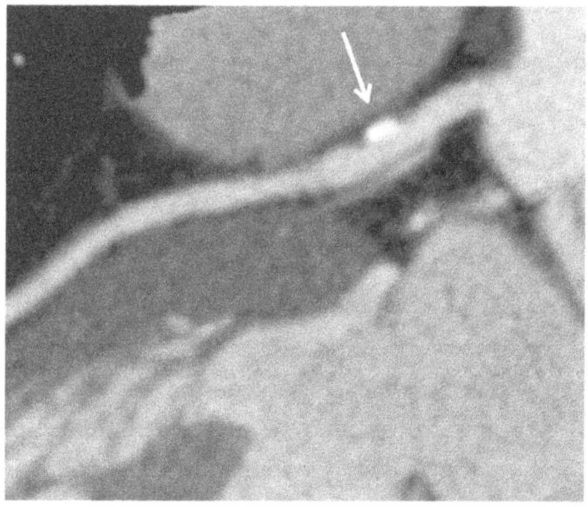

FIGURE 20.3

Computed tomography scan shows mixed calcific and noncalcific plaque (*arrow*) producing less than 50% stenosis in the proximal left anterior descending coronary artery.

leaving the stent in place. The administration of aspirin and clopidogrel (Plavix) is aimed at reducing the likelihood of clot formation on the stent.

21

Myocardial Infarction

A 52-year-old insurance adjuster is brought to a small rural community hospital in an ambulance. His wife, who accompanied him, states that they were on vacation in a remote lodge and that during dinner he started to complain of excruciating chest pain in the region of the sternum. The patient indicates that the pain is retrosternal and describes it as "crushing" and "like an elephant is sitting on my chest." He reports that the pain came on gradually and has gotten progressively more severe, so that it is currently an "11 out of 10." The pain radiates to the left arm and jaw. The pain does not alter with change in position or worsen with inspiration. These symptoms are accompanied by nausea, one episode of vomiting, and severe shortness of breath. The patient reports that for several years he has been suffering from chest pain that radiates into the left arm, particularly after physical effort or emotional upsets; the pain usually lasts 3 to 4 minutes and subsides spontaneously with rest. He has a past medical history of high blood pressure and type 2 diabetes mellitus. He has never been in the hospital before, and he sees his family physician "infrequently." He has no family history of heart disease, takes a "water pill" for his blood pressure, and manages his diabetes with his diet. He has a 40 pack-year smoking history and has no allergies.

Examination and Further Course

On admission, the patient appears diaphoretic and in distress from significant retrosternal pain. His skin is ashen gray with some mild cyanosis about the lips. His extremities are cold and clammy. He is tachypneic and complaining of nausea. His blood pressure is 120/50 mm Hg, and his pulse rate is 110 bpm. His head, eye, ear, nose, and throat (HEENT) examination is within normal limits. Examination of the neck reveals jugular venous distention. On auscultation of the lungs, fine crackles (rales) are heard one-third of the way up from the lung bases bilaterally. There is scattered wheezing. The cardiac examination reveals tachycardia but otherwise normal heart sounds. There is a II/VI pansystolic blowing murmur that is heard best at the apex and radiating to the left axilla. The remainder of the examination is unremarkable.

The patient is given oxygen, intravenous morphine to relieve the pain and a 325-mg aspirin tablet to chew. An electrocardiogram (ECG) is obtained. The ECG reveals elevated ST segments in several leads. All of the clinical evidence indicates that the patient is suffering a myocardial infarction. Because this small hospital is not equipped to perform percutaneous coronary intervention, intravenous thrombolytic therapy with tissue plasminogen activator (tPA) is begun. After 12 hours, the patient is stable, and arrangements are made to transfer him to a larger hospital with an interventional cardiologist on staff for evaluation for possible coronary angioplasty and stent placement.

Diagnosis

The diagnosis is myocardial infarction with ST segment elevation due to occlusion of a coronary artery.

Discussion

Ischemic heart disease, or heart disease caused by insufficient blood supply to the heart muscle, is one of the most frequent conditions encountered in patients older than 40 years of age. It is the leading cause of death in the United States.

The function of the coronary arteries is to carry blood to the myocardium and thus maintain its nutrition. When the lumen of a coronary artery becomes narrowed by atherosclerosis and then occluded by a thrombus, the portion of the myocardium supplied by the affected artery suffers from lack of oxygen (hypoxia), becomes damaged, and subsequently dies. This myocardial infarction results in the classic symptoms exhibited by our patient and, left untreated, may result in a fatal cardiac arrhythmia, such as ventricular fibrillation.

Anatomy of the Coronary Arteries

An important factor in the life of individuals with coronary artherosclerosis is the state of the coronary circulation. The right and left coronary arteries are middle-sized muscular arteries that arise from the right and left aortic sinuses of the ascending aorta, just distal to the aortic semilunar valves. The main arteries run in the epicardial fat of the atrioventricular (coronary) and interventricular sulci; they are partly concealed by fat and in some locations also by thin layers of ventricular myocardium, so that dissection is necessary for their demonstration.

Typically, the right coronary artery (RCA) supplies the right atrium and the right ventricle, with the exception of the left part of the sternocostal surface of the right ventricle, which is supplied by the left coronary artery (LCA). The LCA supplies the left atrium and left ventricle, with the exception of the posterior surface of the left atrium and the right part of the diaphragmatic aspect of the left ventricle, which are supplied by the RCA. The blood supply to the interatrial and interventricular septa is important because parts of the conducting system of the heart are located there. Whereas the interatrial septum is usually supplied from the RCA, both right and left coronary vessels participate in the arterial supply of the interventricular septum through their interventricular branches, with the left commonly carrying the greater share (Fig. 21.1).

The Role of Papillary Muscles

The papillary muscles are bundles of cardiac muscle that project from the ventricular wall or the septal wall into the lumen of the right or left ventricle. The papillary muscles are, in turn, attached to

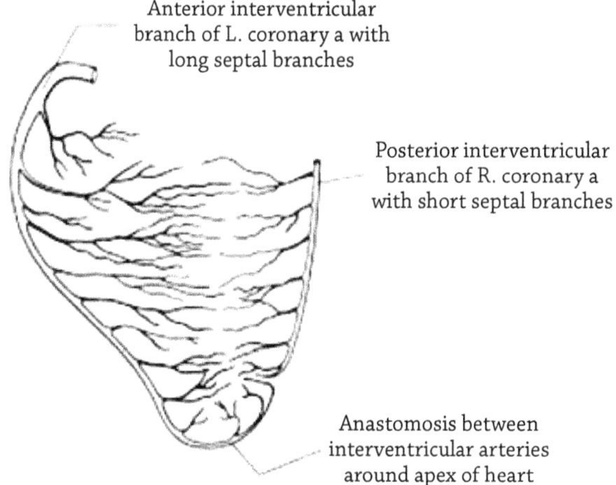

FIGURE 21.1

Arterial supply of the interventricular septum. Notice that in this type the anterior two-thirds of the septum are supplied by the anterior interventricular branch of the left coronary artery, and the posterior third is supplied by the posterior interventricular branch of the right coronary artery. Notice also the site of anastomosis between the two interventricular branches of the coronary arteries around the apex of the heart and the communications of the septal branches. a., artery; L., left; R., right. (Modified from James and Burch.)

the free edges of the tricuspid and mitral valves in the right and left ventricle, respectively, by chordae tendinae, cords of dense connective tissue. The function of the papillary muscles and the chordae tendinae is to control the closure of the tricuspid and mitral valves during systole, preventing them from prolapsing into the right and left atrium, respectively. If a papillary muscle or a chordae tendinae is damaged, allowing prolapse of the valve, the valve will become incompetent and thereby allow regurgitation of blood from the ventricle into the atrium during ventricular systole. This regurgitation results in a systolic murmur.

This patient presented with a mild systolic murmur at the apex radiating to the left axilla. This suggests regurgitation from the left ventricle into the left atrium, possibly from infarction of one or more papillary muscles of the left ventricle resulting in prolapse of the mitral valve.

Are Coronary Arteries End Arteries?

End arteries are arteries that do not anastomose (communicate) with other arteries or arterial branches of the same artery. Obstruction of an end artery interferes with the blood supply to that part of the organ supplied by the artery and leads to necrosis (tissue death) of that portion of the organ. Vital organs that are supplied by end arteries include the retina, inner ear, brain, liver, gall bladder, and kidney. These organs are nourished by arteries that do not anastomose or anastomose only to a degree insufficient to keep the segment viable that is supplied by the obstructed artery. The area of necrosis is known as an *infarct*.

From the frequent occurrence of myocardial infarction, it might be deduced that collateral circulation is absent or inadequate in the heart. However, the branches of the coronary arteries are not true end arteries, because numerous anastomoses take place between the right and left coronary arteries (intercoronary anastomoses) and between branches of the same artery (intracoronary anastomoses).

Collateral Circulation

The common sites of anastomosis between the two coronary arteries are in the coronary sulcus, the posterior interventricular sulcus, and the interventricular septum (Figs. 21.1 and 21.2). The RCA typically anastomoses with the circumflex branch of the LCA within the coronary sulcus. The anterior interventricular artery (a branch of the LCA) is commonly called the left anterior descending artery (LAD) and typically anastomoses with the posterior interventricular artery (a branch of the RCA) in the posterior interventricular sulcus. Branches of the anterior and posterior interventricular arteries may also anastomose within the interventricular septum. There may also be anastomoses between branches of the same coronary artery. For example, the two main branches of the LCA, the anterior interventricular and circumflex branches, can often be seen to communicate around the left (obtuse) border of the heart. Commonly, however, these communications are anatomically patent but small and functionally insignificant. The extent of functional collateral circulation in the heart is variable from one person to another and within the same person over time.

Depending on the degree of obstruction and the size of the obstructed arterial branch, interference with the coronary circulation may be asymptomatic or may result in functional insufficiency, leading to angina pectoris (cardiac pain) or myocardial necrosis of variable extent. If the occlusion of a coronary branch is slow and gradual, anastomoses may enlarge and carry an adequate circulation to the heart muscle. This probably explains why a person may display a significant occlusion of a coronary artery on angiography but nonetheless be asymptomatic.

Sites of Coronary Occlusion

The most common location for coronary occlusion is the LAD branch of the LCA (about 70% of all cases). Next in frequency is the RCA, then the circumflex branch of the LCA. In most cases, the occlusion involves only the proximal portion of the involved blood vessels (Fig. 21.2).

Variations in Dominance of Coronary Arteries

Of great practical importance is the variation in the pattern of coronary arterial distribution from individual to individual, known as *dominance*. The coronary artery that gives rise to the posterior interventricular artery determines the dominance. In about 70% of the population, the RCA gives rise to this artery and the heart is said to be *right dominant*. In such cases, the RCA supplies most of the diaphragmatic surface of both ventricles and part of the interventricular septum. In about 10% of the population, the circumflex branch of the LCA gives rise to the posterior interventricular artery and the

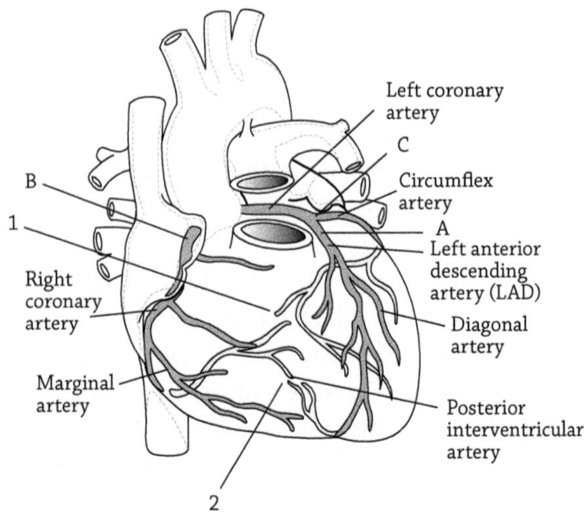

FIGURE 21.2

Location of two typical intercoronary anastomoses and three sites of predilection for coronary occlusion. Anastomosis 1 depicts the communication in the posterior part of the coronary sulcus between the right coronary artery (RCA) and the circumflex branch of the left coronary artery (LCA). Anastomosis 2 shows the communication in the posterior interventricular sulcus between the posterior and anterior interventricular branches of the RCA and LCA. Notice the three most common locations of coronary occlusion. They are, in descending order of frequency, the anterior interventricular branch of the LCA (site A), the RCA (site B), and the circumflex branch of the LCA (site C). Occlusion occurs in all three sites, most commonly close to the origin of the vessels. a., artery; L., left; R., right.

heart is said to be *left dominant*. In the remaining 20% of the population, the posterior interventricular artery receives contributions from both right and left coronary circulations and the heart is said to be *codominant*.

The anastomoses between the anterior and posterior interventricular arteries make up an important part of the collateral circulation of the heart. For this reason, a right-dominant heart is likely to have better collateral circulation than a left-dominant heart, because the anastomoses between the interventricular arteries in a right-dominant heart provide a pathway for RCA-LCA collateral flow. In a left-dominant heart, the anastomoses between the interventricular arteries provide a pathway for LCA-LCA anastomosis. Therefore, if there is an occlusion of the LCA, the circumflex branch, or the LAD in a left-dominant heart, there is little opportunity for collateral flow from the RCA to supply the myocardium compromised by the occlusion.

Surgical Procedures Used to Produce Improved Circulation

Coronary artery bypass graft (CABG) surgery has been used to treat occlusions of the coronary vasculature since the 1960s. A great saphenous vein autograft (graft from the same person) is used to connect the ascending aorta with portions of the RCA or LCA distal to the occlusion, bypassing the diseased section of the artery. Another popular method of bypassing the area of blockage makes use of the internal thoracic artery (frequently called the *internal mammary artery*). This artery is dissected from the anterior chest wall in sufficient length to reach beyond the occlusion of the coronary artery. It is left attached proximally at its origin from the subclavian artery, and its anterior intercostal branches are ligated. Its severed end is grafted into the diseased coronary artery distal to the blockage.

The technique of dilating a blocked vessel by insertion of a small balloon (balloon angioplasty) into the stenosed area is discussed in chapter 20.

22

Coarctation of the Aorta

A 28-year-old construction worker comes to the outpatient department with complaints of headache, nosebleed, occasional dizziness, and palpitations. He reports that for the past 5 months he has had increasing shortness of breath on exertion that, to a certain extent, has interfered with his working capacity. He reports a 2-year history of high blood pressure that is poorly controlled despite three different medications. He is concerned about the headaches and dizziness that are making it difficult for him to work. On further questioning, he does report occasional leg cramps that have made exercise difficult. The cramps are experienced in both legs and typically resolve with rest. He has no family history of high blood pressure or heart disease and is a nonsmoker.

Examination

On physical examination, the patient is a healthy-appearing male in no apparent distress. His blood pressure is 170/100 mm Hg in both arms. Notably, he has an easily palpable radial pulse but diminished pulses in the femoral arteries bilaterally. The pulses in both femoral arteries are quite weak and delayed compared with the radial pulse. The precordium is palpated to assess the point of maximal impulse (PMI) of the left ventricle. It is shifted to the left. On auscultation, there is a continuous systolic murmur over the heart that is also apparent in the interscapular area to the left of the midline. The remainder of the physical examination is normal. Radiographic examination of the thorax shows normal lungs, but the left ventricle is moderately enlarged. The aortic knob, the transitional area between the aortic arch and the descending aorta, is not clearly visualized, and there is a definite bilateral notching of the inferior margins of the posterolateral portions of ribs four to nine. The patient is admitted to the hospital.

On reexamination, previous findings are confirmed, and the following evidence of collateral arterial circulation in the thorax is elicited. Pulsations are visible and palpable in the interscapular area and inferior to both scapulae. Similar pulsations can be demonstrated adjacent to the clavicle and along both sides of the sternum in the area of the internal thoracic artery. On close inspection, tortuous and enlarged blood vessels can be seen under the skin of the back and sides of the thorax.

On the basis of a history of hypertension, the findings of elevated blood pressure in the upper extremities and diminished pressure in the lower extremities, the weak femoral pulse, the presence of demonstrable collateral arterial circulation over the thorax, and the typical radiographic findings of notched ribs, a tentative diagnosis of stenosis or constriction at the isthmus of the aorta (coarctation) is made. In view of the poor prognosis if this condition is left untreated, surgery is recommended.

A preoperative aortogram of the thoracic aorta is ordered to obtain a clear picture of the anatomical condition, particularly the site, width, and length of the aortic constriction. Although a magnetic resonance imaging (MRI) study would provide much of this information without the use of contrast medium, the traditional aortogram was selected because it also provides valuable information, unavailable by MRI, about the intercostal arteries soon to be encountered in the thoracotomy. A catheter is introduced into the radial artery and is advanced retrograde under fluoroscopic control as far as the ascending aorta. Contrast medium is rapidly injected, and multiple radiographs are taken after injection.

The radiographs show a circumscribed stenosis at the typical site of the aortic isthmus beyond the origin of the left subclavian artery. The prestenotic segment of the aorta is somewhat wider than normal; the brachiocephalic trunk and the left common carotid and left subclavian arteries are moderately enlarged. The poststenotic segment is also enlarged, proving that the obstruction of the aorta is incomplete. Branches of the right and left internal thoracic arteries are demonstrated by aortogram to be greatly widened and tortuous as part of the collateral circulation; they anastomose with the inferior epigastric arteries. An enlarged subscapular artery and a few tortuous posterior intercostal arteries are also visualized.

Diagnosis

Circumscribed stenosis of the aortic isthmus with well-developed collateral circulation (aortic coarctation) is diagnosed.

Therapy and Further Course

In view of the anatomical findings of a circumscribed obstruction at the typical site, grafting or the use of a vascular prosthesis is ruled out, and an end-to-end anastomosis after resection of the stenotic portion is planned.

With the patient under general anesthesia, the aorta is approached through a left lateral thoracotomy incision. Several enlarged and tortuous vessels of the chest wall are encountered and doubly ligated. The aorta is mobilized above and below the stenosed area, starting just distal to the left subclavian artery. Here, several dilated and fragile posterior intercostal arteries are seen and ligated. After identification of the left vagus nerve and its recurrent laryngeal branch, the ligamentum arteriosum is ligated and divided. After the aorta is sufficiently freed, it is clamped on either side of the constricted portion, and the area of coarctation is excised. Enough vascular tissue is resected to provide for normal caliber at the site of the anastomosis. Then the cut ends of the aorta are approximated, evened, and sutured together. The clamps are slowly opened, and the suture lines are checked for leaks. The chest wall is closed, leaving a catheter in place for drainage.

The lumen of the aorta in the excised specimen at the constricted site consists only of a small opening not more than 2 mm in diameter, narrower than expected from the outside appearance of the aorta. The obstruction in the interior of the aorta is caused by a diaphragm-like infolding of the media with some secondary intimal thickening. The aortic end of the ligamentum arteriosum, which was removed with the narrowed segment of the aorta, is nonpatent.

The patient's postoperative course is uneventful, and he is discharged from the hospital after 1 week. During this period, pulsations in the femoral artery gradually increase in intensity, and there is also a gradual diminution of blood pressure in the upper extremity and a concomitant increase to normal in the lower extremity. The patient is seen in 6 months and again 1 year after the operation. He is well satisfied with the result and has returned to his former work. His blood pressure in the upper and lower extremities remains normal.

Discussion

Coarctation of the aorta is a congenital cardiovascular anomaly that accounts for 5% to 8% of cardiovascular congenital defects. It is two times more common in males than in females. In females with coarctation, there is a frequent association with Turner's syndrome; 5% to 10% of patients with Turner's syndrome have coarctation. Coarctation (from the Latin word *coarctare*, "to constrict") is a pathological condition in which the lumen of the aortic arch, or of the descending aorta just beyond the arch, is significantly constricted on a congenital basis. It is most often diagnosed soon after birth but, on occasion, may go undiagnosed into early adulthood, as in this case. Coarctation of the aorta may occur as an isolated defect or in association with other cardiac defects, with ventricular septal defect and bicuspid aortic valve being the most common.

The isthmus of the aorta is that region of the aortic arch between the left subclavian artery and the region of the ductus arteriosus. It is normally constricted at birth but enlarges soon thereafter as the ductus arteriosus becomes obliterated. This is also the typical site of coarctation of the aorta. It may occur proximal to the ductus (preductal), in which case the ductus arteriosus often remains patent; more commonly, it occurs just distal to the ductus (postductal), in which case the ductus closes, as in this patient (Fig. 22.1). Other variants rarely occur, such as an aortic stenosis proximal (not distal)

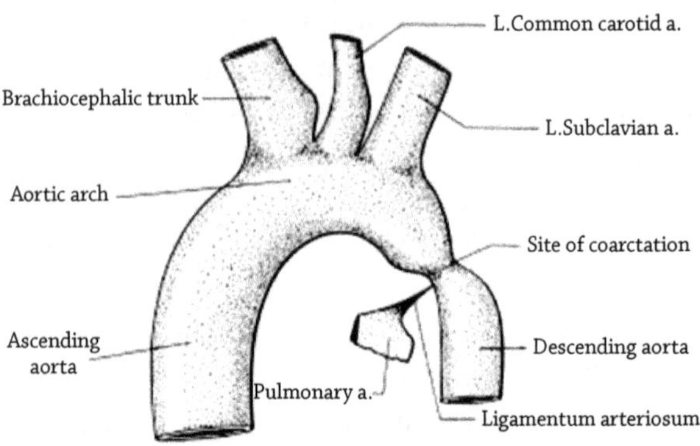

FIGURE 22.1

Coarctation of the aorta beyond the origin of the left subclavian artery at the site of attachment of the ligamentum arteriosum. The aortic arch and its branches are dilated. a., artery; L., left.

to the origin of the left subclavian artery. As noted earlier, the ligamentum arteriosum is ligated and divided to provide more mobility of the aorta. Because the left recurrent laryngeal nerve, a branch of the left vagus nerve, passes under the aortic arch immediately distal to the ligamentum arteriosum, it is necessary to identify this nerve and to keep it out of harm's way. Injury to this nerve would cause weakness or paralysis of the laryngeal muscles, resulting in hoarseness.

Cause of Coarctation

The cause of coarctation is not well understood but is likely multifactorial, and it is probable that there is more than one type of coarctation and more than one cause. In some cases, coarctation is not apparent on prenatal imaging but develops postnatally, concurrent with closure of the ductus arteriosus. There is some evidence that this may be caused by ectopic ductal smooth muscle in the wall of the aorta which responds to increased oxygen saturation just as the smooth muscle in the ductus arteriosus does. In other cases, prenatal imaging reveals the coarctation as a structural defect in the aorta. It has been suggested that such coarctation may be secondary to reduced flow from the left ventricle during development. The concomitant presence of cardiac defects such as ventricular septal defect and aortic valve defect lends some support to this hypothesis.

Explanation of Signs and Symptoms

The patient's symptoms are the result of increased blood pressure in the prestenotic portion of the aorta and its branches, most likely caused by the additional resistance offered to the propulsion of the blood at the site of the stenosis. This conclusion is also borne out by the objective finding of hypertension in both brachial arteries. As a result of the greatly increased arterial pressure in the prestenotic portion of the aorta, the aortic arch and its branches are enlarged and the left ventricle becomes hypertrophied and dilated, leading to gradual failure of the heart with respiratory distress on exertion (also present in this patient). The signs of decreased pressure in the poststenotic part of the aorta and its branches include weak and delayed pulses at the femoral arteries. The femoral artery pulse is palpable inferior to the midpoint of the inguinal ligament.

Collateral Circulation

It is the presence of extensive collateral circulation that permits blood to bypass the constriction, allowing for the survival of the patient to adulthood (Fig. 22.2). In addition to the direct radiographic evidence of enlarged and tortuous vessels in the region of the thoracic wall, there are visible and palpable pulsations in the interscapular area and all along the thoracic wall, particularly at both sides of the sternum. On close inspection, dilated arteries can also be seen under the skin of the thorax. The passage of contrast medium into the aorta distal to the stenotic region demonstrates that the coarctation does not produce complete occlusion of the lumen of the aorta.

The poststenotic portion of the aorta receives blood by direct filling through a narrowed aperture in the aorta at the constricted

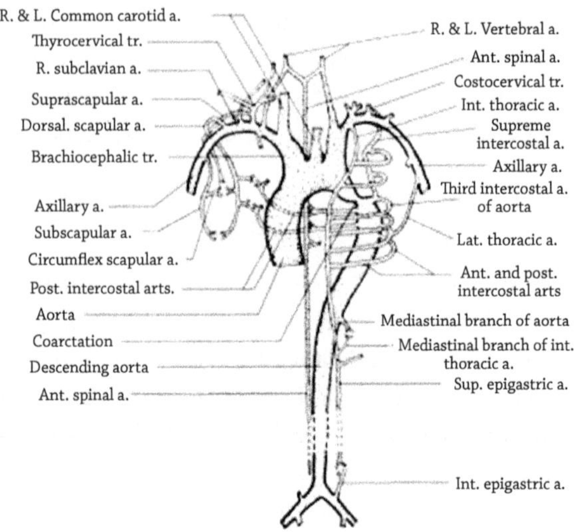

FIGURE 22.2

Various sites of collateral circulation in a case of aortic coarctation. a., artery; ant., anterior; arts., arteries; inf., inferior; int., internal; L., left; lat., lateral; post., posterior; R., right; sup., superior; tr., trunk.

site and by collateral flow into branches distal to the constricted area. Fortunately for this patient, in this location there are ample collateral pathways. These collateral pathways can be divided into four groups:

1. *The scapular and cervical anastomosis:* Scapular and cervical branches from the subclavian and axillary arteries carry blood from the aorta proximal to the coarctation to posterior intercostal arteries which arise from the aorta distal to the coarctation. The subclavian branches include the transverse cervical, deep cervical, suprascapular, and dorsal scapular arteries. The axillary branches are the subscapular artery and its circumflex scapular branch. Some of these channels can be seen or their pulsations felt in this patient in the interscapular region.

2. *The internal thoracic (mammary) anastomosis:* This was clearly demonstrated in this patient on the aortogram of the aortic

circulation. The internal thoracic artery, a branch of the subclavian artery, anastomoses by way of its anterior intercostal arteries with the posterior intercostal aortic branches. The musculophrenic and mediastinal branches communicate with phrenic and mediastinal branches of the descending aorta. Finally, the superior epigastric artery, one of the two important terminal branches of the internal thoracic artery, anastomoses with the inferior epigastric from the external iliac, thus bypassing the constricted area of the aorta.

3. *The intercostal anastomosis:* This has already been discussed in relation to the communications between the anterior and posterior intercostal branches of the internal thoracic artery and the aorta, respectively. It also includes the communications between the supreme (highest) intercostal artery from the costocervical trunk of the subclavian artery and the posterior intercostal artery for the first, second, and third spaces.

4. *The spinal anastomosis:* The anterior spinal artery, which is derived from the vertebral artery, a branch of the subclavian, communicates with segmental spinal branches of the posterior intercostals from the descending aorta and the lumbar and lateral sacral arteries, thus establishing a further collateral channel in coarctation of the aorta.

A key radiographic finding suggestive of coarctation of the aorta, evident on routine chest radiography, is notching of the inferior borders of the ribs. This is caused by enlargement of the intercostal arteries as part of the collateral circulation described earlier. The enlargement of the arteries leads to resorption of the overlying bone, which is seen as notching. These dilated arteries may occasionally cause difficulties for the surgeon because they often become quite friable; some may have to be ligated and excised, as in this case.

The delay of the femoral pulse compared with the radial pulse, observed in this patient, is evidence that the major portion of the blood coursing through the femoral artery arrived in that artery by way of collateral channels rather than directly through the stenotic area. Because these collateral channels may provide adequate blood flow to the lower limbs, there may be easily palpated pulses in the lower limb, such as in the posterior tibial artery at the posterior side of the medial malleolus or in the dorsalis pedis artery on the dorsum of the foot. With exercise, the increased oxygen demand in the muscles of the lower limb may exceed the ability of the collateral circulation to meet the oxygen demand, resulting in cramping in these muscles (claudication). The systolic murmur demonstrable over the cardiac and left interscapular areas is caused by obstruction to the free flow of blood across the coarctation, which creates turbulence in the flow during systole.

Causes of Fatal Outcome in Untreated Cases

A final question needs to be discussed: Why is surgery, which may on occasion be fatal, indicated in this case, when the clinical complaints of the patient are relatively insignificant? If aortic coarctation is left untreated, most patients will die before the age of 40 years. The average life expectancy of all patients with coarctation is 35 years. What is the cause of death in these cases? The harmful effects of coarctation are derived from the hypertension in the upper part of the body, which may eventually lead to heart failure. The prestenotic area of the aorta will dilate and may rupture. Cerebral vessels derived from vertebral and internal carotid arteries likewise dilate as a result of the hypertension and may also rupture, leading to fatal cerebral hemorrhage. Finally, bacterial infection may occur at the site of coarctation or at the aortic valve, and this complication is a frequent accompaniment of aortic coarctation.

23

Obstruction of the Superior Vena Cava

A 57-year-old man presents to the emergency room complaining of increased shortness of breath. He had been well until 2 months earlier, when he noticed an occasional dry cough. The coughing spells increased in frequency and have been accompanied by a significant decrease in exercise tolerance. The patient routinely walked a brisk 2 miles every day but is now unable to walk more than 2 blocks without stopping. It has also been difficult for him to lie flat, and currently he sleeps with the head of the bed slightly elevated. Despite this intervention, he awoke this evening and was acutely short of breath, prompting him to call 911. He has noted increased fatigue, weight loss, and night sweats over the same time frame and has an appointment to see his family physician next week. His collar size has increased, although he has not gained weight, and he is unable to wear his watch or wedding band.

Examination

On examination, the patient shows mild cyanosis of the face and neck. When the patient is in the supine position, the cyanosis deepens. The eyes are prominent, and the eyelids are slightly swollen. There are numerous tortuous superficial veins over the neck, both arms, axillae, and anterior chest wall. In contrast to the face and upper limbs, the skin of the lower limbs is of normal color. However, both upper limbs are edematous when compared with the lower limbs. Prominent axillary adenopathy is noted. He has prominent jugular venous distention.

On further physical examination, the lungs are clear to auscultation, but he has diminished breath sounds at the right base with decreased tactile fremitus. The examination of the heart is normal.

There are no other significant findings. His neurologic and mental status examinations are also normal. Radiographic study of the chest shows a widening of the mediastinal shadow in the region of the right upper mediastinum. This is confirmed by a computed tomography (CT) scan of the chest with contrast, which reveals a mass in the mediastinum accompanied by enlarged paratracheal lymph nodes. It is evident on the CT scan that there is an obstruction of the superior vena cava (SVC).

Venography is performed to determine whether an interventional stent could be placed in the SVC as a temporizing measure. After injection of contrast medium into the cubital vein, the termination of the right subclavian vein appears to be constricted and is accompanied by numerous collateral channels. Complete obstruction is present in the right brachiocephalic vein proximal to its formation by the confluence of the internal jugular and subclavian veins. No contrast medium enters the heart during the radiographic exposure; rather, it is diverted to dilated and tortuous collateral veins in the upper part of the thorax. The medium is seen to enter an enlarged internal thoracic vein that descends and joins with greatly dilated abdominal veins. There is no filling of the terminal portion of the azygos vein. Studies of venous pressure show three times the normal pressure in the veins of the upper limbs, although the pressure in the veins of the lower limbs is normal. A stent is not placed at this time.

Diagnosis

Malignant obstruction of the SVC is diagnosed.

Therapy and Further Course

A tissue biopsy is obtained to plan definitive treatment.

Discussion

The swelling of the face, cyanosis, and increased pressure in the veins of the upper limbs, as well as the distention and tortuosity of the

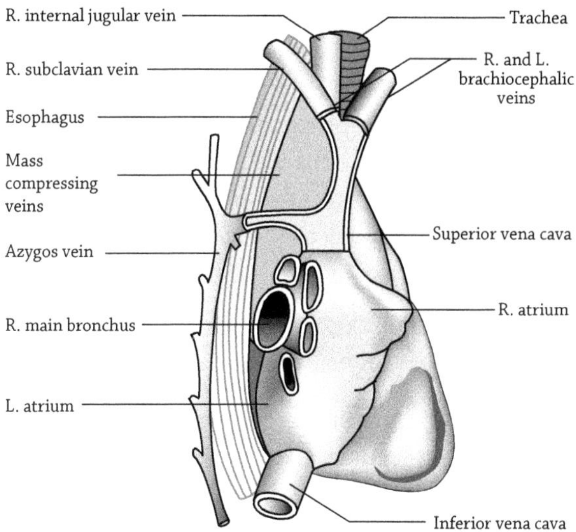

FIGURE 23.1

Compression of the right brachiocephalic vein and the superior vena cava. L., left; R., right.

veins of the neck, arms, and upper trunk, are caused by an obstruction of the venous channels that drain the blood from the upper part of the body (Fig. 23.1). Because the obstruction is relatively acute in onset and the CT scan demonstrates a mass, a malignant cause can be assumed. Indeed, most cases of SVC syndrome (70–90%) are the result of mediastinal malignancies. The malignancies associated with SVC syndrome are most commonly bronchogenic cancer and non-Hodgkin's lymphomas, especially large cell type. Complications of SVC stenosis and thrombosis after the placement of intravascular devices such as central lines are increasingly frequent and often occur in conjunction with treatment of malignancy.

In this patient, the right brachiocephalic vein and the SVC are definitely involved. The distention of the visible veins increases when the patient is in the supine position or bending forward because the direction of blood flow and the absence of valves in the veins of the mediastinum allow blood to accumulate in the most gravity-dependent locations. Bending forward increases intrathoracic pressure, which impedes venous return, causing distention of peripheral veins.

Although the most common causes of obstruction are neoplasms that either press on or invade the SVC, an aneurysm of the ascending aorta could also lead to compression of the SVC, because the ascending aorta is immediately to the left of the SVC.

Collateral Venous Pathways in Obstruction of the Superior Vena Cava

In this case, in which the proximal portion of the right brachiocephalic vein, the SVC, and the termination of the azygos vein are obstructed, collateral venous channels are available. These channels allow the return of venous blood to the right atrium from the upper part of the body. The termination of the azygos vein is also obstructed, so that all blood that normally drains into the SVC must return to the heart by way of the inferior vena cava (IVC) (Fig. 23.2).

The visible dilatation and tortuosity of the superficial veins of the neck, arms, and trunk indicate that these channels are involved in the bypass from the SVC to the IVC. They comprise anastomoses between the veins of the thoracic wall, which normally drain into the axillary and internal thoracic veins, and tributaries of the femoral vein. One of the numerous veins belonging to this group is designated the *thoracoepigastric* vein. It connects the lateral thoracic vein with the superficial epigastric vein. The lateral thoracic vein drains into the axillary vein, and the superficial epigastric vein drains into the great saphenous and through it into the femoral vein (Fig. 23.2). The axillary vein eventually drains to the SVC, through the subclavian and brachiocephalic veins, and the femoral vein drains into the IVC through the external iliac and common iliac veins. Veins belonging to this group are particularly involved in the bypass if the termination of the azygos vein is also obstructed, as in this case.

A second collateral system bypassing the obstruction is represented by the internal thoracic venous system. Here again, reversal

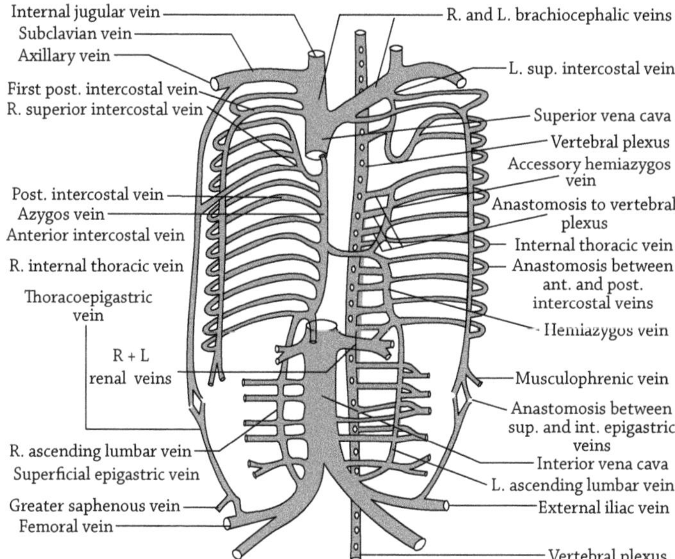

FIGURE 23.2

Diagrammatic representation of the four main collateral systems that function effectively in obstruction to the superior vena cava: (1) the superficial venous system, represented by the thoracoepigastric vein; (2) the internal thoracic system with the anastomosis between the superior and inferior epigastric veins; (3) the vertebral plexus; and (4) the azygos route and its anastomoses with other systems. ant., anterior; inf., inferior; L., left; R., right; post., posterior; sup., superior.

of blood flow is facilitated by the absence or scarcity of valves. Named communicating vessels of this system are the superior epigastric vein, musculophrenic vein, anterior intercostal veins, and perforating cutaneous branches. These veins, all tributaries of the internal thoracic vein, anastomose directly or indirectly with the inferior epigastric vein, which drains into the external iliac vein (Fig. 23.2).

A third channel is represented by the vertebral plexus of veins, an aggregate of veins extending from the head to the sacrum on the outside of the spinal column anteriorly and posteriorly (external plexus) as well as inside the vertebral canal (internal plexus). These veins are characterized not only by rich anastomoses with segmental veins, such as the intercostals, but also by longitudinal anastomoses and by cross-communications between right and left across the midline and by anastomoses from inside the vertebral canal to the outside. Reversal of blood flow is facilitated by the absence of valves in this plexus (Fig. 23.2).

Azygos Route

The azygos route, although its normal drainage into the SVC is blocked, can still contribute to the collateral circulation through reversal of its blood flow and because it receives important segmental tributaries from the thoracic wall and from the other bypassing systems, mentioned previously. Usually the azygos vein is formed by the confluence of the right ascending lumbar and subcostal veins. It frequently also connects directly with the IVC. It receives its segmental venous contributions through the lower right posterior intercostal veins directly and through the right superior intercostal vein indirectly; it also commonly receives left segmental contributions through the hemiazygos and accessory hemiazygos veins. All these intercostal veins are channels of anastomosis with the internal thoracic and vertebral routes (Fig. 23.2).

If the SVC were obstructed distal to the point of entrance of the azygos vein, additional collateral channels could be used to shunt blood. The azygos vein would be capable of carrying blood to the lower part of the SVC, in addition to the previously mentioned bypasses to the IVC.

If, instead of the SVC, the IVC were obstructed, the same veins could be employed to channel blood from the IVC to the SVC, a reversal of the blood flow in the previously listed channels.

24

Cancer of the Esophagus

A 73-year-old retired carpenter is admitted to the hospital. He has severe shortness of breath (dyspnea) and great difficulty in swallowing (dysphagia). The patient states that for the past 6 months he has suffered increasing difficulty in swallowing solid foods. Over the past 2 weeks, he has had difficulty swallowing liquids that is frequently accompanied by coughing. His diet has been increasingly limited, and he reports losing 30 pounds. During the past week, he has become increasingly short of breath, and this has affected his daily activity. He can walk only short distances and can barely climb a flight of stairs. The shortness of breath has acutely worsened over the past 24 hours and is accompanied by frequent coughing spells that are productive of greenish, blood-tinged sputum. He reports fever to 101.3° F but denies chills. He has also noticed a swelling on his right collar bone, which is painful on motion.

Examination

On examination, the patient appears quite cachectic and is tachypneic (rapid respiratory rate). His pulse is rapid, and his temperature is 101° F. He appears mildly cyanotic, suggesting that his oxygenation is poor. There is a hard, fixed mass in the right supraclavicular area, approximately 3 cm by 4 cm in size. Rhonchi and gurgling sounds are audible diffusely on auscultation of the chest. There is increased tactile fremitus over the right lower lobe. The remainder of the physical examination is unremarkable. Laryngoscopic examination reveals the left vocal fold in a semiabducted position on respiration and phonation.

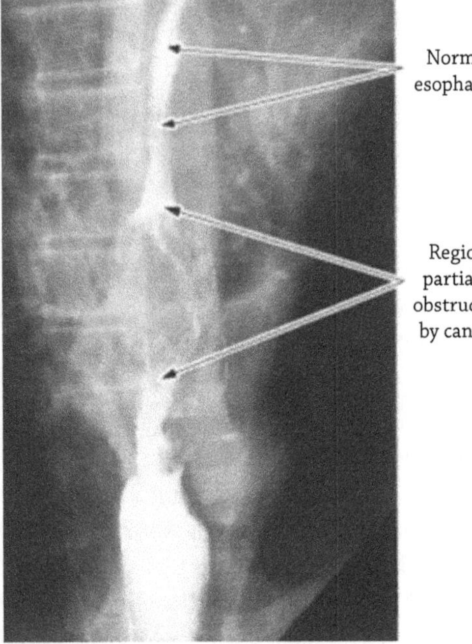

FIGURE 24.1

Radiograph of the esophagus with swallowed barium coating the mucosal lining. Notice the poorly filled, irregular region that indicates cancer of the esophagus.

Radiographic examination of the chest shows widening of the mediastinum with destruction of the lateral half of the right clavicle corresponding to the soft tissue tumor in this area (Fig. 24.1). Brief fluoroscopic examination of the esophagus with dilute barium demonstrates an obstruction at the level of the bifurcation of the trachea and a communication between the esophagus and the trachea. There is consolidation of the right and left lower lobes with air-bronchograms consistent with bilateral pneumonia. Attempted esophagogastroduodenoscopy (EGD) reveals an obstructing mass in the mid-esophagus that prevents further advancement of the scope. Biopsies reveal poorly differentiated squamous cell carcinoma of the esophagus.

Diagnosis

Cancer of the esophagus with obstruction and perforation into the trachea is diagnosed.

Treatment and Further Course

After discussion with the patient and his family, he is given oxygen and narcotics as well as intravenous fluids. On the fourth day, he becomes comatose and dies.

At autopsy, a large, cauliflower-like tumor is found in the esophagus that obstructs the lumen of the esophagus. The esophagus above the obstruction is greatly dilated. At the level of the tracheal bifurcation, the mass has perforated the trachea, which shows an ulcerous communication with the esophagus (Figs. 24.2 and 24.3). The tumor mass surrounds and compresses the trachea over an area 3 cm long. The left recurrent laryngeal nerve is likewise embedded in the mass. The mediastinal lymph nodes, particularly in the posterior mediastinum, are greatly enlarged and adherent to each other. The dependent portions of both lungs show signs of bronchopneumonia. There are nodular metastases of varying size in both lungs and scattered over the visceral pleura. There also are round tumors in the liver. On microscopic examination, the area of destruction of the right clavicle is found to be a cancerous metastasis.

Discussion

We are dealing here with the terminal course of an esophageal cancer that has obstructed the esophagus at the level of the tracheal bifurcation. Cancer of the esophagus is typically either squamous cell carcinoma, usually in the proximal esophagus, or adenocarcinoma, usually in the distal esophagus. Dilatation of the esophagus above the obstruction, which was found in this case, is common in cases of esophageal stenosis and represents the result of mechanical stretching of the organ by the ingested food and liquid above the site of the impasse.

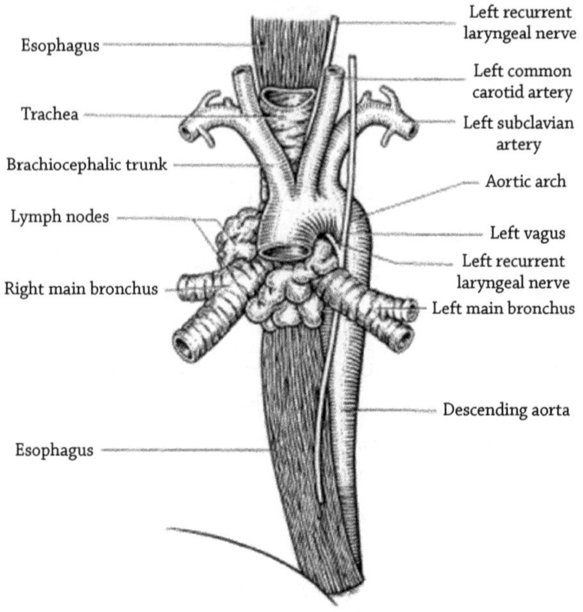

FIGURE 24.2

Anterior view of the esophagus, trachea, and aorta shows the changing relationship of the aorta to the esophagus and the course of the left recurrent laryngeal nerve in relation to the aorta, trachea, and esophagus. Notice the enlarged and cancerous lymph nodes and the dilatation of the upper thoracic portion of the esophagus.

Topographic Anatomy of the Esophagus as Applied to Cancer

The complications of the esophageal cancer caused by invasion of organs and structures in its neighborhood are exemplified in this case by compression of and erosion into the trachea and compression of the left recurrent laryngeal nerve. The esophagus does not have a serosal coat and is separated from the trachea by only a small amount of areolar tissue, explaining the frequent involvement of the trachea in esophageal cancer. The compression of the trachea by the tumor mass explains the severe dyspnea and cyanosis (purple

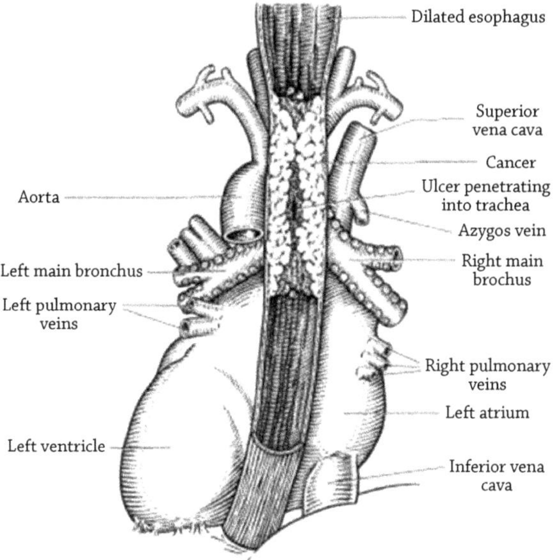

FIGURE 24.3

Posterior view of the esophagus with the esophagus partly opened. The extensive obstructing cancer is shown, as well as the erosion into the trachea and the enlargement of the esophagus above the obstruction. Notice the close relationship of the esophagus to the left atrium.

discoloration due to inadequate oxygenation of the blood). The invasion and ulcerous penetration of the trachea caused the bronchopneumonia, the tracheal hemorrhages, and the blood-tinged sputum. Tracheal and esophageal branches of the thoracic aorta are responsible for the blood supply of the two organs.

The patient's hoarseness and the semiabducted position of his left vocal fold observed on laryngoscopy result from the effect of the cancer on the left recurrent laryngeal nerve. This nerve arises from the vagus where the latter passes over the aortic arch. It then passes to the left of the ligamentum arteriosum, below the arch, and from there runs upward in the tracheoesophageal groove on the left side of the trachea and esophagus (Fig. 24.2). As frequently occurs in esophageal cancer, the mass in this patient compressed the nerve. The recurrent laryngeal nerve innervates all laryngeal muscles, with the exception of the cricothyroid muscle. Lesion of the nerve immobilizes the vocal fold on that side and puts it in a semiabducted position. The recurrent laryngeal nerve also provides sensory innervation to the mucous membrane of the larynx below the vocal folds. The left recurrent laryngeal nerve is more frequently affected by esophageal cancer than the right because of the difference in the course of the two nerves. On the left, the recurrent laryngeal nerve branches from the vagus in the thorax at the level of the aortic arch, as described earlier. On the right, the recurrent laryngeal nerve branches from the vagus in the neck at the level of the right subclavian artery and then passes under this artery to reach the esophagus and trachea and ascend to the larynx. Hence, the right recurrent laryngeal nerve is in close proximity to the esophagus only in the neck, whereas on the left, the nerve is in close proximity to the esophagus in the thorax and the neck. Because esophageal cancer arises more commonly in the thoracic portion of the esophagus, the left recurrent laryngeal nerve is more likely to be affected.

Knowledge of the anatomical relations of the thoracic esophagus allows us to identify other structures and organs frequently penetrated by the growing cancer. In addition to the trachea and main bronchi, the pleural cavity, lungs, aorta, pericardium, and heart may be invaded. Because of the closer relationship of the left bronchus to the esophagus, this bronchus is more frequently involved than the right. On the other hand, the right mediastinal pleura that is more likely to insinuate itself between the esophagus and aorta, forming a retroesophageal recess. It is therefore more commonly affected than the left in the pleural spread of esophageal cancer. Perforation into the aorta may lead to immediate fatal hemorrhage. In the posterior mediastinum, the aorta is at first on the left side and then posterior to the esophagus. Because the left atrium is immediately anterior to the thoracic esophagus, with only the pericardium intervening, the left atrium is the chamber of the heart that may be infiltrated by cancerous growth from the esophagus (Fig. 24.3).

Lymphatic Spread of Esophageal Cancer

Cancer does not spread only by invasive growth to the surrounding tissues and organs. More important even for the final outcome is penetration of the lymphatic and vascular channels that disseminate clusters of tumor cells (tumor emboli) to all parts of the body. This dissemination is well exemplified in this case. The patient had large masses of cancerous lymph nodes in the posterior mediastinum that were demonstrable on radiography. These, together with periesophageal lymph nodes adjacent to the organ and the tracheobronchial nodes, represent the area of regional lymph drainage from the middle portions of the esophagus. The primary tumor invaded the lymph capillaries in the mucosa and spread from there by way of the lymph vessels in the esophageal musculature to the regional lymph nodes. Lymphatic metastases from the esophageal cancer may reach these regional lymph nodes first; they may then, because of rich lymphatic anastomoses, spread to nodes located at considerable distance, ascending as far as the neck or descending to lymph nodes in the abdomen around the celiac artery.

The common involvement of lungs and pleura, also present in this case, might be explained on the basis of direct spread of the primary cancer. More likely, however, is retrograde dissemination of the cancer through the lymphatics of lung and pleura from the cancerous tracheobronchial lymph nodes. It should also be kept in mind that all lymph, and with it cancerous emboli, finally reach the venous circulation through the termination of the thoracic and right lymphatic ducts in the venous angles of the neck. Therefore, lymphatic spread, if not arrested by surgery or radiation, in the end will bring cancerous cells into the venous circulation and from there to the lungs, a common site of metastasis.

Venous Spread of Esophageal Cancer

Invasion of the esophageal veins at the site of the tumor must also be assumed to have taken place and with it spread of cancerous emboli along venous channels. Where do the veins of the esophagus drain? The wall of the esophagus is an important site of anastomoses between systemic veins that drain blood by way of the azygos and hemiazygos veins into the superior vena cava and veins that are tributaries of the portal system, such as the lower esophageal veins. The latter drain into the left gastric vein. Cancerous invasion of and spread via the lower esophageal veins explains the metastatic involvement of the liver in this case.

Some cancer cells may be transported by way of the portal vein and its branches through the sinusoids of the liver, then through hepatic veins into the inferior vena cava and right atrium and ventricle, and from there through the pulmonary arteries into the pulmonary circulation. On the other hand, some cancer cells may spread via the esophageal veins draining into the azygos vein and into the superior vena cava, which drains into the right atrium. Therefore, dissemination of the cancer through superior and inferior venae cavae might readily be an additional explanation of metastatic involvement of the lungs.

Arterial Spread of Esophageal Cancer

The final pathway for metastasis from and through the lung is the general arterial circulation. This terminal phase of cancerous spread is exemplified in this case with the involvement of the right clavicle. Cancer cells reaching the venous circulation can pass through the pulmonary circulation to reach the left side of the heart and then the aorta and its branches to the nutrient vessels of the clavicle.

In summary, the neoplasm in this patient, as is so often the case in terminal cancer, used all available channels for dissemination through the body: direct invasion of structures in the neighborhood (e.g., trachea, recurrent laryngeal nerve); lymphatic spread to regional lymph nodes and lungs; venous spread to the liver and possibly lungs and pleura; and arterial dissemination to the clavicle.

Unit III

Review Questions

The number in parentheses is a reference to the page on which information about the question may be found.

1. Which axillary lymph nodes are in the most likely pathway of lymphatic drainage from the breast?
The anterior nodes receive the initial drainage, and these nodes drain to the central and apical nodes. (144)

2. What three nerves pass through the axilla and are most susceptible to injury in an axillary node dissection, and what do these nerves innervate?
The long thoracic nerve lies against the medial wall of the axilla and innervates the serratus anterior. The thoracodorsal nerve lies against the posterior wall of the axilla and innervates the latissimus dorsi. The intercostobrachial nerve traverses the axilla from medial to lateral and provides sensory innervation to the medial arm. (146–147)

3. Why is a dye injected into the region of the breast tumor before a sentinel lymph node biopsy is done?
The dye is picked up by the lymphatic system and will travel to the axillary lymph node or nodes to which the tissue around the tumor drains. This allows identification of the first lymph nodes to which cancer cells from the tumor would metastasize. The biopsy of this node then provides a good indication of whether there has been any metastasis of the cancer from the breast to the axilla. (148)

4. What muscles form the walls of the axilla?
The anterior wall is composed of the pectoralis major and pectoralis minor muscles. The posterior wall is composed of the subscapularis, teres major, and latissimus dorsi muscles. The medial wall is composed of the serratus anterior muscle overlying the rib cage. (143–144)

5. What is the role of the parasternal lymph nodes in the lymphatic drainage from the breast?
A significant portion of the lymphatic drainage from the medial portion of the breast goes to the parasternal lymph nodes, which are in the anterior intercostal spaces near the internal thoracic (mammary) vessels. These nodes drain to the supraclavicular nodes. There are lymphatic communications between the parasternal lymph nodes of the right and left side that provide a pathway for metastasis from one breast to the other. (145–146)

6. What is the functional and structural unit of the lung?
The functional and structural unit of the lung is the bronchopulmonary segment. This is the region of a lobe that is supplied by one segmental (tertiary) bronchus and one segmental branch of a pulmonary artery. Disease processes may be restricted to a single bronchopulmonary segment. (153)

7. Why is an aspirated foreign body more likely to pass into the right main bronchus than the left?
At the tracheal bifurcation, the right main bronchus takes a more vertical course and is wider. Therefore, an aspirated body is more likely to pass into the right main bronchus. (151–152)

8. At what point does the common aerodigestive tract divide into separate airway and digestive tracts?
The oropharynx is a common aerodigestive tract. At the level of about the C4 vertebra, the opening into the larynx is the upper end of the dedicated airway, and the laryngopharynx is dedicated as a food pathway. The larynx continues downward as the trachea, and the laryngopharynx continues as the esophagus. (154)

9. What vascular structures are used surgically as landmarks to identify the boundaries between bronchopulmonary segments?
Branches of the lobar pulmonary veins lie in the connective tissue planes between adjacent bronchopulmonary segments. These intersegmental veins are used as the landmarks to identify the boundaries between the segments. (153)

10. What is the role of the soft palate during swallowing?
During swallowing, the soft palate is elevated to occlude the opening between the nasopharynx and the oropharynx. This prevents food in the oropharynx from passing upward into the nasopharynx when the pharynx constricts. (154)

11. What is the piriform recess, and what is its role in swallowing?
The piriform recess is that portion of the laryngopharynx that is posterolateral to the larynx. During swallowing, food is diverted from the midline by the epiglottis and directed into the piriform recesses. From there, it returns to the midline to enter the esophagus. This pathway keeps the food out of the airway. (154)

12. What is the role of the vocal folds in the cough reflex?
When the supraglottic mucosa is stimulated, the vocal folds adduct to close the glottis. This prevents a foreign body from entering the infraglottic space. With the glottis closed, the intrathoracic pressure is increased by contraction of abdominal muscles. When the pressure gradient between the infraglottic space and the supraglottic vestibule is high enough, the vocal folds rapidly abduct to open the glottis, and a high-velocity blast of air moves upward to clear the vestibule. (156)

13. What four congenital defects are found in tetralogy of Fallot?
The four elements of tetralogy of Fallot are pulmonary stenosis, overriding aorta, ventricular septal defect, and right ventricular hypertrophy. (159)

14. What embryonic structure is responsible for the formation of the ascending aorta and the pulmonary trunk?
The aorticopulmonary septum forms in the truncus arteriousus and divides it into the ascending aorta and the pulmonary trunk. It normally forms in the center of the truncus arteriousus, thus creating two equal-sized vessels. (160)

15. Why does a child with tetralogy of Fallot squat when having a cyanotic episode?
It is believed that the squatting causes a kinking of the arterial supply to the lower limbs and thus increases the peripheral resistance of the systemic circulation. This increases the left ventricular pressure, reducing the pressure gradient between the right and left ventricle and thereby reducing the shunting of deoxygenated blood into the systemic circulation. (162)

16. What structures pass through the hilum of the lung?
All of the structures of the root of the lung pass through the hilum. These include the bronchus, the pulmonary artery, usually two pulmonary veins, the bronchial artery and vein, and the lymphatics of the lung. The pulmonary veins are the most inferior and most anterior structures passing through the hilum. The bronchus is the most posterior structure passing through the hilum. The position of the pulmonary artery is slightly different on the right and left sides. (167)

17. What is the pathway of lymphatic drainage from the lung?
All lymphatic drainage in the lung is toward the hilum. Pulmonary lymph nodes within the lung drain to the bronchopulmonary lymph nodes in the hilum. These nodes drain to the tracheobronchial lymph nodes at the bifurcation of the trachea, which drain to the paratracheal lymph nodes and thence to the bronchomediastinal lymph trunk. (169–170)

18. What are the portions of the parietal pleura?
The portions of parietal pleura are given names according to their location. The costal pleura is attached to the ribs of the chest wall. The diaphragmatic pleura is attached to the upper surface of the diaphragm. The

mediastinal pleura is attached to the lateral surface of the mediastinum. The cervical pleura is the parietal pleura that ascends above the first rib and is in the neck. (173)

19. Where does the parietal pleura become continuous with the visceral pleura?
The visceral pleura is fused to the surface of the lung. The parietal pleura is continuous with the visceral pleura at the hilum of the lung. This pleural reflection surrounds the structures of the root of the lung: the bronchus, the pulmonary artery, the pulmonary veins, the bronchial arteries and veins, and the lymphatics and nerves of the lung. (173)

20. Why does the lung collapse when there is a pneumothorax?
Normally, there is a negative pressure in the pleural cavity (i.e., less than atmospheric pressure). The pressure inside the lung is atmospheric. This pressure gradient keeps the lung expanded against the elastic recoil of the lung. With a pneumothorax, air enters the pleural cavity and raises the pressure in the cavity. This disrupts the pressure gradient that resists the elastic recoil of the lung, allowing the lung to collapse. (174)

21. How does a tension pneumothorax compromise the circulatory system?
In a tension pneumothorax, the intrapleural pressure rises above atmospheric pressure. This results in a pressure gradient between the two pleural cavities that pushes against the mediastinum and displaces it away from the side with the pneumothorax. This causes a kinking of the vena cavae, resulting in a reduction in venous return. Additionally, the compression of the heart reduces diastolic filling of the ventricles, causing a decrease in cardiac output. (175)

22. What is the anatomical pathway for pain from the heart?
The sensory nerve fibers that convey the sensation of pain from the heart travel with the sympathetic nerves that innervate the heart. They travel in the cardiac nerves to reach the sympathetic chain, then pass through the sympathetic ganglia and white rami communicantes to reach the upper thoracic spinal nerves. They continue through the dorsal roots of

these spinal nerves and have their cell bodies in the dorsal root ganglia. (179–180)

23. To which dermatomes is cardiac pain referred?
Pain arising from the heart is referred to the dermatomes that correspond to the spinal nerve levels through which the sensory fibers from the heart reach the spinal cord. These are the upper thoracic spinal nerves. The corresponding dermatomes are found in the upper chest and the medial side of the arm. (181)

24. What sensory functions are served by the sensory nerve fibers from the heart that travel in the vagus nerve?
The sensory fibers from the heart that are in the vagus nerve carry the sensory information necessary for the control of cardiac reflexes. This sensory information reaches the brain stem but does not ascend to conscious levels. (180)

25. What landmarks are used to locate the femoral artery to gain arterial access for coronary angioplasty?
The femoral artery is the distal continuation of the external iliac artery. Its name changes as the artery passes under the inguinal ligament. The femoral artery can be located immediately inferior to the midpoint of the inguinal ligament. This midpoint can be located by identifying the midpoint between the two bony attachments of the inguinal ligament, the anterior superior iliac spine and the pubic tubercle. (182)

26. What are the origins of the right and left coronary arteries?
Both coronary arteries arise from the ascending aorta. They are the only branches of the ascending aorta. The right coronary artery arises from the wall of the right aortic sinus behind the right cusp of the aortic valve; the left coronary artery arises from the wall of the left aortic sinus behind the left cusp of the aortic valve. (186)

27. What are the two main branches of the left coronary artery?
The left coronary artery arises from the left side of the ascending aorta and passes behind the pulmonary trunk. After passing the pulmonary

trunk, the artery divides into the circumflex branch and the anterior interventricular branch (left anterior descending artery). The circumflex branch enters the coronary sulcus, and the anterior interventricular branch enters the anterior interventricular sulcus. (188)

28. What are the major anastomoses between the right coronary artery and the left coronary artery?
The right coronary artery anastomoses with the circumflex branch of the left coronary artery. The anterior interventricular artery (a branch of the left coronary artery) anastomoses with the posterior interventricular artery (a branch of the right coronary artery). (188–189)

29. What is the function of the papillary muscles and the chordae tendinae?
The papillary muscles are bundles of cardiac muscle that project into the lumina of the right and left ventricles. The chordae tendinae are strands of connective tissue that attach the tips of the papillary muscles to the edges of the cusps of the tricuspid and mitral valves in the right and left ventricles, respectively. The papillary muscles and chordae tendinae control the closure of the tricuspid and mitral valves during ventricular systole. They prevent prolapse of these valves. Infarct of a papillary muscle or rupture of chordae tendinae may result in prolapse of the valve with regurgitation. (186–187)

30. What is the difference between a right-dominant heart and a left-dominant heart?
Dominance in the heart is based on the origin of the posterior interventricular artery. If it arises from the right coronary artery (the most common scenario), the heart is said to be right dominant. If it arises from the circumflex branch of the left coronary artery, the heart is said to be left dominant. Right-dominant hearts have more opportunity for anastomoses between the right and left coronary arteries. (189–190)

31. What is the ductus arteriosus?
The ductus arteriosus is an embryonic blood vessel that is derived from the left sixth aortic arch. The ductus arteriosus connects the aortic arch

with the left pulmonary artery. Prenatally, blood is shunted from the pulmonary artery into the aorta through the ductus arteriosus. After birth, the ductus arteriosus normally closes and then becomes fibrotic. It is then called the ligamentum arteriosum. (195)

32. What is the isthmus of the aorta?
The isthmus of the aorta is the region of the aorta between the origin of the left subclavian artery and the ductus arteriosus (or ligamentum arteriosum). This is the most common site of aortic coarctation. (195)

33. Why is a patient with coarctation of the aorta at increased risk for stroke?
Coarctation of the aorta causes an increase in blood pressure proximal to the coarctation. Because the blood supply to the brain arises from the aorta proximal to the usual site of coarctation, the blood pressure in the cerebral circulation is elevated. This increases the risk of stroke. (200)

34. Why is notching of the ribs seen in patients coarctation of the aorta?
The intercostal arteries serve as collateral pathways between the aorta and the internal thoracic arteries. These collateral channels are used to bypass a coarctation of the aorta. The increased flow in the intercostal arteries causes an increase in the size of these arteries. These arteries are located along the lower borders of the ribs, and as they enlarge, they cause resorption of bone along the lower borders of the ribs, resulting in notching. (199)

35. What is the origin of the azygos vein, and into what vein does it drain?
The azygos vein is formed by the union of the right ascending lumbar vein and the right subcostal vein. It ascends into the thorax, and it drains into the superior vena cava. It receives drainage from the intercostal veins on the right, and it receives drainage from the left intercostal veins via the hemiazygos vein. (206)

36. What are the most common causes of compression of the superior vena cava (SVC) and the resultant SVC syndrome?
The most common causes of SVC syndrome are mediastinal malignancies and their associated enlarged lymph nodes. Lymphomas and lung cancer are common sources of these malignancies. (203)

37. What organ is immediately anterior to the esophagus in the neck and is a frequent site of invasion by esophageal cancer?
The trachea is immediately anterior to the esophagus. There is only a thin layer of connective tissue separating these organs. (210)

38. What nerve is found in the tracheoesophageal groove, and what is the effect of its compression by esophageal tumors?
The recurrent laryngeal nerve lies in the tracheoesophageal groove. The nerve ascends from the aortic arch on the left and from the subclavian artery on the right. The nerve innervates all of the muscles of the larynx except for the cricothyroid. Lesion of the nerve results in hoarseness and a semiabducted vocal fold. (211–212)

39. Which chamber of the heart is immediately anterior to the esophagus?
The left atrium is immediately anterior to the esophagus, with only the pericardium intervening between them. Cancer of the esophagus may invade the left atrium. Similarly, enlargement of the left atrium may compress the esophagus. (212)

40. Into what veins do the esophageal veins drain?
The esophageal veins drain into the azygos vein and hemiazygos vein and then into the superior vena cava. They also drain into the left gastric vein, which drains into the portal vein. Cancer of the esophagus may spread in either direction. The esophageal veins serve as an important anastomosis between the portal venous system and the systemic venous system. (214)

UNIT IV

Abdomen

25

Indirect Inguinal Hernia

A 22-year-old man comes to the outpatient department with the complaint that occasionally, particularly when he stands or strains, a "bulge" appears in his right groin. Off and on, he has moderate pain in this area that is increased by activity, particularly lifting or straining hard during a bowel movement. He is otherwise healthy with no known allergies and is taking no medications.

Examination

On inspection with the patient standing, a bulge is noticeable in the right inguinal area that increases in volume on coughing. On palpation, the swelling seems to extend upward into the inguinal canal; however, its upper end cannot be felt. With the patient supine, the lump disappears. When the examiner invaginates the skin of the scrotum and inserts his little finger into the superficial inguinal ring, he feels a definite impact when the patient coughs. With straining, the bulge again becomes demonstrable and is noticeable also when the patient is in a horizontal position. It can be reduced by the examiner. With the examiner's fingers pressed firmly over the area of the deep inguinal ring, the mass does not descend into the inguinal canal when the patient coughs. Examination of the left side does not reveal any abnormality.

Diagnosis

Right-sided, reducible, indirect inguinal hernia is diagnosed.

Therapy and Further Course

The treatment of choice for a symptomatic inguinal hernia is surgery. The alternative options of open surgery and laparoscopic surgery are discussed with the patient. Because of the shorter operative time for the open surgery, the patient's preference for local anesthesia, and the lower rate of complications and recurrence, this procedure is agreed upon. The surgery is performed 1 week later.

With the patient sedated, local anesthesia is provided through nerve blocks of the ilioinguinal and iliohypogastric nerves. Injections of anesthetic are made just medial to the anterior superior iliac spine, just lateral to the pubic tubercle, and along the intended incision line. The skin and superficial fascia are divided by an incision above and parallel to the inguinal ligament down to the aponeurosis of the external oblique muscle. Blood vessels encountered in the superficial fascia are divided and coagulated by electrocautery.

The inguinal canal is opened by incising the aponeurosis of the external oblique muscle in the direction of its fibers. This incision extends the length of the canal and includes the superficial inguinal ring. The ilioinguinal nerve is identified and carefully isolated and retracted. Both portions of the divided external oblique aponeurosis are reflected by blunt dissection. With reflection of the anterior wall of the canal, the spermatic cord and hernial sac within the coverings of the cord are visualized. The hernia sac is typically anteromedial to the elements of the spermatic cord. By blunt dissection, the coverings of the cord are removed from the hernial sac, and the sac is isolated. The walls of the sac are then carefully incised without injury to its contents. The contents in this case consist of a loop of small intestine (Fig. 25.1). The intestine is gently replaced into the peritoneal cavity. The sac is then separated by dissection from the structures of the cord, which lie lateral and posterior to the sac. After the sac has been widely opened and carefully inspected for any further contents, it is ligated at its proximal end and excised. A polypropylene patch is placed behind the spermatic cord in the floor of the inguinal canal and is sutured in place. The spermatic cord is then

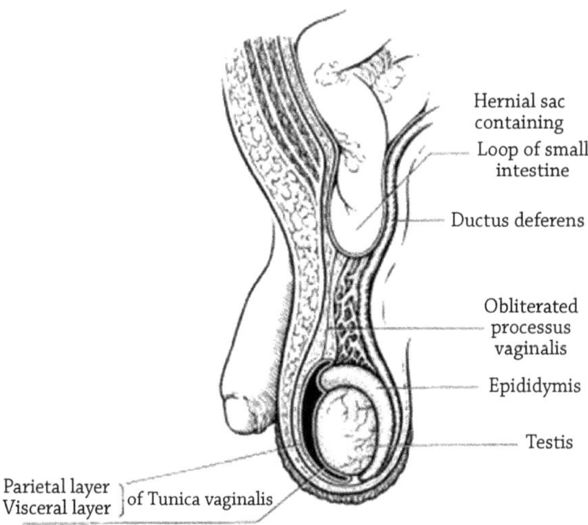

FIGURE 25.1

Section through an indirect inguinal hernia with the hernial sac containing a loop of small intestine. Notice the partial obliteration of the processus vaginalis.

replaced in its normal position, and the two ends of the polypropylene patch are placed around the spermatic cord over the deep inguinal ring. The divided portions of the external oblique aponeurosis, including the superficial inguinal ring, are reunited. The superficial fascia and skin incisions are closed in layers.

The patient is discharged home on the same day. He is told to restrict physical activity for 4 to 6 weeks. On reexamination, he shows no signs of recurrence and has no complaints.

Discussion

An indirect inguinal hernia is a hernia in which an outpouching of the peritoneal sac enters the inguinal canal at the deep inguinal ring and, if complete, leaves it at the superficial inguinal ring. In other words, the hernial sac, formed by peritoneum and containing abdominal contents, takes the same course through the abdominal wall as the spermatic cord. An indirect inguinal hernia has an oblique and longer pathway through the abdominal wall than the direct type. A direct inguinal hernia enters the abdominal wall directly posterior to the superficial inguinal ring and therefore penetrates the inguinal canal through its posterior wall medial to the deep ring.

The layers of the abdominal wall are represented in the layers of the spermatic fascia that cover the testis and the spermatic cord. The innermost layer of the wall is the parietal peritoneum. Outside of that is the extraperitoneal layer, where the testis develops. Outside of that is the transversalis fascia. This fascia is evaginated at the deep inguinal ring to become the internal spermatic fascia. The next three layers are muscular layers; from within outward, they are the transversus abdominis, the internal oblique, and the external oblique. Each of these muscle layers has an associated layer of deep fascia covering it.

In the inguinal region, the transversus abdominis layer and the internal oblique layer are fused together. Some of the internal oblique muscle fibers along with the fascia of the internal oblique are evaginated to become the cremaster muscle and fascia, which make up the middle layer of the spermatic fascia. The cremaster muscle is able to elevate the testis within the scrotum and thereby help to regulate the temperature of the testis, which must be maintained a few degrees below body temperature to allow spermatogenesis to occur.

The fascia of the external oblique is evaginated at the superficial inguinal ring to become the external spermatic fascia, the outermost layer of spermatic fascia. Outside of the external oblique layer are the superficial fascia and skin of the abdomen, which continue as the dartos fascia and skin of the scrotum.

A predisposing factor for development of an indirect inguinal hernia is the persistence of the processus vaginalis. The processus vaginalis is a diverticulum or outpouching of the parietal peritoneum that, during embryonic development, precedes the testis in its migration into the scrotum, evaginating before it all layers of the abdominal wall that are encountered in its descent. Whereas the lower portion of this peritoneal diverticulum remains patent as the tunica vaginalis testis, the upper part typically becomes obliterated. This obliteration normally takes place during the first postnatal year.

Indirect Inguinal Hernia and Inguinal Canal

A patent processus vaginalis is a predisposing factor to indirect inguinal hernia; however, hernia does not occur in all such cases. Hernia requires the protrusion of a viscus or part of a viscus through the deep inguinal ring into this preformed sac. The deep inguinal ring is an evagination of the transversalis fascia. It is the site where the transversalis fascia is continued as an outpouching over the spermatic cord and testis, forming its innermost sheath, the internal spermatic fascia. The deep ring is located about 1 to 2 cm above the midpoint of the inguinal ligament. This midpoint can be located halfway between the two attachments of the inguinal ligament, the anterior superior iliac spine and the pubic tubercle. In this case, when the examiner compresses the deep inguinal ring at this site, the hernia sac does not enter the canal. This is evidence that the hernia is passing through the deep ring and, therefore, is an indirect inguinal hernia.

Because the normal inguinal canal represents a weakness of the anterior abdominal wall, we must consider what counteracts the formation of a hernia even in the presence of a partially or totally open processus vaginalis. The obliquity of the canal constitutes a natural obstacle to the formation of a hernia. An increase in intraabdominal pressure, such as when coughing, straining, or lifting, actually forces the walls of the canal closer together.

Herniation through the deep inguinal ring into the open processus vaginalis occurs only after the ring has become wide enough to permit some contents of the peritoneal cavity to extrude through the ring into the canal in conjunction with the spermatic cord. The hernial sac lies within the substance of the cord, ensheathed by the internal spermatic fascia and the cremaster muscle and fascia. These form the coverings of the cord within the inguinal canal. The ductus deferens lies posterior to the sac (Fig. 25.2).

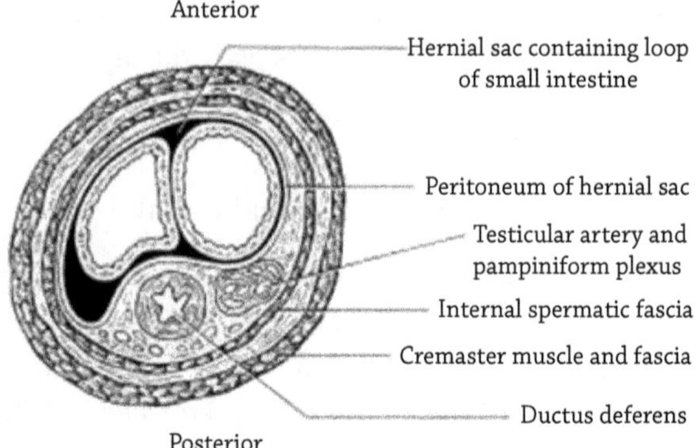

FIGURE 25.2

Cross section through the spermatic cord and hernial sac containing a loop of small intestine. Notice that the hernia forms part of the contents of the cord and is surrounded by its coverings. Also notice the typical location of the sac anterior to the ductus deferens.

The aponeurosis of the external abdominal oblique muscle forms the anterior wall of the inguinal canal. This aponeurosis must be incised surgically to open the anterior wall of the inguinal canal. The superficial inguinal ring is a triangular gap in the aponeurosis of the external oblique. At the superficial inguinal ring, the external oblique fascia (the fascia that covers the external oblique aponeurosis) continues onto the spermatic cord as the external spermatic fascia. This fascia forms the outermost sheath of a hernia that emerges through the superficial ring. The superficial ring lies superolateral to the pubic tubercle. Its lateral (inferior) crus attaches to the pubic tubercle, and its medial (superior) crus inserts on the pubic crest.

Anatomy of Surgical Complications

Endangered Nerves

During surgery in this case, as in every case of inguinal hernia, the ilioinguinal nerve is particularly endangered because it lies in the operative field and passes through the superficial inguinal ring. It is derived from the anterior ramus of the first lumbar (L1) spinal nerve and supplies the skin of the anterior portion of the scrotum and the adjacent region of the thigh with sensory fibers. If it is divided within the canal, numbness of the scrotum and inner aspect of the thigh results. If it is included in a suture or embedded in scar tissue, postoperative neuritic pain will ensue and can be quite severe.

The ilioinguinal nerve and the more superiorly located iliohypogastric nerve, both of which lie in the operative area, carry motor nerve fibers that innervate the lowermost portions of the internal oblique and transversus muscles. Section of these nerves at this level would interfere with the nerve supply to these muscles, leading to weakness of the posterior wall of the inguinal canal, which might result in recurrence of the hernia.

Endangered Blood Vessels.

Postoperative hemorrhage is probably the most common complication of inguinal hernia. The superficial epigastric artery and vein, which ascend in a medial direction across the midportion of the inguinal ligament, are divided and coagulated in this operation. They are branches of the femoral artery and the great saphenous vein, respectively. The superficial external pudendal artery and vein, which are branches of the same vessels, may also be encountered superficial to the spermatic cord.

A major vessel that lies in close relation to the deep inguinal ring is the inferior epigastric artery, one of the two main branches of the external iliac artery. If this vessel is inadvertently cut during a hernia repair and not ligated, severe bleeding will result. The inferior epigastric artery has an important relationship to the deep inguinal ring and therefore to the point of entrance of an indirect inguinal hernia into the inguinal canal. The inferior epigastric artery lies medial to the deep inguinal ring but forms the lateral boundary of the inguinal (Hesselbach's) triangle, which is the site of entrance of a direct inguinal hernia. This means that the inferior epigastric artery lies between the point of exit of an indirect inguinal hernia (the deep inguinal ring) and the point of exit of a direct inguinal hernia (Hesselbach's triangle). The three boundaries of the inguinal (Hesselbach's) triangle are the inferior epigastric artery superolaterally, the rectus abdominis medially, and the inguinal ligament inferiorly.

Injury to the Ductus Deferens.

Another undesirable accident in herniorrhaphy is inadvertent cutting of the ductus deferens when the hernial sac is dissected free. The ductus deferens lies in the posterior part of the spermatic cord and therefore is posterior to the hernia sac; it can be recognized by its hard and cordlike feel when it is rolled between the thumb and index finger. Division of the ductus deferens will result in sterility on that side. An attempt at reuniting the divided ends should be made. Damage to the testicular artery and pampiniform plexus should likewise be avoided, because it will cause hemorrhage and may also result in infertility on one side.

Reducible, Incarcerated, and Strangulated Hernias

The hernia in this case is a reducible hernia: Although the hernia sac has passed through the inguinal canal, it is possible for the sac to return to the abdominal cavity spontaneously, as it did when the patient was in the supine position. An incarcerated hernia is one that cannot be reduced; it can lead to bowel obstruction, but the blood supply to the viscus remains unaffected. A strangulated hernia is an incarcerated hernia in which the blood supply and lymph drainage of the herniated viscus are impaired or occluded. Depending on the degree of vascular occlusion, the intestinal loop will lose its viability within hours unless the hernia is attended to immediately. Strangulated hernia is a surgical emergency. Incarcerated hernias are also considered emergencies because of the risk that they will strangulate.

26

Biliary Colic, Acute Cholecystitis, and Cholecystectomy

A 53-year-old woman presents to the hospital with a complaint of severe pain in the right upper abdominal region. She states that the pain came on suddenly about 2 hours after dinner and is rapidly increasing in severity. It is described as sharp and constant, radiating around the costal margin to her shoulder blade. She has taken an "antacid" without relief. She reports that she has had repeated attacks of severe pain in the right upper quadrant of the abdomen and suffers from indigestion and "gas pain on my stomach," particularly after eating fatty foods. She reports no fever or chills. She is nauseated and vomited bilious fluid once without relief. She has had no change in her bowel habits and reports no itching or change in the color of her skin. She is postmenopausal and has had three pregnancies.

Examination

The patient's temperature is 101.3° F. The remainder of her vital signs are within normal limits. She is 5 feet 2 inches tall and weighs 174 lb. Her calculated body mass index (BMI) is 32, which places her in the obese category. On head, eye, ear, nose, and throat (HEENT) examination, her sclera are anicteric (no jaundice is evident). Her mucous membranes are dry, suggesting mild dehydration. The heart and lung examinations are normal. There is marked tenderness and some rigidity in the right hypochondriac region. She has a positive Murphy's sign (a pause in inspiration with palpation in the right upper quadrant). Her white blood cell count is 12,900 cells/μL. Ultrasound examination shows multiple stones in the gall bladder,

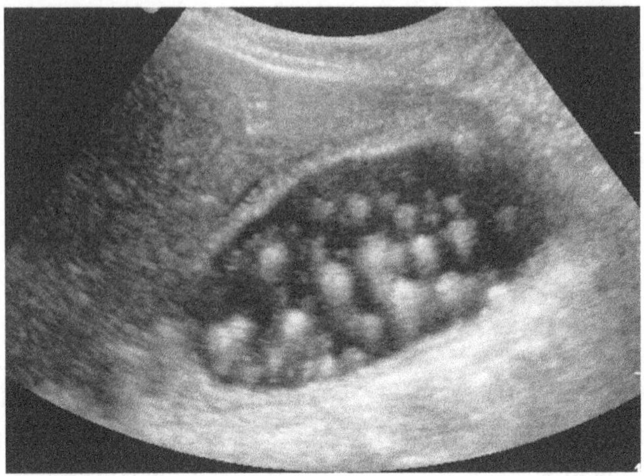

FIGURE 26.1

Ultrasound image of the gall bladder. The gall bladder is the dark, transversely oriented structure that contains multiple whitish gallstones.

a thickened gallbladder wall, and a small amount of pericholecystic fluid (Fig. 26.1).

Diagnosis

The diagnosis is biliary colic and acute calculus cholecystitis (inflammation of the gall bladder accompanied by gallstone formation).

Therapy and Further Course

The patient is given intravenous pain medication and antibiotics and is scheduled for a laparoscopic cholecystectomy the next day. Laparoscopic cholecystectomy reduces the amount of recovery time and pain associated with removal of the gall bladder. According to some sources, 95% of patients can now be considered suitable for this procedure, and most patients are able to ambulate and return home the next day. Endoscopic video equipment, including a tiny video camera attached to the laparoscope with cable connections to transmit images of the operative field to a monitor, as well as specially designed surgical instruments, are inserted into the abdominal cavity through small puncture sites.

The peritoneal cavity must be distended by creating a pneumoperitoneum with insufflation equipment to make room for the laparoscope and the manipulation of the surgical instruments in the operative field. Carbon dioxide is the standard gas used for producing the pneumoperitoneum. Irrigation-aspiration devices are also used to keep the operative field clean and to remove debris. Forceps and electrocautery devices are used to dissect the tissue and to achieve hemostasis of small blood vessels.

A blunt forceps is used to grasp the fundus of the gall bladder and to retract it over the right lobe of the liver toward the diaphragm. Another is used to retract Hartmann's pouch laterally. Hartmann's pouch is an evagination of the wall of the gall bladder at the junction of the neck of the gall bladder and the cystic duct. Retraction of the pouch causes the peritoneal fold of the cystic duct and the cystic artery to be placed on stretch. The cystic artery is located in the cystohepatic triangle (triangle of Calot), which is formed by the cystic duct, the hepatic ducts, and the border of the liver). The cystic artery is dissected free circumferentially from the surrounding tissues. Similarly, the cystic duct junction with the gall bladder is identified, and the cystic duct is circumferentially dissected free of tissue before ligation of both structures with clips. At that point, the fundus of the gall bladder can be retracted to allow dissection of the gall bladder from the gall bladder fossa of the liver. Once it has been completely freed from the liver bed, the gall bladder is typically placed within a bag to contain its contents and is then removed through the umbilical port site. The gall bladder fossa is checked for hemostasis, and the peritoneal cavity is irrigated. The instruments are then removed with direct visualization, and the incisions are closed. The nasogastric tube and Foley catheter are removed in the operating room. The patient's diet can be advanced that same evening, and usually the patient can be discharged the following morning.

Should an open cholecystectomy be required, the following steps are taken. The abdominal wall is opened by a subcostal incision that begins at the tip of the xiphoid process and is directed laterally and downward, paralleling the costal margin about 2 fingerbreadths inferior to it. After the anterior layer of the rectus sheath has been split, the rectus abdominis muscle is divided with cautery in a direction paralleling the skin incision. The incision is continued laterally through the external oblique, the internal oblique, and the transversus abdominis muscles in a direction paralleling the skin incision. The posterior layer of the rectus sheath is likewise divided, as are the transversalis fascia, the extraperitoneal fat, and the peritoneum. During this procedure, an attempt is made to preserve intercostal nerves as they are seen within the rectus sheath deep to the rectus muscle by retracting them out of the way. After the peritoneal cavity has been opened, it is explored with one hand with particular attention to the stomach, duodenum, transverse colon, and dome of the liver. The operative field is walled off with gauze pads, and a retractor is placed to lift the costal margin.

The surgeon then introduces a finger into the epiploic foramen, and between this finger and the thumb palpates the common bile duct within the hepatoduodenal ligament for evidence of stones, thickening, and dilatation. With the gall bladder retracted by its fundus, an incision is made into the hepatoduodenal ligament close to its free border. By blunt dissection, the cystic duct is exposed at its junction with the neck of the gall bladder and doubly clamped and divided. Next, the cystic artery is identified, doubly ligated, and divided between ligatures. Invariably, the cystic artery is located in the triangle of Calot (cystohepatic triangle). The peritoneal attachment of the gall bladder to the liver is incised to free the gall bladder. The gall bladder is separated from its bed using the cautery and removed from the operative field. Venous bleeding from the gall bladder bed is controlled with electrocautery. The incisions are closed in layers. Postoperatively, the patient is given intravenous fluids initially, and diet is advanced as tolerated. Good pain control is essential. Typically, patients are in the hospital 3 to 4 days before discharge.

Discussion

Common risk factors for the development of gallstones include female sex, increased age, obesity, and pregnancy. In addition, there is a strong genetic component to the disease that is associated with mutations in bile duct cholesterol transport proteins. Gallstone formation is promoted when components of the bile are present in concentrations that approach the limits of their solubility. This problem is exacerbated with the concentration of bile by the gall bladder. The gall bladder can become supersaturated with these substances, which then precipitate from solution as microscopic crystals. Over time, the crystals grow, aggregate, and become a nidus for the formation of macroscopic stones. Usually, occlusion of the cystic duct by a gallstone is the precipitating event leading to acute cholecystitis.

Transient obstruction of the cystic duct by a stone produces the classic symptoms of epigastric pain (so-called biliary colic), indigestion, nausea, and vomiting that occur particularly after fatty meals and that subside spontaneously when the stone either passes through the duct or is expelled back into the gall bladder. The acute exacerbation of pain, with superimposed infection as found in this case, is caused by impaction of a stone in the cystic duct (Fig. 26.2).

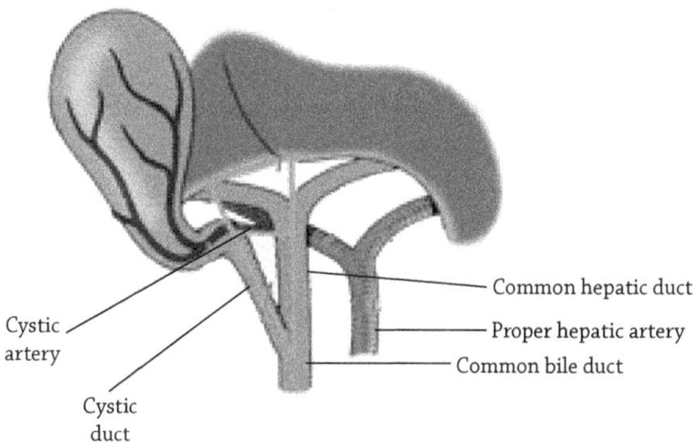

FIGURE 26.2

Extrahepatic biliary passages and blood supply in the typical arrangement. Notice the triangle of Calot containing the cystic artery.

Anatomy of Biliary Pain and Rigidity

Typical for biliary colic is the sudden onset of sharp, severe pain that starts in the epigastric and umbilical regions. The pain then becomes localized in the right hypochondriac area and radiates toward the inferior angle of the scapula and inferior to it.

The pain in the right hypochondriac area is caused by direct inflammation of the parietal peritoneum contacted by the gall bladder and stimulation of the sensory nerve endings in this parietal peritoneum. Innervation of the centrally located parietal peritoneum on the undersurface of the right dome of the diaphragm is provided by the right phrenic nerve. If this region is irritated by an inflamed gall bladder, pain is sometimes referred to the ipsilateral neck and shoulder region in the region of the cervical C4 and C5 dermatomes. These are spinal cord segments represented in the phrenic nerve. The pain in the scapular region is referred pain, which is common in diseases involving the viscera. Pain arising in sensory nerve endings in the viscera, in this instance the gall bladder, is referred to areas of the body surface that send sensory impulses to the same segment of the spinal cord. Sensory fibers from the gall bladder run in plexuses along the biliary duct, closely intermingled with sympathetic efferent fibers. They pass through the celiac ganglion, the greater splanchnic nerve, the sympathetic chain ganglia, and, via white rami communicantes, to spinal nerves and their dorsal roots and ganglia. This is where their cell bodies are located. Central fibers from the dorsal root ganglia terminate in the seventh to ninth thoracic spinal cord segments. It is to the dermatomes innervated by these spinal cord segments that the radiating pain to the scapular and infrascapular areas is localized.

The muscular rigidity that is found over the diseased area is a state of involuntary contraction of the muscles of the anterior abdominal wall, particularly the rectus abdominis, which is a reflex response to stimulation of the nerve endings in the parietal peritoneum in the region of the gall bladder. This, presumably, is a protective mechanism intended to protect the diseased organ.

Topography of the Abdomen

In this case history, two different topographic terminologies, both common in clinical descriptions, are used. The simpler one divides the abdomen into four quadrants by a midsagittal and a horizontal plane laid through the umbilicus. A second, more complex terminology, defines nine regions, created by two vertical and two horizontal planes. The two vertical planes pass through the midpoints of the inguinal ligaments. The upper horizontal plane, the *subcostal plane*, is at the lowest point of the tenth rib, which corresponds to the level of the third lumbar vertebra. The lower horizontal plane, the *intertubercular plane*, passes through the two iliac tubercles and corresponds to the level of the fifth lumbar vertebra. The regions outlined are the right and left hypochondriac, the right and left lumbar, the right and left inguinal, the epigastric, the umbilical, and the hypogastric (Fig. 26.3).

Anatomical Relationships of the Gall Bladder and Liver

The gall bladder is located in its own bed on the visceral surface of the liver. It forms the boundary between the right lobe and the quadrate lobe of the liver. There is connective tissue but no peritoneum intervening between the liver and the gall bladder. In other words, the peritoneum that covers the visceral surface of the liver passes over the sides and inferior surface of the gall bladder and does not cover the area in direct contact with the liver. A comprehensive knowledge of the anatomical relationships around the liver and their common variations can prevent many complications of surgery in this region. Cautious dissection will help in identifying the important structures and protecting them from injury.

The liver is connected to the diaphragm by the coronary ligament. The coronary ligament is the reflection of the peritoneum from the visceral peritoneum on the liver to the parietal peritoneum on the abdominal surface of the diaphragm. The coronary ligament is rhomboid in shape and surrounds the bare area of the liver. The bare area is in direct contact with the diaphragm without any

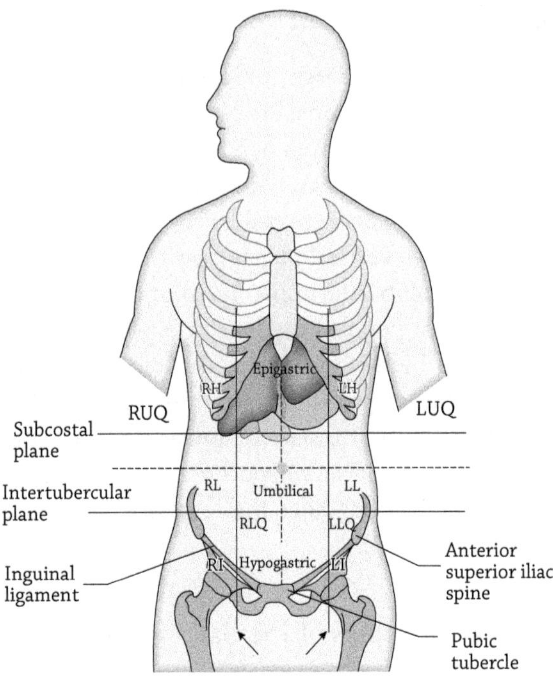

FIGURE 26.3

The four quadrants and the nine regions of the abdomen. LLQ, left lower quadrant; LUQ, left upper quadrant; RLQ, right lower quadrant; RUQ, right upper quadrant.

intervening peritoneum. The right and left extremities of the coronary ligament are named the right and left triangular ligaments, respectively. The hepatic veins exit from the liver in the bare area and enters the inferior vena cava.

The visceral peritoneum reflects off the visceral surface of the liver to form the lesser omentum, a double layer of peritoneum that connects the liver to the stomach and the duodenum. The lesser omentum is divided into two portions: the hepatogastric ligament, which attaches to the lesser curvature of the stomach, and the hepatoduodenal ligament, which attaches to the first part of the duodenum. The hepatoduodenal ligament has a free border on its right which forms the anterior wall of the epiploic foramen of Winslow. One of the maneuvers performed during open cholecystectomy is palpation of the hepatoduodenal ligament close to its free border. Between the two layers of the hepatoduodenal ligament, near its free margin, lie three important structures: the common bile duct farthest to the right, the proper hepatic artery to the left of the common bile duct, and the portal vein between and posterior to the other two. Other structures surrounding this triad are autonomic nerve fibers and lymphatic vessels. If a stone is lodged in the common bile duct, it can be palpated within the duct in the free edge of the lesser omentum.

Secretion and Storage of Bile

Bile is secreted by the hepatocytes of the liver into the biliary canaliculi. These biliary canaliculi coalesce to form the right and left hepatic ducts, which in turn fuse to form the common hepatic duct. The common hepatic duct is joined by the cystic duct to form the common bile duct, which then joins the major pancreatic duct and enters the second portion of the duodenum. Within the duodenum, bile serves to emulsify fats and thus aids in the digestion of fat by pancreatic lipase. During periods between meals, the sphincter of the ampulla of the common bile duct (sphincter of Oddi) is closed, preventing the passage of bile into the duodenum. The bile being secreted by the liver backs up into the gall bladder through the cystic duct. In the gall bladder, water is absorbed from the bile, concentrating it. When food is released by the stomach into the duodenum, cholecystokinin, which causes relaxation of the sphincter of Oddi and contraction of the smooth muscle of the gall bladder, is released. This causes bile stored in the gall bladder to be propelled into the duodenum. If the cystic duct is occluded by a stone, the forceful contraction of the smooth muscle of the gall bladder and the duct, attempting to propel the bile past the obstruction, causes the painful biliary colic which the patient experiences after a meal.

Anomalies of the Cystic Duct

In performing a cholecystectomy, it is the task of the surgeon to identify the cystic duct and then doubly clamp, ligate, and divide it. With the liver and gall bladder retracted, the cystic duct, about 3 to 4 cm long, runs posteriorly, inferiorly, and to the left within the lesser omentum and joins the common hepatic duct to form the common bile duct. Most important to the surgeon are variations in the length and course of the cystic duct and in the site of junction with the common hepatic duct (Fig. 26.4). If the cystic duct is unusually long, it may run alongside the common hepatic duct for a variable length of the latter's course, often attached to it by connective tissue. The cystic duct, instead of joining the common hepatic duct on its right side, may pass in front or behind the common hepatic duct, uniting with it on its left side. If the anomalies mentioned are not recognized, the common hepatic duct may be mistaken for the cystic duct and may be clamped, ligated, or even partially resected. Blind clamping or ligation of bleeding blood vessels may also lead to injuries or occlusion of the common hepatic duct. The result of complete occlusion of the common hepatic duct is severe jaundice, which is fatal unless the patient undergoes surgery to reestablish patency.

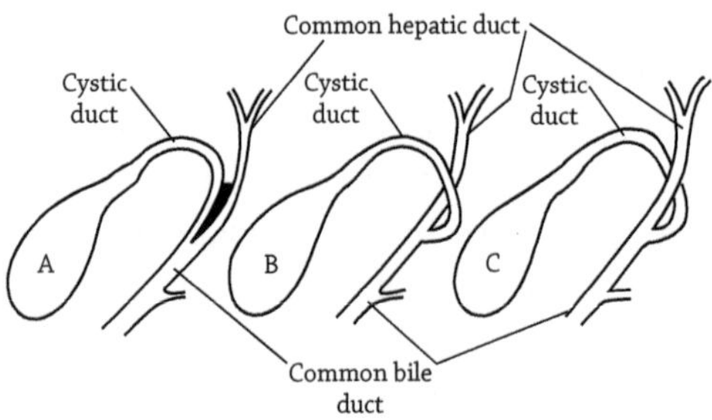

FIGURE 26.4

A, An unusually long cystic duct is attached to the common hepatic duct by connective tissue. **B,** This cystic duct joins the common hepatic duct on its left side by passing in front of it. **C,** This cystic duct joins the common hepatic duct on its left side by passing behind it.

Anomalies of the Cystic Artery

Recognition of vascular anomalies, particularly of the cystic artery, is of equal clinical importance. In the typical arrangement, the cystic artery arises from the right hepatic artery to the right of the common hepatic duct. After a course that varies in length, the cystic artery divides into a superficial and a deep branch, one going to the peritoneal and the other to the attached surface of the gall bladder. Variations in this arrangement of the blood supply are fairly common. The superficial and deep branches may arise separately rather than from a common stem, resulting in a double cystic artery. This is reported to occur in 10% to 15% of cases. The cystic artery may also arise from the proper hepatic artery or from the left hepatic artery. Other, rarer origins of the cystic artery are from the gastroduodenal artery or from a hepatic artery that is a branch of the superior mesenteric artery.

If the surgeon is unfamiliar with the possible multiplicity of the cystic artery or its abnormal course, profuse unexpected hemorrhage may result, which can be temporarily controlled by compression (between index finger and thumb) of the proper hepatic artery within the layers of the lesser omentum (Pringle maneuver). If the right hepatic artery is mistaken for the cystic artery and ligated instead of the cystic artery, necrosis of the liver occurs, with serious consequences possibly including death. Significant intraoperative hemorrhage from injury to abnormal blood vessels during laparoscopic cholecystectomy often requires conversion to open surgery. It is best avoided by carefully identifying all blood vessels at the time of cholecystectomy and being aware of the possibility of aberrant blood vessels.

27

Bariatric Surgery for Morbid Obesity

A 53-year-old male physician presents to a surgical colleague for evaluation for bariatric surgery. The patient has struggled with his weight for 25 years. Despite regular efforts at weight loss, his body weight has increased over the past 2 years from 275 to 310 pounds, and his body mass index (BMI)—the weight in kilograms divided by the square of the height in meters—has risen from 38.4 to 43.2. Numerous weight loss attempts have included diet and exercise in addition to psychotherapy and hypnosis. The patient also has struggled with poorly controlled type 2 diabetes mellitus, severe osteoarthritis of the knees, and obstructive sleep apnea. He has no surgical history, has no allergies, and is a nonsmoker. He takes insulin for his diabetes and uses nasal continuous positive airway pressure (CPAP) for his sleep apnea. He has a significant family history of obesity.

Examination

On physical examination, the patient is morbidly obese (defined as a BMI >40) with a BMI of 43.2. He is afebrile, and the remainder of his vital signs are significant for hypertension (180/100 mm Hg), made difficult to assess because of the special cuff size required. His heart sounds are distant, and respiratory efforts are poor. His abdominal examination is made difficult because of his obesity, but there are no masses. No skin lesions are noted in the intertriginous region (areas where skin surfaces come in contact). The lower extremity examination is significant for reddish-brown skin discoloration over the medial aspect of both ankles, consistent with mild venous stasis dermatitis.

Diagnosis

The diagnosis is morbid obesity.

Therapy and Further Course

Because all other attempts at weight loss have been unsuccessful and because of the continued risk to the patient's health caused by his morbid obesity, laparoscopic bariatric surgery (Roux-en-Y gastric bypass) is recommended and agreed to.

With the patient under general anesthesia, initial port placement and insufflation of the abdomen is achieved. After inspection of the abdomen with the laparoscope and lysis of any adhesions, the first step in the surgery is identification of the jejunal limb of the bypass. The greater omentum is identified and gently lifted toward the upper abdomen to expose the suspensory ligament (of Treitz) at the duodenojejunal junction. The jejunum is measured 50 cm from the ligament of Treitz using an intestinal grasper. A stapler is applied perpendicular to the jejunum and parallel to the mesenteric vascular arcade to divide the bowel, creating a biliopancreatic limb (proximal limb) and a Roux-limb (distal limb) of the jejunum. Vascular clips are applied to divide the jejunal mesentery with good hemostasis and to allow the Roux-limb sufficient mobility to reach over the transverse colon toward the gastric pouch. The Roux-limb is measured 75 cm distally (for patients with a BMI <50) or 150 cm distally (for those with a BMI >50) for the construction of the jejunojejunostomy. After this step, the gastric pouch is created.

To accomplish creation of the pouch, the patient is transferred to a steep reverse Trendelenburg (head up) position to facilitate exposure of the upper abdomen by using gravity to move the viscera into the pelvis. The upper portion of the stomach is then exposed by retracting the liver anteriorly. A window is created in the nonvascular area of the gastrohepatic ligament immediately anterior to the caudate lobe of the liver. The opening in the gastrohepatic ligament provides access to the lesser

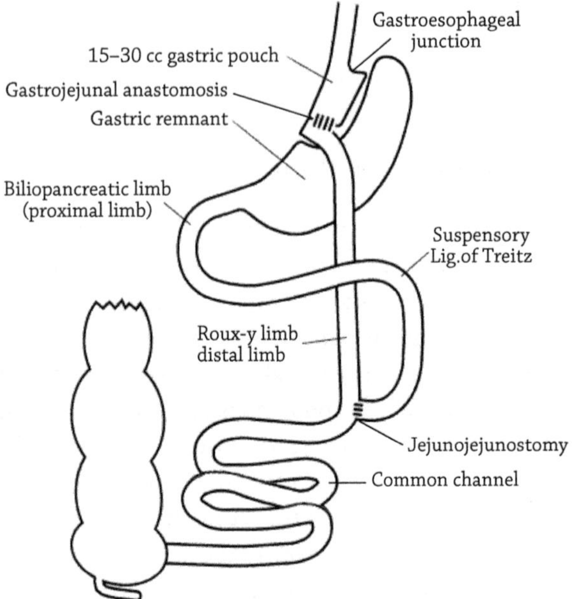

FIGURE 27.1

Schematic diagram of Roux-en-Y gastric bypass. Lig.,ligament.

sac (omental bursa) behind the stomach. The gastroesophageal junction is then identified, and a stapler is applied to the lesser omentum 1 cm distal to the gastroesophageal junction. After division of the lesser omentum, a stapler is applied across the gastric cardia toward the incisura to create a gastric pouch. After good hemostasis of the staple lines is ensured, the Roux-limb is brought toward the gastric pouch and an end-to-side gastrojejunal anastomosis is performed. An omental "patch" is usually placed around the pouch to protect against an anastomotic leak. Additionally, a drain is often placed adjacent to the pouch to control a leak should it occur.

The patient is discharged from the hospital the next day. Because bariatric surgery is a risk factor for pernicious anemia, he is prescribed vitamin B_{12} supplementation and referred for counseling on diet modification.

Discussion

Obesity is an epidemic, not only in the United States, where an estimated one-third of the adult population is obese, but also worldwide. Approximately 5% of the U.S. population is considered to be morbidly obese (BMI ≥40). Morbid obesity has numerous comorbidities, as demonstrated by this patient's history. These include increased risk of cardiovascular and pulmonary diseases, diabetes, osteoarthritis, and stroke, with resulting reduced life expectancy and significant health care expenditure.

Bariatric surgical procedures are accepted methods to achieve weight loss in severely obese individuals for whom all other attempts at weight loss have failed. They work by restricting caloric intake through surgical alteration of the gastrointestinal tract to modify the capacity of the stomach (a restrictive procedure) or to bypass the absorptive surface of the small intestine (a malabsorptive procedure). Restrictive procedures include adjustable gastric banding, in which an adjustable synthetic band is wrapped around the stomach, and gastric stapling. However, the gold standard for weight-loss procedures is the Roux-en-Y gastric bypass operation, which is a combined restrictive and malabsorptive procedure. It is named in honor of Dr. Phillibart Roux, a nineteenth century French surgeon who introduced the idea of bypass surgery, and for the Y shape of the anatomy of the jejunum created by the surgery. Advanced laparoscopic techniques have allowed the procedure to be performed with diminished pain and faster recovery time. However, the associated surgical complications, for both the open and the laparoscopic procedures, can be severe and potentially life-threatening, so that potential candidates for bariatric surgery should be referred to centers of excellence that have a documented record of positive outcomes.

The Digestive Pathway

To understand the rationale for Roux-en-Y bariatric surgery, it is necessary to understand the roles of the various digestive organs in the absorption of nutrients. Digestion begins in the mouth with the maceration and moistening of food and the addition of digestive enzymes in the saliva. The esophagus transports the food to the stomach, where gastric enzymes, primarily pepsinogen, hydrochloric acid, and gastric intrinsic factor, are added. Food is then released into the duodenum, where bile from the liver and many pancreatic enzymes are added. The food continues into the jejunum and ileum, where some additional enzymes are added and almost all of the nutrient absorption occurs. In the colon, much of the remaining water is absorbed to produce feces, which are stored in the rectum and released through the anal canal. The Roux-en-Y procedure is designed to substantially reduce the storage capacity of the stomach, so that the patient must eat less, and to reduce the functional length of the jejunum, so that there is less surface area for absorption of nutrients.

Because gastric intrinsic factor, which is secreted by the parietal cells of the stomach, is necessary for the absorption of vitamin B_{12}, substantial reduction in gastric size is likely to result in a vitamin B_{12} deficiency. For this reason, our patient was started on supplementation of this vitamin.

As a result of bypass surgery, this patient now has a small stomach pouch in the cardia region of the stomach which is about the size of an egg. This allows him to eat only a very small volume of food before having a feeling of fullness. Because of the construction of the gastrojejunostomy between the stomach pouch and the Roux (distal) limb of the jejunum, all of the duodenum and approximately 50 cm of the jejunum are bypassed, thus reducing the amount of absorptive surface. Because the pancreatic enzymes and bile are secreted into the duodenum, which after the surgery is no longer a part of the pathway for food leaving the stomach, it is necessary to get these secretions into the jejunum where the food is. It is for this reason that the proximal (biliopancreatic) limb is joined with the distal (Roux) limb at the jejunojejunostomy. The peristaltic contraction of the proximal limb prevents retrograde flow of the food across the jejunojejunostomy.

The Mesenteries of the Stomach

In the description of the surgical procedure, both mesenteries of the stomach are mentioned. The *greater omentum* is derived from the original dorsal mesogastrium (dorsal mesentery of the stomach). In the adult, this mesentery is attached to the greater curvature of the stomach, which was the embryonic dorsal wall of the stomach, and is draped in front of many organs of the peritoneal cavity. During embryonic development, because of the 90-degree rotation of the foregut, the mesentery becomes very long and folds upon itself to become the greater omentum. The greater omentum is directly continuous with the gastrosplenic ligament, the portion of the dorsal mesogastrium that connects the greater curvature of the stomach with the spleen. To gain access to the small intestine, it is necessary for the surgeon to retract the greater omentum superiorly.

The *lesser omentum* is derived from the original ventral mesogastrium. In the adult, the lesser omentum connects the liver to the lesser curvature of the stomach and to the first part of the duodenum. The portion of the lesser omentum that connects the liver to the duodenum is termed the *hepatoduodenal ligament*. This is the part of the lesser omentum that is near its free edge on the right. It is quite thick because it contains multiple structures, including the common bile duct, the proper hepatic artery, and the portal vein. The much larger part of the lesser omentum, which connects the liver to the lesser curvature of the stomach, is termed the *hepatogastric ligament*. This part of the mesentery is quite thin and is mostly free of any contents, except near the border of the stomach, where the left and right gastric arteries and veins are contained within it. The lesser omentum forms part of the anterior wall of the lesser sac (omental bursa) and separates the lesser sac from the greater sac. The surgeon perforates the nonvascular portion of the hepatogastric ligament to gain access into the lesser sac in order to have wider access to the gastroesophageal junction, allowing the creation of the gastric pouch.

The Small Intestine

The small intestine is divided into three parts: duodenum, jejunum, and ileum. The duodenum (from the Latin word for "twelve") is approximately 12 inches long and is divided into four parts. The first or superior part begins at the pylorus at the level of the first lumbar vertebra and is horizontally oriented. It turns inferiorly to become the second or descending portion. This part descends to the level of the third lumbar vertebra. Here it turns to the left to become the third or inferior horizontal portion, which crosses from the right side of the vertebral column to the left side. It then turns superiorly to become the fourth or ascending portion. At the end of the fourth portion, at the level of the second lumbar vertebra, there is a sharp turn at the duodenojejunal flexure, where the duodenum ends and the jejunum begins. The duodenojejunal flexure is attached to the posterior abdominal wall by the suspensory ligament of Treitz. The first part of the duodenum begins as a peritoneal organ and then becomes retroperitoneal. The second, third, and fourth parts of the duodenum are retroperitoneal.

At the duodenojejunal junction, the intestine becomes peritoneal and gains a mesentery. This marks the beginning of the jejunum. The jejunum and the ileum comprise a continuous peritoneal portion of the small intestine that is suspended from a mesentery in which is found its blood supply, nerve supply, and lymphatic drainage. The ileum ends at the ileocecal junction. The jejunum and ileum together are about 6 to 7 meters long. The first 40% of this length is defined as the jejunum and the last 60% as the ileum. There is no specific anatomical landmark that divides the jejunum from the ileum. The jejunum is mostly in the left upper quadrant of the abdomen, whereas the ileum is mostly in the right lower quadrant. Structural characteristics of the jejunum and ileum change gradually from proximal to distal. As such, the distal jejunum is indistinguishable from the proximal ileum. However, if the proximal jejunum is compared with the distal ileum, some structural differences can be seen. The proximal small intestine is wider and has a thicker muscular wall. It is also somewhat more vascularized and therefore has a deeper color. In addition, there are differences that can be seen at the histological level.

Outcomes

Laparoscopic Roux-en-Y gastric bypass procedures are highly effective in weight reduction in the morbidly obese population. The literature reports an average 60% loss of excess body weight 20 months after surgery. In addition, type 2 diabetes is reversed in a majority of patients, with fasting blood glucose levels returning to normal and the administration of insulin and oral hypoglycemic agents no longer needed.

28

Obstructive Jaundice

A 71-year-old man presents to his family physician with a 2-day history of diffuse pruritus. The patient states that he was well until approximately 2 days ago, when he first noted mild itching, principally on his trunk. The pruritus has progressed so that it is now severe and diffuse. His sleep last night was disturbed, and he is having difficulty concentrating. He denies any nausea, vomiting, or change in bowel habits, although he did notice a change in the color of his stool, reporting that it is "clay-colored." He also reports a 1-month history of vague epigastric discomfort, typically after meals and at night, but does not currently have abdominal pain. He reports that he has lost about 10 pounds over the past month due to a "decreased appetite" and has noted increasing fatigue with routine activities of daily living. He denies alcohol consumption, but he has an 80 pack-year smoking history. He has no significant medical problems or allergies and has never had surgery.

Examination

On physical examination, the patient clearly has skin irritation with numerous excoriations (abrasions from scratching) on both the upper and lower extremities. He otherwise is in no distress. He is afebrile, and the remainder of his vital signs are within normal range. On head, eye, ear, nose, and throat (HEENT) examination, scleral icterus (jaundice) is noted. There is no cervical or supraclavicular adenopathy. He has no jugular venous distention. His lung examination reveals equal breath sounds without rales or rhonchi. On auscultation of the heart, he has normal heart sounds without murmurs or gallops. Inspection of his abdomen reveals mild distention; there is no venous engorgement (caput medusae). Bowel sounds are present and are normoactive. The abdomen is nontender to percussion and palpation. However, there is a nontender, firm mass that is palpable in the right upper quadrant. The liver edge is nonpalpable below the costal margin. There is no evidence of ascites (e.g., shifting dullness). No periumbilical mass is identified. The rectal examination is normal. The skin is examined, and no spider angiomata are identified.

The physician recommends admission to the hospital to evaluate the patient's jaundice. On admission, blood is drawn for a complete blood count (CBC) and serum chemistries. The patient is also scheduled for a right upper quadrant ultrasound examination. The laboratory values demonstrate normal values for white blood cell count, hemoglobin level, and hematocrit. His electrolytes are all within normal limits. However, his total bilirubin level is 9.3 mg/dL (reference value, 0–1.5 mg/dL) with a direct component of 7.0 mg/dL. His alkaline phosphatase level is 649 IU/L (reference value, 39–117 IU/L). The remaining chemistries are not significantly elevated.

The right upper quadrant ultrasound study demonstrates a largely distended gall bladder but no gallstones. There is no gall bladder wall thickening or pericholecystic fluid. Intrahepatic ductal dilatation is noted. The common bile duct is measured at 17 mm (10 mm is the upper limit of normal). No stones are noted in the common bile duct. There is no free fluid in the abdomen (ascites). No hepatic masses are visible. The pancreas is not well visualized because of overlying bowel gas. The ultrasound examination is compatible with a diagnosis of *obstructive jaundice*.

Multidetector spiral computed axial tomography (CT) of the abdomen is recommended for further evaluation. This study provides excellent visualization of the pancreas and also provides important information about the immediately adjacent vascular structures, such as the portal and superior mesenteric veins, as well as the superior mesenteric artery (SMA) and the celiac axis, which determine whether surgical resection of the pancreas can be performed safely, should it become necessary. Additionally, identification of metastatic disease to the liver, to the perihepatic lymph nodes, or elsewhere in the abdomen can be achieved. The patient's

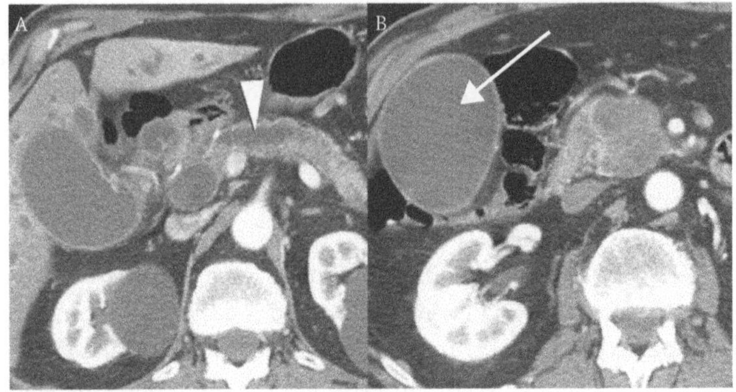

FIGURE 28.1

A, Magnetic resonance image (MRI) shows a dilated pancreatic duct (*white arrowhead*) caused by tumor in the head of the pancreas. **B,** MRI shows dilated gall bladder (*arrow*) caused by obstruction of the common bile duct in the pancreatic head.

CT scan demonstrates a 2.5-cm mass in the head of the pancreas that is obstructing the common bile duct. No evidence of metastatic disease is detected (Fig. 28.1).

Upper endoscopy is then performed, and an endoscopic ultrasound-guided pancreatic biopsy of the mass is performed under direct visualization. Biopsy confirms the suspected diagnosis.

Diagnosis

The diagnosis is adenocarcinoma of the pancreas.

Therapy and Further Course

The patient is scheduled for a pancreaticoduodenectomy, a surgical procedure commonly referred to as a Whipple procedure. This procedure was named after Allen Whipple, an American surgeon who pioneered the technique of pancreatic resection in 1935. A Whipple procedure involves surgical resection of the head of the pancreas, the duodenum, the antrum of the stomach, the common bile duct, and the gall bladder. Before the standard operation, laparoscopy is usually performed to visually confirm the absence of metastatic disease (which is an absolute contraindication to surgical resection). After the abdomen is opened, it is explored to identify any metastatic deposits. The lateral duodenal peritoneal reflection is opened to allow mobilization of the duodenum as far as the inferior vena cava (IVC) medially, facilitating manual examination of the pancreas and palpation of the SMA. In this way, the surgeon can be certain that the tumor does not extend beyond the uncinate process of the pancreas.

The posterior aspect of the pancreas can be separated by gentle dissection from the IVC and the right kidney. The regional lymph nodes as well as those in the porta hepatis are examined, and any suspicious nodes are biopsied by frozen section. The root of the mesentery of the transverse colon is also examined for tumor extension or nodal metastases. By lifting of the transverse colon, the transverse mesocolon can be examined and the middle colic vessels identified and traced to where they join the superior mesenteric vessels at the inferior margin of the pancreas. The common bile duct is then mobilized and isolated with an umbilical tape. Just distal to the junction of the common bile duct with the cystic duct, the common hepatic duct can be divided, allowing immediate identification of the portal vein. The portal vein is identified, and the right index finger is placed on the anterior surface of the vein and gently advanced inferiorly, creating a plane of dissection between the pancreas and the portal vein. If this maneuver can be performed successfully, then the remainder of the operation can proceed.

The gastroduodenal artery is identified and compressed. It is important, before ligation, to ensure that there is still a pulse in the proper hepatic artery (i.e., that the gastroduodenal artery is not the source of the proper hepatic artery). Once this is confirmed, the gastroduodenal artery is ligated at its origin from the common hepatic artery. The surgeon can then take steps to ensure that no other vascular anomalies (e.g., take-off of the right hepatic artery from the SMA) exist, although this can usually be excluded by the preoperative CT scan. Next, the third portion of the duodenum is freed from its retroperitoneal attachments. The superior mesenteric vein is identified crossing anterior to the third portion of the duodenum. Its anterior surface is gently freed under the neck of the pancreas and is usually found to be free of significant venous branches, except for the origin of the right gastroepiploic vein. This venous structure is almost always present and must be carefully identified, ligated, and divided. The first portion of the duodenum is then mobilized and dissected free from the neck of the pancreas. It is divided with a stapler.

At this point, the neck of the pancreas can be divided with the use of electrocautery. The superior mesenteric and portal veins are then dissected away from the neck and uncinate process of the pancreas. The superior pancreaticoduodenal vein, also known as the vein of Belcher, must be identified, doubly ligated, and divided. In addition, more distally on the superior mesenteric vein and near the inferior border of the uncinate process, the first jejunal branch is a constant landmark. This also has to be ligated and divided. The uncinate process of the pancreas is adjacent to the right border of the SMA, and several arterial branches will need to be ligated and divided during this dissection. The transverse colon is then lifted to allow identification of the suspensory ligament of Treitz. The proximal jejunum is divided distal to this ligament. The mesentery to the proximal jejunum and the third and fourth portions of the duodenum are then divided between clamps, allowing mobilization of the remainder of the specimen.

The proximal jejunum is passed behind the superior mesenteric vessels over to the right side of the abdomen, and the specimen is removed from the operative field. The pancreas is then anastomosed to the jejunum (pancreaticojejunostomy), and, about 3 or 4 cm distal to the pancreaticojejunostomy, the common hepatic duct is anastomosed to the jejunum (hepaticojejunostomy). This is followed by an end-to-side gastrojejunostomy to complete the reconstruction and reestablish intestinal continuity. The abdomen is then closed.

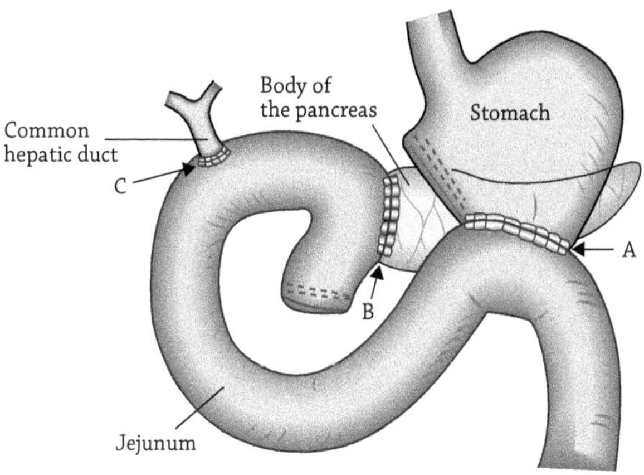

FIGURE 28.2

Schematic diagram of the Whipple procedure, which includes a gastrojejunostomy (A), pancreaticojejunostomy (B), and hepaticojejunostomy (C).

Discussion

Bilirubin, a yellow pigment, is a product of the breakdown of hemoglobin. The liver metabolizes bilirubin and excretes it in the form of bile. The bile passes through the biliary duct system into the duodenum, where it aids in the digestion of fats and is excreted with the feces. The common bile duct passes through the head of the pancreas in its path to the duodenum. In this patient, a tumor in the head of the pancreas resulted in obstruction of the common bile duct, which led to an elevated bilirubin level in the blood and resultant jaundice. Jaundice can result from prehepatic abnormalities (e.g., excessive breakdown of hemoglobin) that overwhelm the liver's ability to metabolize bilirubin; from hepatic abnormalities (e.g., hepatitis) that compromise the liver's ability to metabolize bilirubin; or from posthepatic abnormalities (e.g., obstruction of the bile duct) that compromise the liver's ability to excrete bile. Bile duct obstruction is the cause in this patient. The deficit of bile in the feces accounts for the patient's report of "clay-colored" feces. Alkaline phosphatase is an enzyme that is found in many tissues, and there are particularly high amounts in the liver. Biliary obstruction can cause elevation of the serum alkaline phosphatase levels.

Duodenum and Pancreas

The initial steps of the Whipple procedure involve mobilization of the duodenum and the head of the pancreas. In essence, this reestablishes the embryonic position of these organs. In the adult, almost all of the duodenum and almost all of the pancreas are in a retroperitoneal position (secondary retroperitoneal). Initially, in the embryo, these organs are peritoneal and possess a mesentery. The duodenum, like almost all of the gut tube, is suspended from the dorsal mesentery, which is the pathway through which it receives its blood supply. The pancreas forms in the dorsal mesentery from two evaginations of the duodenum. These evaginations become the pancreatic ducts. Subsequently, the duodenum, along with its mesentery and contained pancreas, fuses with the posterior wall of the abdomen. The visceral peritoneum on the surface of the duodenum, the mesentery of the duodenum, and the parietal peritoneum of the posterior abdominal wall in the region of this fusion are replaced with fascia. This fascia (sometimes referred to as *fusion fascia*) forms the cleavage plane that the surgeon uses to mobilize the duodenum and the head of the pancreas.

When the surgeon opens the lateral peritoneal fold of the duodenum, he or she is beginning to restore the embryonic relationship that existed before the organ fused. The plane of the fusion fascia is entered, and the duodenum is lifted away from the body wall, including the right kidney, which was a retroperitoneal structure in the embryo and remain as such in the adult (primary retroperitoneal). Similarly, the embryonic mesentery with its contained pancreas is also lifted away from the body wall, including the IVC which was also a retroperitoneal structure in the embryo (primary retroperitoneal). The cleavage plane along which this separation is made represents the plane of fusion in the embryo. Because there are no vessels or other structures crossing through the peritoneal cavity in the embryo, there will be no significant structures crossing the plane of fusion fascia, allowing the mobilization of the organs. The vessels and ducts associated with these organs (e.g., portal vein, hepatic artery, common bile duct) are mobilized along with the organs.

Biliary Duct System

The bile excreted by the liver enters biliary canaliculi in the liver that drain into the right and left hepatic ducts. These two ducts merge to form the common hepatic duct. The cystic duct from the gall bladder merges with the common hepatic duct to form the common bile duct. The common bile duct passes behind the first part of the duodenum and through a groove in the head of the pancreas. It then merges with the major pancreatic duct (of Wirsung) to form the hepatopancreatic ampulla (of Vater), which opens into the second part of the duodenum. In the Whipple procedure, the gall bladder, cystic duct, and common bile duct are removed, and the common hepatic duct is anastomosed to the jejunum to provide a pathway for the flow of bile from the liver into the digestive tract.

The Portal Triad

The common bile duct is accompanied by the proper hepatic artery and the portal vein within the edge of the lesser omentum. The common bile duct is to the right of the proper hepatic artery, and the portal vein is posterior to both the duct and the artery. These three structures approach and enter the porta hepatis together. Collectively, these structures are referred to as the portal triad. During the Whipple procedure, the common bile duct must be identified and separated from the proper hepatic artery and the portal vein before the common hepatic duct is divided. The proper hepatic artery is typically one of the two terminal branches of the common hepatic artery; the other terminal branch is the gastroduodenal artery. Recall that the surgeon compressed the gastroduodenal artery while checking for a pulse in the proper hepatic artery. This was done because sometimes the proper hepatic artery has an aberrant origin from the gastroduodenal artery. The portal vein passes behind the neck of the pancreas, where it takes its origin from the union of the superior mesenteric vein and the splenic vein.

Blood Supply to the Pancreas and Duodenum

The pancreas receives its blood supply from several arteries. The body and tail of the pancreas, which are not removed in this procedure, receive their supply from branches of the splenic artery. The head and neck of the pancreas, which are removed, receive their blood supply from two sources, the superior pancreaticoduodenal artery (a branch of the gastroduodenal artery) and the inferior pancreaticoduodenal artery (a branch of the SMA). Both of these arteries send branches into the head of the pancreas, one from above and the other from below. These branches supply the pancreas and also pass through the head of the pancreas to reach the duodenum, which surrounds the head of the pancreas in the shape of the letter C. Because the duodenum receives its blood supply by way of vessels that pass through the head of the pancreas, the duodenum must be removed along with the head of the pancreas. The anastomotic connections between the branches of the superior and inferior pancreaticoduodenal arteries form an important collateral pathway between the celiac trunk and the SMA. By way of this collateral pathway, if there is a partial occlusion of the celiac trunk, all of the organs normally supplied by the celiac trunk can get an adequate blood supply from the SMA, and vice-versa. The ligation of the gastroduodenal artery deprives not only the superior pancreaticoduodenal artery but also the right gastroepiploic artery of its blood flow. (The latter is the other branch of the gastroduodenal artery.) The right gastroepiploic artery provides blood supply to the stomach along its greater curvature. This blood supply is replaced by flow from the left gastroepiploic artery, a branch of the splenic artery. The right and left gastroepiploic arteries anastomose along the greater curvature of the stomach.

Reestablishment of the Digestive Pathway

Because of the removal of the duodenum, it is necessary to establish a new pathway for the passage of food through the digestive tract. The gastrojejunostomy establishes a pathway for food to pass from the stomach to the jejunum. Because the bile from the liver and the pancreatic enzymes essential for digestion enter the digestive tract in the duodenum, it is necessary to establish new pathways for the entry of these substances into the digestive tract. The hepaticojejunostomy provides the pathway for bile from the common hepatic duct to enter the jejunum. The pancreaticojejunostomy provides the pathway for pancreatic enzymes to enter the jejunum.

29

Superior Mesenteric Artery Syndrome

A 28-year-old medical secretary comes to the physician's office complaining of recurrent episodes of nausea and vomiting of bile-stained, partially digested food. In addition, she reports frequent bloating, belching, and epigastric discomfort. These symptoms appear about 1 to 2 hours after meals. She reports no hematemesis. Vomiting typically relieves the symptoms, at least partially, until her next meal. She has had no recent change in bowel habits. She denies a history of heartburn or peptic ulcer disease. She takes no medications or over-the-counter drugs such as aspirin or ibubrofen. Of note, she suffered a marked 25-pound weight loss after hospitalization for injuries suffered in a motor vehicle accident. This weight loss seems to have precipitated her symptoms, which have gradually worsened and she has lost even more weight because of the difficulty she has eating.

On inquiry, she states that since adolescence she has had alternating periods of well-being and abdominal discomfort accompanied by vomiting. Since the recent aggravation of her symptoms, she has felt extremely fatigued and has lost her appetite. She further states that when she has these attacks of pain and vomiting, she can obtain relief by lying on either side or in the knee-to-chest position.

Examination

On physical examination, she is 5 feet 8 inches tall and weighs 115 pounds, placing her body mass index at 17.5 (underweight). Her vital signs are normal. She has a prominent lumbar lordosis. On abdominal examination, her abdomen is scaphoid in appearance. No scars, pulsations, or masses are evident on inspection. The bowel sounds are normoactive; there are no bruits. The abdominal wall is flaccid. There is minimal tenderness to palpation in the epigastrium without guarding. The liver and kidneys can be palpated easily; the liver span is normal as determined by percussion. There are no palpable masses.

Initial flat and upright radiographs of the abdomen reveal a nonspecific bowel gas pattern, and she is referred for additional studies. Radiographic study of the upright patient under the fluoroscope after a radiopaque meal shows rapid emptying of the stomach, excluding pyloric stenosis. The first three portions of the duodenum fill rapidly and are considerably dilated. Under active peristalsis, the duodenum finally empties part of the barium into its fourth portion, but there is marked indentation of the barium filling at the site of transition between the third and fourth portions of the duodenum at the level of the third lumbar vertebra (L3). Radiographic examination 6 hours after the barium meal shows a marked and abnormal residue of barium in the duodenum. Computed tomographic (CT) angiography of the abdomen reveals that the angle between the aorta and the superior mesenteric artery (SMA) is 22 degrees (the normal angle is approximately 45 degrees).

Diagnosis

SMA syndrome with occlusion of the duodenum is diagnosed.

Therapy and Further Course

It is recommended that conservative, nonsurgical therapy be attempted for the purpose of increasing her weight. She is admitted to the hospital, and enteral feeding with a nasojejunal tube is initiated. After her throat is anesthetized with a lidocaine spray, a nasojejunal tube is placed under fluoroscopic observation. Her caloric intake is supplemented with parenteral feeding. After a week of treatment with no appreciable weight gain, a repeat CT angiogram is done, and no change is seen. It is then decided to correct the problem surgically. She is taken to the operating room, and a laparoscopic duodenojejunostomy is performed. Six months later, she has regained her normal weight and feels comfortable. She reports that she no longer suffers from epigastric pain and is able to eat normally.

Discussion

Anatomy of the Duodenum

The duodenum is described as having four parts. The first part begins at the pylorus and extends horizontally to the right at the L1 level. This part of the duodenum begins as a peritoneal structure and becomes retroperitoneal about halfway along its length. All of the remainder of the duodenum is retroperitoneal. The second part of the duodenum, sometimes referred to as the descending portion of the duodenum, takes a vertical course and descends from L1 down to the L3 level. This vertical portion of the duodenum is to the right of the vertebral column. The third portion of the duodenum, sometimes referred to as the inferior horizontal portion, extends horizontally at the L3 level from the right side to the left side of the vertebral column. As it crosses in front of the vertebral column, it also crosses in front of the inferior vena cava and then the abdominal aorta. The fourth part of the duodenum, also referred to as the ascending portion, has a vertical course on the left side of the vertebral column and ascends from the L3 to the L2 level. At that point, it takes a sharp turn, known as the duodenojejunal flexure, and becomes peritoneal again, after which it is called the jejunum. The suspensory ligament of Treitz attaches the duodenojejunal flexure to the posterior abdominal wall at the right crus of the diaphragm. Therefore, the duodenum describes a C shape, and within the concavity of the C is found the head and neck of the pancreas.

As indicated previously, the second portion of the first part of the duodenum and all of the second, third, and fourth parts of the duodenum lie behind the parietal peritoneum. The root of the transverse mesocolon arises from the parietal peritoneum in front of the second part of the duodenum, and the root of the mesentery of the

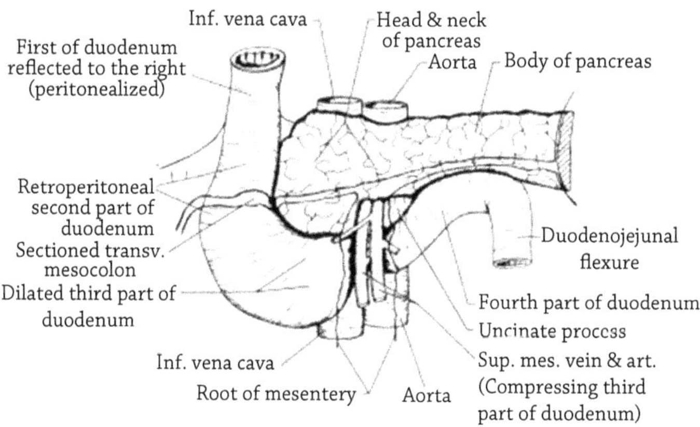

FIGURE 29.1

Front view of the duodenum in a case of superior mesenteric artery (SMA) occlusion of the third portion of the duodenum. Notice the prestenotic dilatation of the duodenum and the compression of its third portion by root of mesentery and superior mesenteric vessels. Observe that the SMA arises from the aorta posterior to the neck of the pancreas but crosses in front of the uncinate process. The crossing of the root of the transverse mesocolon over the second portion of the duodenum and the anterior surface of the pancreas is also shown. Inf., inferior; Sup. mes. vein & art., superior mesenteric vein and artery.

small intestine arises from the parietal peritoneum in front of the third part of the duodenum. (Figs. 29.1 and 29.2).

As stated earlier, the third part of the duodenum is covered anteriorly by the parietal peritoneum except for a small area where the superior mesenteric vessels cross it. It is separated from the vertebral column by the inferior vena cava to the right of the column and the abdominal aorta in front of the column. The transverse mesocolon, with the transverse colon suspended from it, crosses superior to the third part of the duodenum by passing over the second or descending portion. The transverse mesocolon divides the duodenum into supracolic and infracolic portions. The pancreas is likewise located superior to the third part of the duodenum.

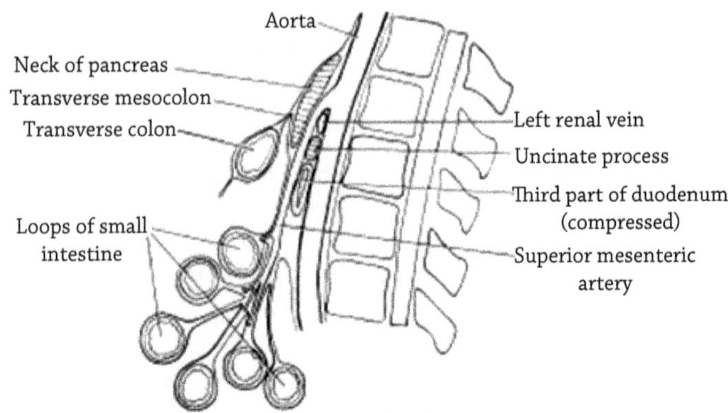

FIGURE 29.2

Midsagittal section shows the superior mesenteric artery stretched over the third portion of the duodenum and the left renal vein by low-lying loops of small intestine in a case of severe weight loss and depletion of mesenteric fat. Notice the compression of the third portion of the duodenum. The normal relationship of the artery as it passes behind the neck but in front of the uncinate process of the pancreas is also shown.

Superior Mesenteric Artery and Vein

The SMA arises from the front of the aorta as the second of the unpaired visceral arteries (the celiac trunk is the first, and the inferior mesenteric artery is the third), usually at the level of the lower portion of the L1 vertebra and therefore superior to the third part of the duodenum. The artery is accompanied by its vein as it passes over the third part of the duodenum to enter the mesentery and supply the small and large intestines from the distal duodenum to the left colic flexure. The superior mesenteric vein drains the same area of intestine and courses to the right of the artery (Figs. 29.1 and 29.2).

The SMA has an interesting relationship to the pancreas. It arises from the aorta behind the neck of the pancreas but then crosses in front of the uncinate process of the pancreas. In its course, the artery is surrounded by the superior mesenteric nerve plexus. Because the artery runs posterior to the neck of the pancreas, it is also posterior to the transverse mesocolon, which arises from the anterior surface of the pancreas. It is worthwhile to keep in mind that, whereas the origin of the SMA is superior to the third portion of the duodenum, the origin of the inferior mesenteric artery is either behind or inferior to this part of the duodenum.

Changing Position of the Duodenum

The duodenum, with the exception of its first portion, is a retroperitoneal structure; its position is therefore less variable than organs having a mesentery. Nevertheless, the duodenum is relatively mobile in vivo. Its location varies with body posture, being lowest in the upright position and highest in the prone position. It also changes with the degree of its filling and the state of contraction of the anterior abdominal wall. It descends with age. Therefore, the level of the L3 vertebra, or the disk inferior to it, represents only an average as a landmark for locating the third portion of the duodenum, with the range extending from L2 to L5.

An understanding of the adult location of the third part of the duodenum in a retroperitoneal and retrovascular position depends on knowledge of the embryological development of the gut tube. During embryonic development, the midgut portion of the gut tube forms an anteriorly convex loop in the midsagittal plane and is suspended from the posterior wall of the abdomen by a mesentery. The tube rapidly increases in length and herniates into the umbilical cord. While it is in the umbilical cord, and during the process of retracting back into the abdominal cavity, the intestinal loop undergoes a counterclockwise rotation of 270 degrees, as viewed from the front, with the SMA acting as the axis of rotation. As the distal part of the intestinal loop turns over the proximal portion, the SMA comes to lie in front of the third part of the duodenum but posterior to the transverse colon. At a later stage, the duodenum, together with certain other portions of the intestinal tract, loses its mesentery by peritoneal fusion and, except for its first portion, becomes fixed to the posterior abdominal wall in a retroperitoneal position.

Pathogenesis of Superior Mesenteric Artery Syndrome

The cardinal point of this discussion is, of course, the pathogenesis (i.e., mode of origin and development) of the clinical entity exemplified by our patient. Whereas normally the superior mesenteric vessels pass gently over the third part of the duodenum, in this case we must visualize the third part of the duodenum as being markedly compressed, as in a vise, between the aorta and the lordotic vertebral column posteriorly and the taut superior mesenteric vessels anteriorly. This may happen if, due to substantial weight loss in a patient with insufficient abdominal muscular support, the intestines drop inferiorly to an unusual degree. Additionally, the loss of mesenteric fat reduces the cushion that this fat provides between the vessels and the duodenum. Therefore, marked traction is exerted on the superior mesenteric vessels at the site of the mesenteric root, which can lead to acute or intermittent chronic obstruction of the duodenum at this level.

Explanation of Symptoms

How do we explain the patient's symptoms in the acute stages of her illness? From her history, we learn that she has had acute periods of illness characterized by nausea, vomiting, belching, and pain in the right upper abdomen since adolescence. This is consistent with intermittent compression of the third part of the duodenum as the cause of the described symptoms. Vomiting temporarily relieves the overloading of the stomach and duodenum proximal to the site of the compression. The recent aggravation of all symptoms was caused by the severe loss of weight and increased flaccidity of her abdominal musculature. The weight loss resulted in diminution of the fat cushion in the mesenteric root which had protected the duodenum from complete and lasting compression. The accompanying loss of fat in the pelvis and retroperitoneal structures and the weakening of the abdominal musculature led to further sagging of the intestines into the pelvis and an increase of drag on the vessels. This further decreased the acute angle between the aorta and the SMA, a process that has been compared with the action of a nutcracker clamping down on the third part of the duodenum. The patient reports that the pain and discomfort occur after meals (postprandial), when the stomach empties its contents into the duodenum. The pain is relieved by assuming the decubitus or knee-to-chest position, because this position allows gravity to pull the intestinal mesentery, with its contained superior mesenteric vessels, away from the aorta, thereby relieving the compression of the duodenum.

Contributing Developmental Abnormalities

Certain developmental events can contribute to SMA syndrome. A mobile cecum and an ascending colon suspended by a mesocolon, which result from failure of this mesentery to fuse to the posterior wall, will exert traction on their supply arteries, which are branches of the SMA, thus increasing the pull on this artery and the degree of compression of the duodenum. Occasionally, a rigid, arteriosclerotic SMA is thought to be a contributing factor.

Duodenal Arterial Supply from the Superior Mesenteric Artery

As already stated, the SMA contributes to the blood supply of the duodenum. At the level of the pancreatic notch, the SMA gives off the inferior pancreaticoduodenal artery, which then divides into two branches, the anterior and posterior inferior pancreaticoduodenal arteries. These form arcades between the pancreas and the descending part of the duodenum by communicating with the superior pancreaticoduodenal artery, a branch of the gastroduodenal artery. They thus establish an important anastomosis between the celiac artery and the SMA. The branches that supply the duodenum pass through the head of the pancreas to reach the duodenum.

Left Renal Vein Exposed to Compression

Another important blood vessel located in the angle between the aorta and the SMA that may likewise be compressed by the downward traction of the superior mesenteric vessels is the left renal vein. As this vein passes from the left kidney toward the inferior vena cava, it crosses the aorta deep to the origin of the SMA above the third part of the duodenum. It has been asserted that increased acuteness in the previously mentioned angle may cause compression of this renal vein and circulatory changes in the left kidney, sometimes resulting in albuminuria (Fig. 29.2). This may also explain the increased frequency of varicocele of the left testicle, because the left testicular vein drains into the left renal vein proximal to the site of compression, whereas the right testicular vein is a direct tributary of the inferior vena cava.

Rationale for Therapeutic Course

Initially, a nonsurgical approach was taken to attempt to relieve the problem. It was hoped that if the patient gained weight, the deposition of fat into the region of the root of the mesentery might provide sufficient cushion to relieve the compression of the duodenum. Because the compression of the duodenum precludes consumption of a sufficient volume of food to provide the calories necessary for this weight gain, a nasojejunal tube was inserted to bypass the duodenum and allow the food to be introduced directly into the jejunum. This was supplemented with additional calories through parenteral feeding. When this approach did not yield results, the problem was corrected surgically by a laparoscopic procedure performed to anastomose the proximal portion of the duodenum to the jejunum (duodenojejunostomy), thus permanently bypassing the obstructed third portion of the duodenum. This allowed the patient to eat normally and the stomach to empty normally after meals.

30

Omphalocele

A 34-year-old woman is pregnant with her third child. Her two previous pregnancies were normal, and she had vaginal deliveries at term. Her 7-year-old son and 3-year-old daughter are both in good health, developing normally, and meeting all developmental milestones. The patient's prenatal visits with her obstetrician were uneventful, and an ultrasound that was done at 10 weeks of gestation appeared normal.

Examination

Blood tests that were taken at 18 weeks of gestation revealed an elevated serum α-fetoprotein level. This finding prompted a level II ultrasound examination, which was performed at 19 weeks of gestation. This study revealed a fetal abdominal wall defect with abdominal viscera protruding out of the abdomen. Ultrasound imaging of the heart, kidneys, respiratory tract, and gastrointestinal tract did not reveal any additional defects. Ultrasound monitoring of the fetus was scheduled at regular intervals for the duration of the pregnancy.

Diagnosis

The diagnosis is fetal ventral body wall defect, possibly omphalocele or gastroschisis.

Therapy and Further Course

It is explained to the mother that her fetus has a defect in the abdominal wall. It is not yet certain whether it is omphalocele or gastroschisis. It is explained that often gastroschisis occurs as an isolated defect, but there is a high correlation between omphalocele and other defects, particularly of the heart. Although the level II ultrasound study did not reveal any apparent cardiac, renal, or other gastrointestinal defects, the possibility nonetheless continues to exist. There is also the risk that a chromosomal abnormality, most commonly trisomy 13, 18, or 21, might exist, and therefore an amniocentesis is recommended. The obstetrician explains to the mother that it may be necessary to deliver the baby by cesarean section, but there is also a good possibility that a vaginal delivery will be possible. This will depend on the size of the defect that is evident as the pregnancy progresses.

An amniocentesis is performed for karyotyping, and no chromosomal abnormalities are found. In successive ultrasound images, it becomes apparent that the fetus has a small omphalocele, because intestine is seen in the base of the umbilical cord. With gastroschisis, the typical finding would be detection of intestinal loops floating freely in the amniotic fluid. Ultrasound imaging is continued through the remainder of the pregnancy to determine whether the omphalocele will reduce spontaneously. As the mother approaches term, the small omphalocele is still present. It is determined that a vaginal delivery would be safe. Because outcomes of infants with omphalocele are better after vaginal delivery than after cesarean delivery, it is decided to allow an attempt at vaginal delivery.

One week before the mother's due date, she is admitted to a hospital that has a neonatal intensive care unit (NICU) and a pediatric surgeon on staff. Labor is induced, and the baby is delivered vaginally without difficulty. The omphalocele has an intact membrane surrounding it, and care is taken to not disrupt the membrane. The omphalocele is seen to contain loops of small intestine, but no other organs are seen within it (Fig. 30.1). The omphalocele is covered with sterile gauze and kept moist with warm sterile saline. A complete examination of the newborn reveals no murmurs or other evidence of cardiac defects, respiratory defects, renal defects, neural tube defects, or other gastrointestinal defects. A nasogastric tube is inserted to decompress the stomach and provide additional space within the abdomen.

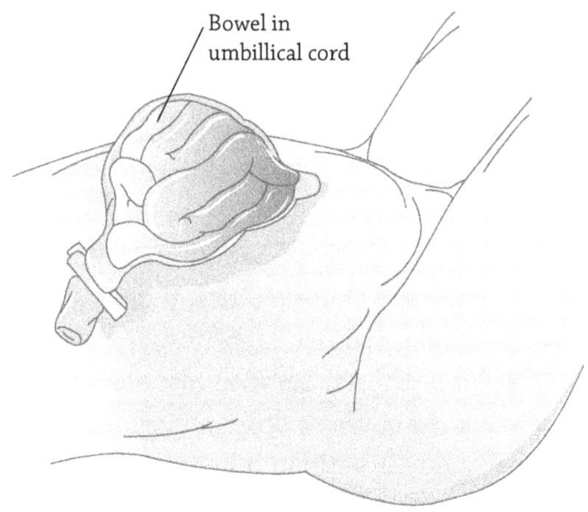

FIGURE 30.1

Newborn with omphalocele. Notice the loops of intestine within the umbilical cord.

The next day, the baby is prepared for surgery. An endotracheal tube is placed to provide respiratory assistance, because the increased abdominal content (and, consequently, increased pressures) after reduction of the omphalocele may interfere with diaphragmatic action. A primary repair of the abdominal defect is performed. The remnants of the umbilical arteries and umbilical vein distal to the omphalocele are identified and ligated. The content of the omphalocele is gently moved into the abdomen. Care is taken to ensure that the space within the abdomen is sufficient to contain the viscera without compression of the blood supply. The musculature, fascia, and skin of the abdominal wall are closed.

Postoperatively, the baby is taken to the NICU. Blood oxygen levels are monitored, and over the course of the next 2 days, the baby is weaned from the respirator. Feedings are begun, and the abdomen is monitored for normal bowel sounds, which are present. After 24 hours, bowel movements are seen. Two weeks after surgery, the infant is released to home with instructions to the parents for care of the surgical wound.

Discussion

Omphalocele is reported to occur in approximately 1 of every 4000 live births. There is a high occurrence of chromosomal abnormalities (about 30%) in babies with omphalocele. These abnormalities are frequently trisomies in chromosomes 13, 18, or 21 or Beckwith-Wiedemann syndrome. Survival rates for these babies are quite poor. Even in those without chromosomal abnormalities, there is a high incidence of other congenital abnormalities (approximately 50%), including cardiac, renal, and limb defects. Survival rates for these infants are also poor, usually related to these other abnormalities. The baby in this case has an omphalocele without other associated abnormalities. Survival rates for such infants is very high (approximately 97%), and their prognosis for a normal life is excellent.

Omphalocele Versus Gastroschisis

Omphalocele is a ventral body wall defect at the umbilical ring in which abdominal viscera are found within the umbilical cord. The viscera are covered by parietal peritoneum as well as the amniotic membrane that covers the umbilical cord. Therefore, the viscera are not free within the amniotic cavity and not in contact with the amniotic fluid. Sometimes, the membranes covering the omphalocele rupture, either in utero or during delivery. In such cases, the exposed viscera are subject to damage from the amniotic fluid and desiccation after birth. The risk for infection in these babies is increased. The viscera found within the omphalocele are quite variable. In small omphaloceles, such as in this case, only portions of the small intestine are in the defect. In large omphaloceles (often referred to as giant omphaloceles), liver, stomach, and other organs, in addition to small intestine, may be found in the umbilical cord. The more abdominal viscera found in the omphalocele, the less fully developed the abdominal cavity is, and the more complicated the reduction of the omphalocele becomes (see later discussion). Survival rates for babies with giant omphaloceles are lower than for those with small omphaloceles.

Gastroschisis is a ventral body wall defect located outside the umbilical ring, usually to the right of the umbilicus. In these defects, the extra-abdominal viscera are covered by neither parietal peritoneum nor amniotic membrane. The organs are free in the amniotic cavity and are bathed in amniotic fluid. The inflammation of the bowel associated with their contact with amniotic fluid typically leads to a period of delayed and impaired function of the digestive system after reduction of the gastroschisis. These babies also are confronted with risks of dehydration, hypothermia, and infection. Nonetheless, because there is a much lower incidence of chromosomal syndromes and coexisting congenital defects of other organ systems, the overall mortality rate for babies with gastroschisis is much lower than for those with omphalocele. Omphalocele and gastroschisis are compared in Table 30.1.

Normal Development of the Midgut

The midgut is the portion of the embryonic gut tube that receives its blood supply from the superior mesenteric artery. The midgut

TABLE 30.1 Comparison of Omphalocele and Gastroschisis

	Omphalocele	*Gastroschisis*
Location of abdominal wall defect	At umbilical ring	Outside umbilical ring (most often to the right)
Location of viscera	Within the umbilical cord	Outside the umbilical cord (free within the amniotic cavity)
Contact with amniotic fluid	Not in contact with amniotic fluid	In contact with amniotic fluid with resulting inflammation
Associated defects	Commonly has associated chromosomal defects and other congenital defects	Usually does not have associated defects

develops into most of the duodenum, the jejunum and ileum, the cecum and appendix, the ascending colon, and most of the transverse colon. During the sixth week of embryonic development, the midgut starts to lengthen appreciably. At this stage of development, the abdominal cavity is still quite small, and much of the space within it is occupied by the liver and kidneys. Because there is inadequate space within the abdominal cavity to accommodate the enlarging midgut, the midgut begins to expand into the umbilical cord in the form of a loop of intestine. This intestinal loop takes the superior mesenteric artery with it into the umbilical cord. The artery passes down the center of the loop formed by the midgut and provides arterial branches to the intestinal loop.

While the intestinal loop is in the umbilical cord, it begins to rotate around the axis formed by the superior mesenteric artery. This rotation is in a counterclockwise direction if viewed from the ventral side. The intestinal loop remains in the umbilical cord during weeks 6 to 11 of development. Usually, in week 11, the loop begins to retract from the umbilical cord and return into the abdomen, which is now large enough to accommodate it. During this retraction, the counterclockwise rotation continues, so that by the time the loop has fully retracted (week 12), it has undergone a 270-degree rotation. This rotation is what dictates the adult locations of the colon and small intestine. If the intestinal loop fails to fully retract from the umbilical cord, the baby will be born with intestine in the umbilical cord (small omphalocele). It appears that this is what occurred in our patient. The persistence of the intestinal loop in the umbilical cord can interfere with the normal development of the ventral body wall, resulting in an abnormally large umbilical ring. This can allow other organs (e.g., stomach, liver) to migrate into the umbilical cord, resulting in a giant omphalocele.

Reduction of Omphalocele

Because in babies with omphalocele the abdominal viscera are not in the abdominal cavity during most of development, the size of the abdominal cavity is smaller than normal. Depending on how small the abdominal cavity is and how much visceral volume needs to be reduced, the reduction procedure may need to be modified. The two major concerns are that if the blood supply to the viscera is squeezed, visceral ischemia or necrosis may result, and if the diaphragm's ability to descend is compromised, the baby's respiration will be compromised. In this case, the omphalocele was small and the space in the abdomen was adequate to accommodate the viscera. Nonetheless, the baby was kept on a respirator postoperatively to assist with respiration if diaphragmatic excursion became compromised.

If the omphalocele is too large to be brought into the abdomen without compression, a primary closure cannot be done, and the reduction must be done in stages. A silo is constructed from Dacron-reinforced Silastic sheeting. The silo is sutured to the rectus abdominis fascia on each side of the omphalocele and completely encloses the omphalocele. Then, over a period of days or weeks, the silo is reduced in size, gradually returning the viscera to the abdominal cavity. This allows time for growth of the abdominal wall, which gradually increases the volume of the abdominal cavity, thus allowing the viscera to be accommodated. The baby is maintained on respiratory support throughout this procedure. Once all of the viscera have been reduced into the abdomen, the abdominal wall defect is closed surgically.

Gastroschisis

Gastroschisis has a lower incidence than omphalocele, with estimates ranging from 1 in 5000 to 1 in 8000 live births. Gastroschisis is typically not accompanied by chromosomal defects nor by other congenital defects. This fact accounts for the higher survival rate among babies with gastroschisis even though the damage to the intestine may be greater in gastroschisis due to the inflammatory effect of amniotic fluid. Typically, the rupture of the body wall that allows the escape of abdominal viscera occurs late in development. Because the abdomen has housed the viscera during most of gestation, the abdominal cavity is usually larger in babies with gastroschisis than in those with omphalocele, making the reduction of the viscera an easier process.

The underlying cause of gastroschisis is not well understood. Some theories attribute it to defective fusion of the lateral body folds during the fourth week of development; the resulting abnormalities in mesoderm formation in this region lead to a weakness of the abdominal wall. Other theories attribute it to abnormal regression of embryonic blood vessels in the region of the wall where the defect appears. Some have suggested that the regression of the right umbilical vein is responsible, whereas others have attributed it to regression of the right vitelline artery. There is no good evidence to support any of the extant theories, and the cause of gastroschisis remains elusive.

α-Fetoprotein Screening

α-Fetoprotein is a glycoprotein that is normally produced in the fetal liver. It is the major serum protein during the first trimester and is analogous to albumin. Its concentration increases steadily in fetal serum until about week 13, after which levels rapidly decrease. α-Fetoprotein is found in steadily increasing quantities in maternal serum after 12 weeks. An assay of maternal serum α-fetoprotein levels is done at about week 16 to week 18 as a screening test. Fetal body wall defects that are not covered by integument permit the leakage of α-fetoprotein into the amniotic fluid and thence into maternal serum, resulting in dramatically increased levels in maternal serum. Such defects include neural tube defects such as spina bifida and anencephaly and ventral body wall defects such as omphalocele and gastroschisis. It was this screening test that raised the suspicion of a possible fetal defect in our patient and led to the ultrasound imaging that revealed the defect.

31

Appendicitis

A 22-year-old male university student and collegiate athlete in excellent health presents to the college infirmary with a 24-hour history of abdominal pain. He states that he awoke the previous night with a severe attack of "indigestion," which he described as a dull, crampy pain around the umbilicus. He felt mildly nauseated but did not vomit. In the morning, he felt hot and uncomfortable and decided to stay in bed. He had no appetite, and the nausea persisted. By evening, the pain had moved to the right lower quadrant of his abdomen. He reports that the pain is now sharp and constant. It has increased in severity from 4 to 9 on a scale of 10, with 10 being the worst level of pain. The pain increases with movement and is relieved somewhat when he is still. He reports that he has never had a pain like this before, and this fact prompted his trip to the infirmary. He has not eaten, and his last bowel movement, which was normal, was 2 days earlier. He denies dysuria, urgency, or frequency. The infirmary makes the decision to transfer him to the hospital.

Examination

The patient is examined, and his vital signs are taken. His heart rate is 90 bpm and regular, and his blood pressure is 110/70 mm Hg. He has a slightly increased temperature of 99.6° F. He appears mildly uncomfortable, and his skin is warm and dry. The patient lies on his back with his right thigh flexed. He now localizes his pain in the right lower quadrant of the abdomen. On inspection, his abdomen is mildly distended. There are no visible scars or hernias. His bowel sounds are hypoactive. He has percussion tenderness in the left lower quadrant that is referred to the right, in addition to direct percussion tenderness on the right. On palpation of the abdomen, marked localized

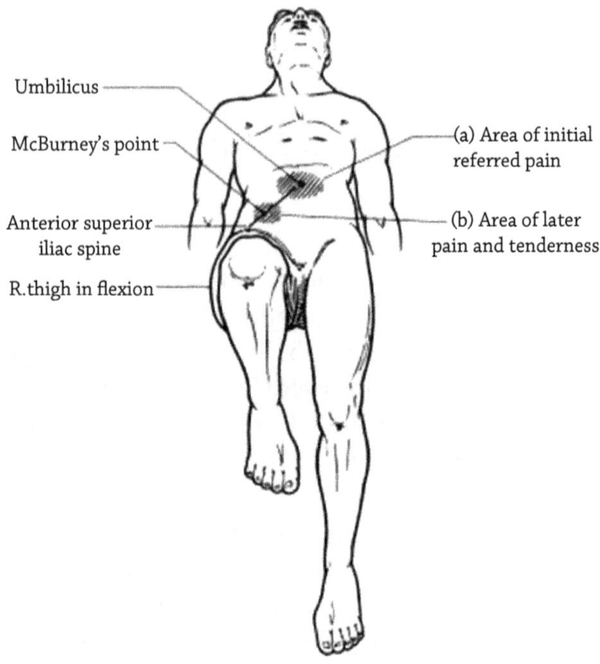

FIGURE 31.1

The two areas of pain in a patient with appendicitis: (a) initial referred pain in the umbilical and paraumbilical region; (b) later pain in the right lower quadrant caused by irritation of the parietal peritoneum. McBurney's point is at the site of greatest tenderness. The right thigh is flexed to relieve tension. R., right.

tenderness and some rigidity in the right iliac fossa are noted. Pressure with the fingertip shows that the area of greatest tenderness is located near McBurney's point (Fig. 31.1). Rectal examination reveals a definite difference in sensitivity on palpation of the right and left sides of the rectovesical pouch; the right side is distinctly more tender.

Diagnosis

The typical history of acute onset of abdominal pain with loss of appetite, nausea, and constipation and the migration of pain from the umbilical region to the right lower quadrant make the diagnosis of acute appendicitis most likely. This diagnosis is supported by the localized peritoneal findings elicited on the abdominal examination, including the percussion tenderness and localized, involuntary rigidity (guarding). The rectal examination also supports the diagnosis.

Therapy and Further Course

In view of the diagnosis of acute appendicitis, and to forestall complications such as perforation and peritonitis, surgery is advised and performed. A right lower muscle-splitting (McBurney) incision through the abdominal wall is chosen to obtain access to the appendix. In this incision, the external and internal abdominal oblique muscles and the transversus abdominis muscle, along with their aponeuroses, are split in the direction of their fibers. Next, the transversalis fascia, the extraperitoneal fat, and the parietal peritoneum are incised, and the appendix is visualized. In this case, the appendix is found to be greatly inflamed and distended, and its visceral peritoneal covering is quite red. The appendix crosses the psoas major muscle and reaches into the true pelvis with its tip hanging over the pelvic brim. It is raised and manipulated into view.

The mesoappendix, or mesentery of the appendix, is clamped and divided, and the appendicular vessels and their branches are ligated. Next, the base (root) of the appendix is clamped, crushed, and ligated, and the appendix is amputated distal to the ligature. The stump of the appendix is cauterized. The peritoneum and the other components of the abdominal wall are closed in layers.

With administration of intravenous fluids and antibiotics, the patient progresses satisfactorily and is discharged from the hospital 2 days after operation.

Discussion

The cause of acute appendicitis is not known but probably is multifactorial. Factors thought to contribute to the pathogenesis include luminal obstruction, dietary factors, and familial factors. Infection and inflammation develop in the distended portion and may lead to death of tissue, perforation, and abscess formation.

Anatomy of Pain Transmission in Appendicitis

The changing pattern of pain in this case—shifting from the region of the umbilicus to the right lower quadrant—illustrates the difference between visceral and somatic pain. The initial pain in the umbilical region originates in visceral sensory fibers in the wall of the inflamed appendix. These sensory impulses from the appendix travel in visceral sensory nerve fibers, which are closely intermingled with sympathetic efferent fibers. They travel from the organ, through the superior mesenteric plexus and ganglion, to reach the thoracic splanchnic nerves. These provide entry into the sympathetic chain ganglia, and from there the impulses reach the spinal nerves via white rami communicantes. From the spinal nerves, they enter the dorsal roots to reach the spinal cord. The cell bodies of the visceral sensory nerve fibers are located in the dorsal root ganglia. The pain arising in the appendiceal wall is referred to areas of the body surface that send sensory impulses to the same segments of the cord that receive pain impulses from the appendix; namely, the ninth through twelfth thoracic nerves. The tenth thoracic spinal cord segment supplies the area around the umbilicus, with overlap from the ninth and eleventh segments. Therefore, the visceral pain arising from the appendix is perceived to arise from the abdominal wall in the periumbilical region, which corresponds to dermatomes T9 to T11. Because these nerve fibers reach the spinal cord through both right and left spinal nerves, the pain is perceived in the midline.

The later pain in the right lower quadrant is caused by contact of the inflamed appendix with the overlying abdominal wall, which results in stimulation of somatic sensory fibers supplying the parietal peritoneum. The eleventh intercostal nerve (T11), the subcostal nerve (T12), and the first lumbar nerve (iliolumbar and ilioinguinal) carry somatic sensory (pain) fibers from this area. Because only the right spinal nerves at these levels are carrying these impulses, the pain is perceived on the right side. It is important to note that if the appendix is in an alternative position, it will contact the abdominal wall in a different location, and the somatic pain will be perceived in that location. Tenderness on palpation and involuntary muscle contraction, which expresses itself as rigidity of the right lateral abdominal wall, are likewise the result of irritation of the parietal peritoneum.

McBurney's Point

McBurney's point is classically defined as a point located two-thirds of the way along a line drawn from the umbilicus to the anterior superior iliac spine (Fig. 31.1). As originally conceived by McBurney, this point is supposed to correspond to the site of origin of the appendix, but variability in the position of the umbilicus, in the degree of descent of the cecum, and in the location of the origin of the appendix makes this point a somewhat questionable landmark.

Positive Psoas Test and Rectal Findings

This patient exhibits a preference for flexion of the right thigh. This is related to the fact that the appendix and the right psoas major muscle are in close relationship. The psoas major muscle is the major flexor of the thigh at the hip. The patient prefers flexion of the thigh to relieve tension on the inflamed area (Fig. 31.1). The opposite movement, hyperextension of the thigh, puts the psoas muscle and its inflamed fascia on stretch; this movement is painful and is resisted by the patient (psoas test in appendicitis).

On rectal examination, the difference in sensitivity to palpation between the right and left sides is a result of inflammation of the peritoneum in the rectovesicle pouch in the region of the appendix. The rectovesicle pouch in the male is the recess of the peritoneal cavity between the rectum and the bladder. It is the most inferior extent of the peritoneal cavity in the male. The increased tenderness on the right side of this pouch is caused by irritation or inflammation of the parietal peritoneum in this area when the appendix reaches this region.

Anatomy of the Right Lower Abdominal Muscle-Splitting Incision

The approach to the appendix in this case was a right lower abdominal muscle-splitting incision through the abdominal wall. The fibers of the external abdominal oblique muscle run from lateral above to medial below ("as if you put your hand in your front pocket"). In the inguinal region, the muscle fibers of both the internal abdominal oblique and the transversus abdominis muscles typically run transversely. At higher levels of the abdominal wall, fibers of the internal oblique muscle run at right angles to the external oblique fibers (i.e., from medial above to lateral below). The iliohypogastric and ilioinguinal nerves lie deep to the internal oblique muscle and may be damaged by this incision.

In a female patient, disease of the female internal genitalia (e.g., infection of the uterine tube or other parts of the female adnexa) must be considered as the possible source of signs and symptoms very similar to those of appendicitis, and these cannot be ruled out by physical examination. If disease of the female pelvic organs is a diagnostic possibility, the McBurney incision should not be done, because it is a small incision that cannot be extended sufficiently to give adequate surgical exposure of the female pelvic organs. Surgical exploration of these organs usually requires a longer incision, such as that allowed by a midline incision.

Laparoscopic appendectomy is an alternative procedure that is being used with increasing frequency and could have been used in this patient. In this procedure, several small incisions are made in the abdominal wall to allow insertion of a camera and surgical instruments. The appendix can be removed with these instruments. This procedure avoids the need for a larger surgical incision and therefore results in less postoperative pain, reduced incidence of wound infection, shorter hospital stay, and more rapid return to work. That being said, studies have demonstrated a higher incidence of intra-abdominal infections with laparoscopic appendectomy.

Location of Appendix and Its Blood Supply

The arrangement of the longitudinal musculature of the cecum assists in locating the origin of the appendix (Fig. 31.2). The three tenia coli converge at the root of the appendix and blend together to form a continuous outer longitudinal layer of muscle on the appendix. Following any of the three tenia along the cecum will lead to the root of the appendix. The anterior tenia coli is the best guide to this point. In our case, the position of the appendix facilitated its removal. A retrocecal position of the appendix is fairly common and could make the operation more difficult.

The appendicular artery and vein and their branches and tributaries are enclosed in the mesentery of the appendix (mesoappendix) and must be identified and ligated before the appendix is removed. The appendicular artery usually is a branch of the ileocolic artery from the superior mesenteric artery and passes posterior to the terminal portion of the ileum before entering the mesentery of the appendix. The appendicular artery and its branches

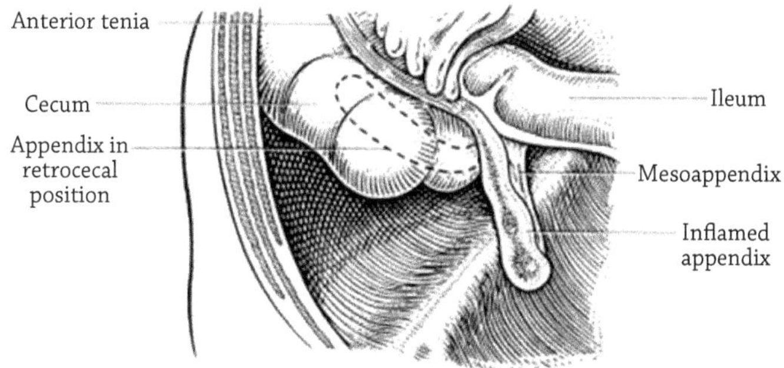

FIGURE 31.2

The diagram shows an appendix vermiformis that is inflamed and distended in its distal portion with its tip hanging over the pelvic brim. Notice how the anterior tenia acts as a guide to the origin of the appendix. Notice also how a retrocecal appendix might be difficult to approach surgically.

are end arteries (i.e., arteries that do not anastomose with other arteries). Therefore, if it or one of its branches is blocked by pressure from a fecal stone or by thrombosis, local necrosis occurs, leading to abscess formation, perforation, and, at worst, generalized peritonitis and death.

32

Ureteral Stone with Hydronephrosis

A 58-year-old male school teacher awoke from his sleep with the sudden onset of abdominal pain. He believed that he had a severe upset stomach with cramping, and he tried to have a bowel movement. The pain was waxing and waning; it was primarily located on his right side in the flank region, and it radiated around to the right anterolateral abdomen. Unable to have a bowel movement, he returned to bed, hoping that the pain would subside. He was unable to get comfortable and was continually changing his position. The pain became constant and increased in intensity. He asked his wife to call for an ambulance, and he was transported to the emergency department of his local hospital. On arrival at the hospital, he reports the pain is "11" on a scale of 1 to 10, with 10 being the worst. He says that it is the worst pain that he has ever experienced. He reports that the pain is now primarily in his right lower quadrant, in the right groin, and radiating into his right testicle. Although he has not vomited, he feels nauseated. The remainder of his medical history is noncontributory. He is taking no medications and has no allergies.

Examination

The patient is a well-nourished, apparently healthy adult man who is in severe pain. His temperature is 98.3° F, his pulse is 92 bpm, his respiratory rate is 22 breaths/min, and his blood pressure is 144/88 mm Hg. His abdomen is soft with mild tenderness in the right lower quadrant with no guarding or other peritoneal signs. There is right costovertebral angle tenderness. There are no palpable masses, and a normal abdominal aortic pulse is palpable. A urine sample is taken for analysis and is positive for occult blood. Microscopic examination of his urine reveals 50 to 75 red blood cells and 5 to 10 white blood cells per high-power field. Intravenous access is established, and morphine is given to control the patient's pain. An antiemetic is administered to relieve his nausea. A complete blood count (CBC) and blood chemistry values are all within normal limits.

Diagnosis

The presumptive diagnosis is ureteral obstruction.

Therapy and Further Course

The patient is taken to the radiology department for a plain kidney, ureter, and bladder (KUB) study and for a noncontrast, spiral computed tomography (CT) scan of the abdomen and pelvis. A calcified stone is identified in the right ureter at the ureterovesical junction, and mild hydronephrosis (enlargement of the renal pelvis and calyces) of the right kidney is noted (Fig. 32.1).

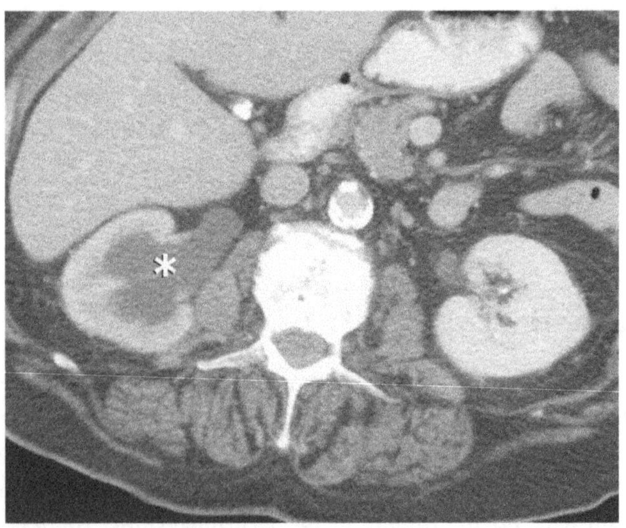

FIGURE 32.1

Magnetic resonance image shows dilated renal pelvis and calyces in the right kidney (*asterisk*).

The patient reports that with the morphine, his pain has completely abated. He is started on oxycodone and acetaminophen and given a prescription for these medications as well as a nonsteroidal antiinflammatory agent. He is released to home, accompanied by his wife, and referred to his urologist for outpatient follow-up care.

He is seen by his urologist the next day. It is decided that he will be given a few days to try to pass the stone. If he is not successful at doing this, then the stone will be retrieved through a ureteroscope. He is instructed to strain his urine, to inspect the strainer for a stone after each urination, and to retain the stone. He is instructed to increase his fluid intake and to remain very hydrated.

On the second day, he recovers a small stone from the strainer. The urologist sends the stone for analysis and determines that it is composed of 80% calcium oxalate and 20% calcium phosphate. The patient is advised that because he has had a kidney stone, there is a 50% probability that he will have another one. He is advised to increase his water intake and to try to achieve a daily urine output of 2 to 2.5 L.

Discussion

Nephrolithiasis is the formation of calculi (stones) in the kidney. In this patient, nephrolithiasis became symptomatic as a ureteral stone, which is the most common presentation. Ureteral stones originate in the kidney and then move into the ureter, although they may increase in size while in the ureter. Renal calculi become symptomatic when they obstruct the flow of urine, in either the kidney or the ureter. The obstruction to the flow of urine results in back pressure, which can cause hydronephrosis (enlargement of the renal pelvis and calyces) (Fig. 32.2; see Fig. 32.1). Long-term hydronephrosis can lead to impairment of kidney function. This patient had a stone composed of calcium salts, as is seen in about 70% to 75% of cases. Other stones may be composed of uric acid (15–20%); struvite (ammonium magnesium phosphate, 5–15%), typically secondary to infection; or cystine (1–2%).

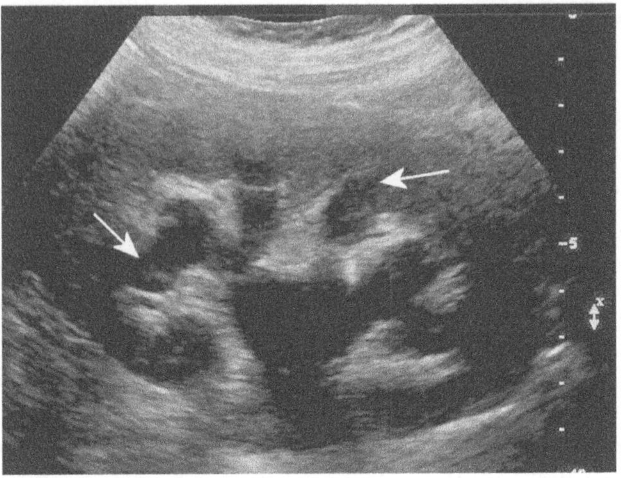

FIGURE 32.2

Ultrasound image of kidney shows dilated renal pelvis and calyces (*arrows*).

Anatomy of the Kidney

Urine is produced in the nephrons, which are located primarily in the cortex of the kidney. The urine that emerges from the nephron passes into a collecting tubule. The pyramids of the kidney are composed of collecting tubules, and at the apex of the pyramid, the collecting tubules open into a minor calyx. The minor calyces coalesce into approximately three major calyces, and the major calyces drain into the renal pelvis. The renal pelvis leaves the kidney at the hilum and continues as the ureter.

Anatomy of the Ureter

As the ureter leaves the kidney, it lies on the anterior surface of the psoas major muscle. It descends through the abdomen, in the retroperitoneal space immediately behind the parietal peritoneum, on the anterior surface of this muscle. Immediately anterior to the bifurcation of the common iliac artery, the ureter crosses over the pelvic brim to enter the pelvis. The ureter then crosses the most proximal portion of the external iliac artery and continues down the posterolateral pelvic wall, crossing anteriorly to reach the bladder. The ureter passes through the bladder wall in an oblique path such that when the bladder wall muscle (detrusor muscle) contracts during micturition, it compresses the ureter to prevent retrograde flow of urine from the bladder into the ureter (vesicoureteral reflux). The ureter has a thick muscular wall (smooth muscle) which contracts in a peristaltic manner to conduct urine toward the bladder.

The ureter has three distinct points of narrowing where ureteral stones are most likely to become impacted (Fig. 32.3). The first is at the ureteropelvic junction, where the renal pelvis transitions to

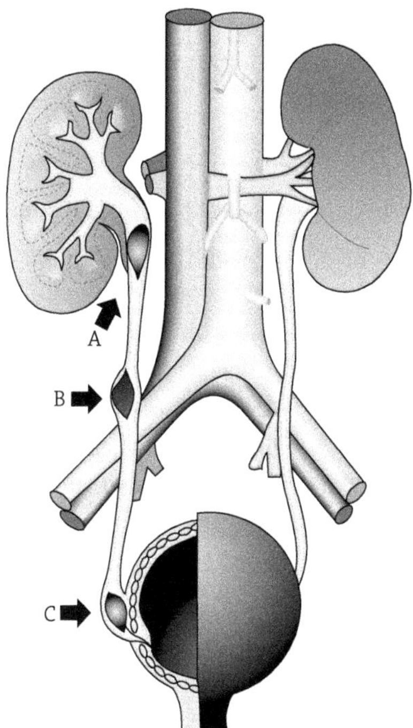

FIGURE 32.3

Diagram shows the three most common sites for impaction of a ureteral stone: the ureteropelvic junction (A), crossing the bifurcation of the common iliac artery (B), and the ureterovesical junction (C).

ureter. The second is where the ureter crosses the pelvic brim at the common iliac artery bifurcation. The third is at the ureterovesical junction, where the ureter passes through the bladder wall. Each point of narrowing is somewhat smaller than the one above. Therefore, if a stone is able to get past the first narrowing, it still may become impacted at the second, and if it is small enough to get past the second point, it still may get impacted at the third. Because the diameter of the ureter is smallest at the ureterovesical junction, it is the most common site for impaction of ureteral stones, as was the case in this patient. If the stone is able to pass the ureterovesical junction and enter the bladder, it will be able to exit the bladder through the urethra, which is much larger than the ureter. The obstruction of the ureter by a stone results in strong, painful contraction of the ureteric smooth muscle (ureteric colic).

Blood Supply of the Ureter

The ureter receives its blood supply from several different sources. The superior portion of the ureter is supplied by branches of the renal artery. More inferiorly, the blood supply comes from branches of the gonadal artery, the abdominal aorta, the common iliac artery, and branches of the internal iliac artery. Because of these multiple sources, it is not possible to retain the blood supply for the entire ureter when doing a kidney transplantation. Therefore, only the upper portion of the ureter is transplanted, along with its blood supply from the renal artery; the kidney is transplanted into the recipient's iliac fossa, close to the bladder so that there is no need for the entire length of the ureter.

Innervation of the Ureter

The ureter receives parasympathetic innervation from the vagus nerve and from sacral parasympathetics (pelvic splanchnic nerves). It receives sympathetic innervation by way of preganglionic fibers in the lesser splanchnic nerve (T10 and T11), the least splanchnic nerve (T12), and the lumbar splanchnic nerves (L1 and L2). Sensory innervation of the ureter parallels the sympathetic innervation and therefore enters the spinal cord at segmental levels T10 to L2. The higher levels innervate the more superior part of the ureter, and the lower levels innervate the more inferior part of the ureter. Pain arising from the ureter is referred to the corresponding dermatomes, thus accounting for the "loin to groin" progression of pain in our patient as the ureteric stone passed through the ureter. Typically, pain caused by a ureteral stone is severe (11 out of 10). However, because the origin of the pain is visceral rather than parietal, peritoneal findings (e.g., guarding) are absent. Also, the patient will move frequently to find a comfortable position, in contrast to a patient with peritonitis, who will remain still.

Treatments

This patient had a fairly small stone which was able to pass spontaneously into the bladder. When a patient has a larger stone that will not pass spontaneously, it may be possible to break the stone into smaller pieces with the use of high-energy sound waves directed at the stone within the ureter or kidney. This procedure is called *extracorporeal shock wave lithotripsy*. Other methods for removing impacted calculi include the use of a ureteroscope, which is passed into the ureter through the bladder. If the stone is in the kidney, percutaneous nephrolithotomy may be used. A puncture wound is made in the posterior abdominal wall, and a nephroscope is passed into the renal pelvis to retrieve the stone.

33

Colon Cancer

A 57-year-old woman presents to her physician's office with complaints of increased fatigue accompanied by decreased exercise tolerance. She has exercised regularly for most of her adult life but has recently found that she feels tired even after a relatively simple workout. She initially attributed these changes to increased stress at work, but her workload has lightened without improvement in her symptoms. She denies fever or night sweats. She denies anorexia, nausea, or a change in bowel habits. Her weight has been stable. Her last menstrual period was 5 years earlier, and she has had minimal menopausal symptoms. She has no significant past medical or surgical history. She takes a baby aspirin daily. She has no allergies and is a nonsmoker. Of note, her family history is significant for both a father and a brother with colon cancer. The patient has not had a screening colonoscopy.

Examination

On physical examination, the patient is a pale, thin woman in no acute distress. Her vital signs are as follows: supine, blood pressure 140/80 mm Hg and pulse 86 bpm; standing, blood pressure 120/65 mm Hg and pulse is 94 bpm.

Examination of the head, eyes, ears, nose, and throat (HEENT) reveals that her sclerae are anicteric (without jaundice) with pale conjunctiva. There is no cervical or supraclavicular adenopathy. The lungs are clear to auscultation, with equal breath sounds bilaterally. Cardiac examination is normal. The abdominal examination reveals no distention and normoactive bowel sounds. The abdomen is nontender in all quadrants with no masses. There is no hepatosplenomegaly. A digital rectal examination reveals no masses, but a stool guaiac test (for occult blood) is positive. Initial laboratory workup shows a normal white blood cell count. However, her hemoglobin concentration is low at 7.5 g/dL (normal, 12–14 g/dL). The indices suggest low iron levels consistent with chronic blood loss.

The patient's history, family history, physical examination, and laboratory data support a diagnosis of iron deficiency anemia, most likely resulting from chronic blood loss. Because she is postmenopausal and her stool is guaiac positive, both upper and lower intestinal endoscopy studies are recommended to identify the source of blood loss. The upper esophagogastroduodenoscopy (EGD) is normal; no evidence of gastritis or peptic ulcer disease is seen. A colonoscopy is then performed and identifies a large (5 cm), sessile polyp in the right (ascending) colon. Biopsy specimens are obtained and are positive for adenocarcinoma of the colon. A subsequent staging workup, including CT scans of the chest, abdomen, and pelvis, is negative for metastatic disease, and surgery is recommended.

Diagnosis

The diagnosis is adenocarcinoma of the ascending colon.

Therapy

In preparation for surgery, the patient is placed in the supine position, and a nasogastric tube and Foley catheter are inserted. A vertical midline incision is made to allow a manual exploration of the abdomen. Care is taken to identify any palpable metastases in the liver or evidence of peritoneal implants of the cancer, which would alter the patient's staging. No metastases are found. The small bowel is then carefully packed away to allow exposure of the right colon. The right colon is palpated gently to confirm the position of the tumor in the ascending colon, approximately 6 cm distal to the ileocecal valve.

The operative approach to the patient with colorectal cancer is distinctly different from that for a patient with benign colorectal disease. With benign disease, the goal of the surgeon is to resect the affected colon back to healthy, well-vascularized colon to ensure successful anastomosis (reconnection) of the two ends of the bowel. The surgeon can dissect and divide the mesentery of the colon at a location where it is easy and most convenient. With malignant disease, however, the colon resection should include radical en bloc removal of the draining lymphovascular complex, with wide enough margins to reduce the risk of local recurrence. To prevent regional lymphatic recurrence and to identify any positive lymph nodes, the major draining mesenteric vessel (in this case, the right colic vessel) should be divided at the point of origin. If the tumor is equidistant from two named mesenteric vessels, both vessels should be ligated proximally.

To resect the right colon, it is first retracted medially so that the avascular region along the lateral paracolic gutter (known by surgeons as the line of Toldt) can be visualized. This avascular line is then incised from the cecum to the hepatic flexure. This allows the right colon to be lifted and rotated medially. Further division of some of the underlying connective tissue allows identification of some of the underlying structures, including the right kidney and the duodenum. The dissection is extended across the ileocecal junction and completed by mobilization of the terminal ileum.

Next, the right ureter is identified before any deeper dissection is performed. The right ureter is usually located where it passes into the pelvis at the bifurcation of the right common iliac artery. Once the ureter is identified, it is pushed gently away from the operative field. The hepatic flexure is gently grasped and retracted inferiorly. It is mobilized away from the liver by dividing any peritoneal adhesions. The right portion of the gastrocolic ligament is also divided to provide more mobility of the right part of the transverse colon. Because the gastrocolic ligament can fuse to the mesentery of the transverse colon, care should be taken to ensure that the transverse mesocolon is not entered inadvertently, which could cause unnecessary injury to the middle colic vessels. Once the hepatic flexure has been freed, the vascular arcades within the colonic mesentery can be inspected.

The ileum is transected with a stapler about 10 cm proximal to its junction with the cecum. The transverse colon is transected in a similar fashion, taking care to ensure that the arcade of the middle colic vessels is intact. The medial leaf of the mesentery of the ileum is then divided, and the vessels within the ileal mesentery are ligated. The ileocolic artery, the right colic artery, and the right branch of the middle colic artery are identified and doubly ligated, and the specimen is removed. A side-to-side anastomosis of the ileum and transverse colon is performed with staplers, and the defect in the mesentery is then closed. The operative field is checked for hemostasis, and the abdominal cavity is irrigated with warm saline. The abdominal wall is then closed.

Discussion

The large intestine begins at the ileocecal valve and ends at the anus. The portions of the large intestine are the cecum and appendix; the ascending, transverse, descending, and sigmoid colon; and the rectum and anal canal. The large intestine is distinguished from the small intestine by several physical characteristics. It is larger in diameter. The small intestine has an inner circular layer and a continuous outer longitudinal layer of smooth muscle, whereas most of the large intestine has an inner circular and a discontinuous outer longitudinal layer. The longitudinal muscle in most of the large intestine is consolidated into three strips of smooth muscle called the *tenia*. Only the appendix, rectum, and anal canal have a continuous outer longitudinal layer of muscle. Because the tenia are shorter than the colon, the wall of the colon is thrown into a series of outpouchings known as the *haustra*. The colon is also characterized by the presence of subserosal accumulations of fat called the *appendices epiploica*.

Blood Supply to the Large Intestine

The large intestine is supplied by branches of the superior and inferior mesenteric arteries (SMA and IMA, respectively). The SMA gives rise to the ileocolic artery, which supplies the distal ileum, the cecum, and the proximal ascending colon. The appendicular artery, a branch of the ileocolic artery, supplies the appendix. Also branching from the SMA are the right colic and middle colic arteries. The right colic artery supplies the ascending colon, and the middle colic artery supplies the transverse colon (Fig. 33.1). The IMA gives rise to the left colic artery, which supplies the descending colon, and several sigmoidal arteries, which supply the sigmoid colon. After the last sigmoidal artery arises from the IMA, the IMA continues as the superior rectal artery to supply the rectum.

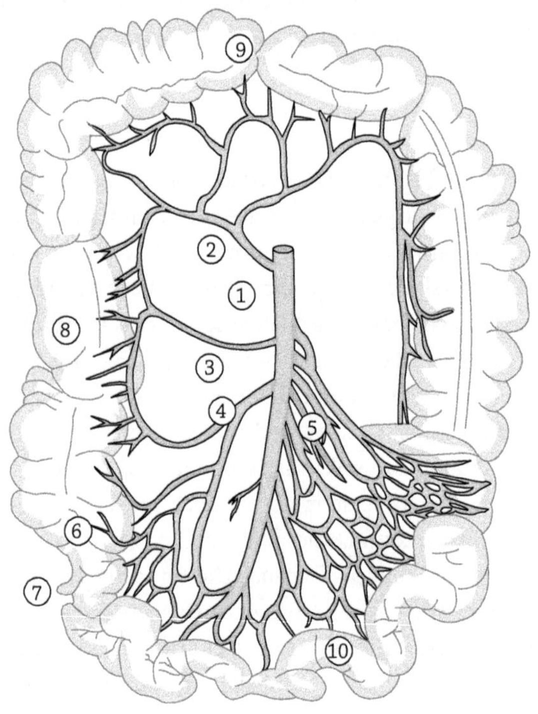

FIGURE 33.1

Distribution of the superior mesenteric artery. 1, Superior mesenteric artery; 2, middle colic artery; 3, right colic artery; 4, ileocolic artery; 5, intestinal arteries; 6, cecum; 7, appendix; 8, ascending colon; 9, transverse colon; 10, small intestine.

As each of these arteries approaches the colon, it divides into branches that travel proximally and distally near the border of the colon. The distal branch of one artery anastomoses with the proximal branch of the next artery: The ileocolic artery anastomoses with the right colic artery, which anastomoses with the middle colic artery, which anastomoses with the left colic artery, which anastomoses with the sigmoidal arteries, which anastomose with one another and with the superior rectal artery. This series of anastomoses creates a continuous vessel along the border of the colon, called the *marginal artery* (of Drummond). This anastomotic pathway provides collateral circulation among the arteries that supply the colon.

From the marginal artery, there are multiple small arteries, the *vasa recta*, which enter the wall of the colon. These vasa recta comprise the ultimate final pathway for arterial supply. Because the vasa recta do not anastomose with one another, occlusion of a vas recta will result in a segment of ischemic colon. The points of entry into the colonic wall of the vasa recta tend to coincide with the sites of diverticula in colonic diverticular disease, presumably because of a weakness in the wall at these sites. The venous drainage and the lymphatic drainage of the colon follow the pathway of the arteries.

Watershed Area of Colon

The marginal artery, described earlier, is sometimes incomplete. The most frequent site of discontinuity is the anastomosis of the left colic artery with the middle colic artery at the region of the splenic flexure. Even when the marginal artery is complete and there is anatomical communication between the left colic and middle colic arteries, the quality of this anastomosis is often poorer than that of the other anastomoses that comprise the marginal artery. For this reason, the collateral blood supply to the region of the splenic flexure is less good than to other regions of the bowel, and this is the most frequent site of ischemic bowel. If there is occlusion of the middle colic artery, most of the transverse colon can be supplied by the anastomosis with the right colic artery, but the region of the transverse colon near the splenic flexure is at risk of ischemia.

Similarly, if the left colic artery is occluded, most of the descending colon can be supplied by anastomoses with the sigmoidal arteries, but the region of the descending colon near the splenic flexure is at risk of ischemia.

For similar reasons, the venous drainage and the lymphatic drainage in the region of the splenic flexure tend to have few anastomoses, and the drainages from this region are toward the middle colic vessels proximal to the splenic flexure and toward the left colic vessels distal to the splenic flexure. Therefore, the splenic flexure is referred to as the watershed area of the colon.

Retroperitonealization of the Ascending Colon

During early embryonic development, almost the entire digestive tube is a peritoneal structure that has a mesentery through which the arterial supply, the venous and lymphatic drainages, and the nerve supply reach the organ (Fig. 33.2). During development, some parts of the gut tube fuse to the posterior abdominal wall to

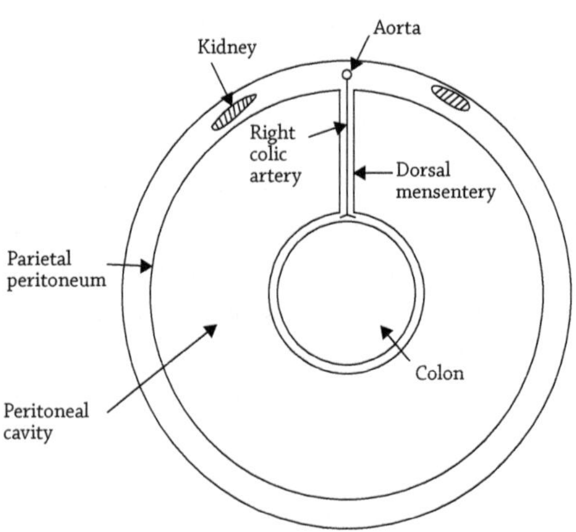

FIGURE 33.2

Cross-sectional schematic of the embryonic relationships of the portion of the gut tube that will become the ascending colon.

become retroperitoneal, and the mesentery, with its enclosed neurovascular contents, also fuses to the posterior wall. This process of retroperitonealization involves most of the duodenum, the ascending colon, the descending colon, and the rectum. Organs that become secondarily retroperitoneal can have their previous embryonic relationship reestablished surgically. When the organ and its mesentery fuse to the posterior body wall, a layer of fascia is established in the fusion plane. This fascial plane can be cleaved by blunt dissection by the surgeon. When this is done, the neurovascular supply to the organ is elevated along with the mesentery (Fig. 33.3).

In the surgical procedure described in this case study, an incision was made along the avascular line in the lateral colic gutter. This avascular line marks the entry into the fascial plane along which the

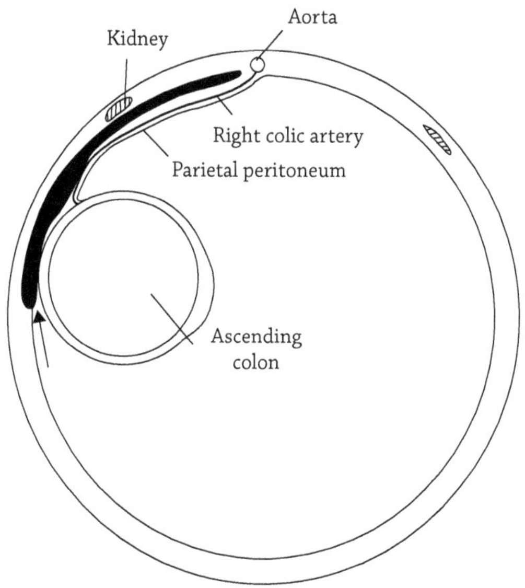

FIGURE 33.3

Cross-sectional schematic of the ascending colon after retroperitonealization. The arrow indicates the avascular region where the incision is made to mobilize the ascending colon from the posterior abdominal wall along the fascial plane of fusion.

ascending colon and its mesentery fused. The peritoneum medial to the adult ascending colon was the embryonic mesentery of the ascending colon and contains the neurovascular supply to the colon. Therefore, all of the neurovascular supply to the ascending colon comes from the medial side, and the lateral side is avascular. As the surgeon elevated the ascending colon by separating the connective tissue in the fascial plane of embryonic fusion, the embryonic mesentery with its enclosed neurovascular structures was reestablished. This allowed identification of the lymphatic pathways for drainage of the ascending colon and a broad resection of these pathways without endangering other structures of the posterior wall such as the ureter, the inferior vena cava, and the iliac vessels.

Typically, the entire ascending colon fuses to the posterior abdominal wall and is immobile. Sometimes this fusion is incomplete and some mobility may be seen. There is considerable variability in the extent of fusion between the cecum and the posterior abdominal wall. Therefore, mobility of the cecum is variable. With cecal mobility there arises the possibility of cecal volvulus and bowel obstruction, a rare occurrence.

34

Portal Hypertension

A 65-year-old man with a past medical history significant for alcohol abuse presents to the emergency room with a history of vomiting a large amount of blood (hematemesis). He states that he was well until about 2 hours earlier, when he began experiencing mild nausea. This progressed over the next hour, and then he vomited a large amount of blood into the toilet bowl. The patient reports that he only vomited one time but called an ambulance for transport to the hospital. He has never had anything like this happen before. He is not nauseated at this time and does not feel lightheaded. He denies abdominal pain. He has not had a bowel movement in the past 24 hours. He reports no history of peptic ulcer disease or gastroesophageal reflux disease, and he has never been told that he has liver disease. He states that he has not used aspirin or nonsteroidal antiinflammatory drugs. He has no allergies to medications and has never had surgery before. Of note, he has a long history of alcohol abuse, drinking one or two six-packs of beer per night up until 1 year ago.

Examination

The patient is in mild distress. His blood pressure is 110/50 mm Hg, and his heart rate is 120 bpm. His respiratory rate is 18 breaths/min, and he is afebrile. Examination of the skin reveals scattered spider angiomata on the trunk. His head, eye, ear, nose, and throat (HEENT) examination is normal. The sclera are anicteric. His neck veins are flat. The lung examination reveals equal breath sounds bilaterally without wheezes, rales, or rhonchi. Cardiac auscultation reveals tachycardia, regular rhythm, normal S_1 and S_2 heart sounds without gallops or murmurs. The abdominal examination is significant for mild distention, but no fluid wave is evident. There are no prominent venous patterns on the abdominal wall. The bowel sounds are hyperactive. The abdomen is nontender to percussion and palpation, and there are no hernias. The tip of the spleen is palpable just below the left costal margin. The liver edge is nonpalpable. There are no masses. Examination of the extremities reveals no palmar erythema or asterixis (tremor of the wrist when extended, as seen in patients with liver failure). A rectal examination is performed and reveals very prominent internal hemorrhoids on Valsalva maneuver. The prostate is smooth and without nodules.

Diagnosis

The diagnosis is upper gastrointestinal hemorrhage.

Therapy and Further Course

With this patient's history of chronic alcohol abuse, there are several possible etiologies for upper gastrointestinal hemorrhage. Esophageal varices are a consideration, as is a bleeding peptic ulcer or gastric ulcer. The first step, however, is to make sure that the patient remains hemodynamically stable. Therefore, two large-bore intravenous lines are inserted, and fluid resuscitation is begun. Blood is drawn and sent for evaluation of the hemoglobin level, hematocrit, and platelet count as well as serum chemistries and a coagulation profile.

A gastroenterology consultation is obtained, and the patient undergoes an emergent upper endoscopic esophagogastroduodenoscopy (EGD). EGD is the best test for the patient at this time, because it can be used not only to establish a clear diagnosis but also for therapeutic intervention. For example, electrocautery can be performed to cauterize a bleeding vessel in an ulcer bed. Likewise, dilated veins (varices) in the distal esophagus can be banded or injected with a sclerosing agent.

In this instance, the EGD identifies gastroesophageal varices without evidence of active bleeding. A diagnosis of portal hypertension is made. It is most likely a consequence of liver cirrhosis due to alcoholic liver disease. Although this patient is not bleeding actively at this time, the incidence of rebleeding from the varices is quite high (80% at 2 years). For this reason, it is recommended that he begin pharmacological therapy with a β-blocker to reduce the risk of future bleeding. In addition, he is referred for therapeutic EGD to begin a schedule for variceal banding.

Cirrhosis of the liver occurs as a result of alcohol injury to the liver. The persistent injury leads to increased fibrosis and architectural distortion of the hepatic sinusoids. The net result is an increase in hepatic vascular resistance, which leads to resistance to portal flow. Extensive portosystemic collateral circulation develops (see later discussion) and can result in serious, life-threatening hemorrhage without timely and appropriate intervention.

Discussion

There are two venous systems in the abdomen: the inferior vena cava (IVC) and its tributaries, and the portal vein and its tributaries. The abdominal organs that are primary retroperitoneal organs, as well as the body wall itself, drain into the IVC. Those organs that are peritoneal, as well as those that are secondarily retroperitoneal, drain into the portal vein. The blood flow from the IVC is directly to the right atrium. The blood flow from the portal vein is to the porta hepatis, where it enters the liver, and through the sinusoids of the liver. After passing through the sinusoids, the blood flows into central veins and then into the hepatic veins. The hepatic veins drain into the IVC. This means that all of the portal venous drainage flows through the liver on its way to the right atrium. If there is an obstruction to flow through the liver, as may occur with liver disease, the pressure in the portal venous system rises. This is known as *portal hypertension*. The blood in the portal system will seek alternative pathways that bypass the liver to get to the heart. These pathways will involve portocaval anastomoses, as discussed later.

The Portal Venous System

The portal vein is formed by the union of the superior mesenteric vein and the splenic vein. This union typically occurs immediately posterior to the neck of the pancreas. The inferior mesenteric vein typically flows into the splenic vein, although it may drain into the superior mesenteric vein or directly into the portal vein. After forming behind the neck of the pancreas, the portal vein ascends to the liver within the hepatoduodenal portion of the lesser omentum. Before reaching the liver, the portal vein receives the right and left gastric veins.

The Splenic Vein

The splenic vein lies on the posterior surface of the neck, body, and tail of the pancreas. It receives venous drainage from the spleen, the pancreas, and the stomach. In this patient, the obstruction to flow in the portal system has caused splenomegaly, as evidenced by the palpable spleen below the left costal margin.

The Superior Mesenteric Vein

The superior mesenteric vein lies on the posterior surface of the neck of the pancreas; it continues inferiorly by passing anterior to the uncinate process of the pancreas, then anterior to the third part of the duodenum, and then along the base of the mesentery of the small intestine. It has the same branches as the superior mesenteric artery, draining the duodenum and head of the pancreas, the jejunum and ileum, the cecum and appendix, the ascending colon, and the proximal two-thirds of the transverse colon.

The Inferior Mesenteric Vein

The inferior mesenteric vein descends from its union with the splenic vein in the parietal peritoneum on the left side of the midline. It gives rise to the left colic vein and several sigmoidal veins and then terminates as the superior rectal vein. It drains the distal one-third of the transverse colon, the descending colon, the sigmoid colon, and the upper portion of the rectum.

The Left Gastric Vein

The left gastric vein arises from the portal vein and joins the left gastric artery to run along the lesser curvature of the stomach. The esophageal branch of this vein runs along the abdominal portion of the esophagus toward the esophageal hiatus of the diaphragm.

Portocaval Anastomoses

Portocaval anastomoses are venous communications between branches of the portal system of veins and branches of the caval system of veins. At these anastomoses, portal venous blood that is impeded from passing through the liver can be shunted into the caval system to reach the right atrium. For this shunting to occur, the direction of blood flow in veins of the portal system must reverse. This is possible because there are no valves in any of the veins of the portal system; the direction of flow is determined only by the direction of the pressure gradient. The normal pressure gradient in the portal system is toward the liver. However, when there is obstruction to flow through the liver, the resulting increased pressure causes a reversal of the direction of the pressure gradient, and thus of the flow.

There are three regions where there are clinically important portocaval anastomoses: in the esophagus, in the rectum, and in the anterior abdominal wall (Fig. 34.1).

Esophagus

The abdominal portion of the esophagus sends its venous drainage through esophageal branches of the left gastric vein, which drains into the portal vein. The thoracic portion of the esophagus sends its venous drainage through esophageal veins that drain into the azygos vein and thence into the superior vena cava. Therefore, the abdominal portion of the esophagus drains to the portal system and the thoracic portion to the caval system. Branches of these two venous systems anastomose within the wall of the esophagus.

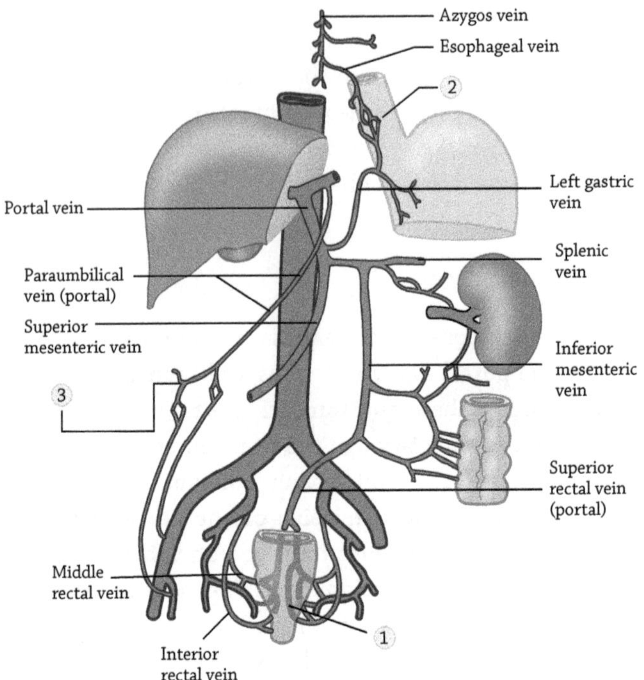

FIGURE 34.1

Major portocaval anastomoses occur in the region of the rectum, in the region of the esophagus, and in the region of the umbilicus. (Courtesy of Kaplan Medical.)

With the development of portal hypertension, the reversal of blood flow in the portal system sends portal blood through the esophageal branches of the left gastric vein into the wall of the esophagus. There, the anastomoses allow the flow to continue into the thoracic esophageal veins, the azygos vein, and then the superior vena cava. Thus, a pathway for shunting of blood from the portal system into the superior vena cava is established.

Because the veins in the wall of the esophagus are carrying much more blood than normal due to shunting of the portal blood, they dilate. The large veins of the esophagus are found in the submucosa, toward the luminal surface of the esophageal wall. When these veins dilate, they bulge the overlying mucosa into the lumen of the esophagus. These enlarged, bulging veins are called *esophageal varices*. Abrasion caused by the swallowing of food can rupture these varices, causing extensive bleeding into the esophagus and down into the stomach. This results in vomiting of blood (hematemesis), as in our patient. Sclerosing or banding of these varices is done therapeutically to prevent such bleeding, and this was recommended to our patient.

Rectum

The upper part of the rectum sends its venous drainage to the superior rectal vein, which drains into the inferior mesenteric vein and then into the portal vein by way of the splenic vein. The lower part of the rectum and the anal canal send venous drainage to the middle and inferior rectal veins. The middle rectal vein drains into the internal iliac vein, and the inferior rectal vein drains to the internal pudendal vein, which drains to the internal iliac vein and then to the IVC by way of the common iliac vein. Therefore, the upper rectum drains to the portal system and the lower rectum and anal canal to the caval system. Branches of these two venous systems anastomose within the wall of the rectum. With the development of portal hypertension, the reversal of blood flow in the portal system sends portal blood through the superior rectal vein into the wall of the rectum. There, the anastomoses allow the flow to continue into the middle and inferior rectal veins and then into the IVC. Thus, a pathway for shunting of blood from the portal system into the IVC is established.

Because the veins in the wall of the rectum are carrying much more blood than normal due to shunting of the portal blood, they dilate. The large veins of the rectum, as in the esophagus, are found in the submucosa, toward the luminal surface of the rectal wall. When these veins dilate, they bulge the overlying mucosa into the lumen of the rectum. These enlarged, bulging veins are called *hemorrhoids* and were found in our patient.

Anterior Abdominal Wall

The ligamentum teres, the postnatal remnant of the umbilical vein, lies in the free edge of the falciform ligament. On the surface of the ligamentum teres there are multiple small paraumbilical veins, which are branches of the portal vein. These veins reach the anterior abdominal wall in the region of the umbilicus. In the superficial fascia of the anterior abdominal wall are the superficial epigastric veins. These veins communicate with abdominal wall tributaries of the external iliac vein inferiorly and the axillary vein superiorly. In the region of the umbilicus, the paraumbilical veins anastomose with the superficial epigastric veins. Thus there is established a portocaval anastomosis. With portal hypertension, blood can flow from the portal vein, through the paraumbilical veins to the superficial epigastric veins, and thence to the superior and inferior venae cavae. This increased flow through the superficial epigastric veins causes them to dilate. Because these dilated veins are in the superficial fascia of the anterior abdominal wall, they can be seen through the skin as a pattern of dilated veins radiating superiorly and inferiorly from the region of the umbilicus. This pattern is termed *caput medusae* because of its resemblance to the snakes radiating from the head of Medusa in mythology (see Fig. 34.1).

Surgical Intervention

When esophageal bleeding due to portal hypertension cannot be controlled with medical treatment or endoscopic banding of the varices, surgical creation of a portocaval shunt can be used to reduce portal hypertension and shunt blood from the esophageal varices into the caval system. One such procedure is the distal splenorenal shunt procedure. The splenic vein is separated from the portal vein and attached to the left renal vein, which is part of the caval system. This allows blood from the esophagus to drain to the splenic vein, by way of gastric venous pathways, and then into the IVC.

An alternative endovascular procedure, which has gained popularity since its first successful use in 1988, is the transjugular intrahepatic portosystemic shunt (TIPS) (Fig. 34.2). After the internal jugular vein

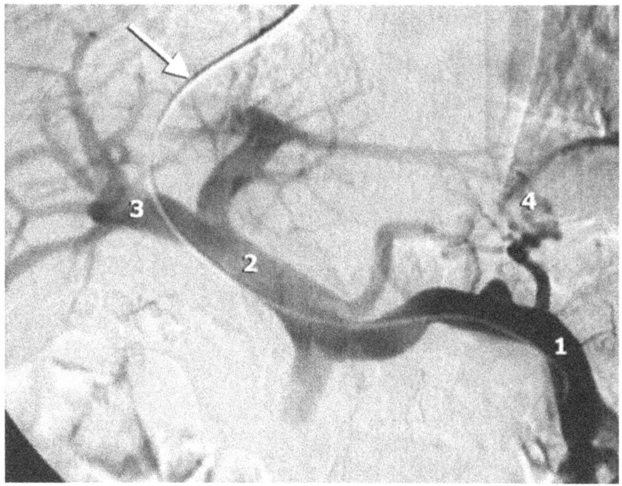

FIGURE 34.2

Portogram from transjugular intrahepatic portosystemic shunt (TIPS) procedure. The catheter (*arrow*) extends from the right hepatic vein, through the liver, and into the portal vein, with its tip in the splenic vein. Contrast medium opacifies the splenic vein (1), portal vein (2), the right portal vein (3), and varices (4).

is entered, a hepatic vein is entered using fluoroscopic guidance, and a shunt is created through the liver to reach the portal vein. A stent is put into place to maintain the patency of the shunt. This allows portal venous blood to reach the IVC through the liver, thus reducing pressure in the portal system.

Unit IV

Review Questions

The number in parentheses is a reference to the page on which information about the question may be found.

1. What characteristics distinguish an indirect inguinal hernia from a direct inguinal hernia?
Both types of inguinal hernia emerge through the superficial inguinal ring. However, an indirect inguinal hernia passes through the deep inguinal ring, and a direct inguinal hernia does not. A direct inguinal hernia passes through the inguinal (Hesselbach's) triangle, which is medial to the deep inguinal ring. An indirect hernia passes lateral to the inferior epigastric artery, whereas a direct hernia passes medial to that artery. An indirect hernia is covered by all three layers of the spermatic fascia after it exits from the superficial ring, whereas a direct hernia is covered only by the external spermatic fascia. (229–230)

2. What is the cremaster muscle? What does it do, and where does it come from?
The cremaster muscle is an evagination of the internal oblique muscle which becomes part of the covering of the spermatic cord. Contraction of the cremaster muscle causes elevation of the spermatic cord and the testis, pulling them closer to the body cavity. The function of the cremaster is to regulate the temperature of the testis by pulling it closer to the body cavity when in a cold environment and lowering if farther from the body cavity when in a warm environment. (230)

3. What is a strangulated hernia?
A strangulated hernia is one in which the blood supply to the herniated viscus becomes impaired or occluded, compromising the organ. If left untreated, this leads to necrosis of the organ. A strangulated hernia is a surgical emergency. (234)

4. What is the processus vaginalis, and how is it related to indirect inguinal hernia?
The processus vaginalis is an evagination of the parietal peritoneum of the anterior abdominal wall that descends through the inguinal canal into the scrotum. The processus vaginalis forms during fetal life and descends through the canal before the testis descends. Normally, the proximal part of the processus vaginalis fuses and degenerates, leaving the distal part covering the testis in the scrotum. This distal remnant is called the tunica vaginalis. If the proximal part of the processus does not fuse and degenerate, it leaves an open pathway between the peritoneal cavity and the scrotum, predisposing the individual for indirect inguinal hernia. (230–231)

5. What landmark is used to identify the cystic artery when performing a cholecystectomy?
The cystic artery is found in the cystohepatic triangle (of Calot). This triangle is formed by the cystic duct, the hepatic ducts, and the border of the liver. The cystic artery is most commonly a branch of the right hepatic artery. (237)

6. What is the anatomical basis for the fact that pain from an inflamed gall bladder sometimes is referred to the right neck and shoulder region?
An inflamed gall bladder can be in contact with, and cause inflammation of, the undersurface of the diaphragm. This region receives sensory innervation from the right phrenic nerve. Because the phrenic nerve arises from spinal nerve levels C3, C4, and C5, pain can be referred to these dermatomes, which are found in the neck and shoulder region. (240)

7. What are the nine regions of the abdomen, and how are they delineated?
The abdomen is divided into nine regions by two vertical lines, the right and left midclavicular or midinguinal lines, and two horizontal lines, the subcostal line at the level of the L3 vertebra and the intertubercular line connecting the iliac tubercles, at the level of the L5 vertebra. The three regions in the midline (i.e., between the midclavicular lines), from superior to inferior, are the epigastric, the periumbilical, and the hypogastric regions. The regions on the right and left, from superior to inferior, are the hypochondriac, the lumbar, and the inguinal regions. (241–242)

8. What is the coronary ligament of the liver?
The coronary ligament is the reflection of peritoneum from the visceral peritoneum of the liver to the parietal peritoneum on the diaphragm. The right and left extremities of the coronary ligament are the right and left triangular ligaments. The region bounded by the coronary ligament is the bare area of the liver. The bare area is in direct contact with the diaphragm without any intervening peritoneum. The hepatic veins leave the liver in the bare area to enter the inferior vena cava. (241–242)

9. What is the portal triad, and where is it located?
The portal triad is composed of the common bile duct, the proper hepatic artery, and the portal vein. These three structures run together in the hepatoduodenal ligament, the right edge of the lesser omentum. The common bile duct is located anterior and to the right, the proper hepatic artery is located anterior and to the left, and the portal vein is posterior to the other two structures. (243, 261)

10. In which part of the digestive system do bile and pancreatic enzymes mix with food?
Bile and pancreatic secretions enter the digestive tract in the second part of the duodenum. The minor pancreatic duct opens independently into the second part of the duodenum, proximal to the ampulla. Food enters the duodenum from the stomach when the pyloric sphincter opens to allow the passage of food. (243)

11. What is the greater omentum, and from what embryonic structure is it derived?
The greater omentum is derived from the dorsal mesogastrium in the embryo. This mesentery becomes very elongated during the rotation of the foregut. The greater omentum is attached to the greater curvature of the stomach, the original dorsal side of the embryonic stomach. The very elongated greater omentum folds upon itself and is draped in front of many of the other abdominal organs. (251)

12. What is the lesser omentum, and what are its two parts?
The lesser omentum is derived from the ventral mesentery of the embryo. It is a mesentery that is stretched between the liver and the stomach and duodenum. The two parts of the lesser omentum are the hepatogastric ligament, which is attached from the liver to the lesser curvature of the stomach, and the hepatoduodenal ligament, which is attached from the liver to the duodenum. The hepatogastric ligament is very thin and translucent. The hepatoduodenal ligament is quite thick and contains the portal triad along with its associated nerve plexus and connective tissue. (251)

13. What is the duodenojejunal flexure?
The duodenojejunal flexure is the point at which the duodenum ends and the jejunum begins. It is at this point that the duodenum emerges from its retroperitoneal position and gains a mesentery to become the jejunum. The duodenojejunal junction is attached to the right crus of the diaphragm by the suspensory ligament of Treitz. (252)

14. What are the four parts of the duodenum?
The duodenum is a C-shaped organ described as having four parts. The first and third parts are horizontally oriented. The first part is at the level of the L1 vertebra and begins at the pylorus; the third part is at the level of the L3 vertebra. The second and fourth parts are vertically oriented. The second part is to the right of the midline and connects the first to the third part; the fourth part is to the left of the midline and ascends from the third part to the level of the L2 vertebra, where it becomes the jejunum. (252)

15. What is the relationship of the superior mesenteric artery to the pancreas?
The superior mesenteric artery arises from the abdominal aorta at the level of the L1 vertebra, behind the body of the pancreas. The artery descends behind the pancreas until it reaches its inferior border, after which it passes anterior to the uncinate process of the pancreas. The artery then continues to descend along the root of the mesentery, sending its intestinal branches into the mesentery to reach the jejunum and ileum. (268–269)

16. What is the source of the blood supply of the duodenum?
The duodenum receives it blood supply from branches of both the celiac trunk and the superior mesenteric artery. The superior and inferior pancreaticoduodenal arteries enter the head of the pancreas from above and below, respectively, and send branches through the head of the pancreas to reach the duodenum, which surrounds the head of the pancreas. The superior pancreaticoduodenal artery is a branch of the gastroduodenal artery, which arises from the common hepatic artery, a branch of the celiac trunk. The inferior pancreaticoduodenal artery is a direct branch of the superior mesenteric artery. (262)

17. What two structures pass between the superior mesenteric artery and the abdominal aorta and are subject to compression?
The two structures that pass through the acute angle between the superior mesenteric artery and the abdominal aorta are the third part of the duodenum and the left renal vein. (270–271)

18. What is omphalocele?
Omphalocele is a developmental defect in which abdominal organs are found outside of the abdominal cavity and within the umbilical cord. Because the organs are within the umbilical cord, which is covered by the amniotic membrane, they are not within the amniotic cavity and are not in contact with amniotic fluid. The site of the defect is at the umbilical ring. (276)

19. What is gastroschisis?
Gastroschisis is a developmental defect in which abdominal organs are found outside of the abdominal cavity and outside the umbilical cord. The organs are free within the amniotic cavity and are in contact with amniotic fluid. The site of the defect is usually to the right of the umbilical ring. (277)

20. What is α-fetoprotein, and how is it used in prenatal screening?
α-Fetoprotein is a glycoprotein that is synthesized in the fetal liver. If there is a body wall defect with an absence of an integumentary covering, this protein can escape from the fetus and enter the amniotic fluid and the maternal bloodstream. An elevated level of α-fetoprotein in the maternal serum is indicative of a defect such as a neural tube defect, omphalocele, or gastroschisis. (280)

21. What is the intestinal loop, and when does it form?
The intestinal loop is a loop of the midgut that forms at about the sixth week of development, when the midgut begins to lengthen. The intestinal loop enters the umbilical cord and remains there until about the eleventh or twelfth week of gestation, when it returns to the abdominal cavity. If it fails to return, omphalocele is the result. (278)

22. Why is the initial pain from an inflamed appendix felt in the region around the umbilicus?
The periumbilical pain from an inflamed appendix is referred pain. The sensory fibers from the appendix travel with the sympathetic innervation to the appendix and then enter the spinal cord through the ninth, tenth, and eleventh thoracic spinal nerves. The brain interprets the pain as coming from the body wall in the region of the T9, T10, and T11 dermatomes. This corresponds to the level of the umbilicus. Because the appendix is bilaterally innervated, the pain is perceived in the midline. (284)

23. Why does pain from an inflamed appendix subsequently migrate to the right lower quadrant?
When the inflammation from the appendix spreads to the overlying parietal peritoneum, the sensory nerve fibers that innervate the body wall in this region carry the pain impulses. The pain is then perceived as coming from the inflamed region of the body wall peritoneum in the right lower quadrant. (284–285)

24. What are taenia coli, and how do they assist in locating the appendix?
Taenia coli are longitudinal strips of smooth muscle found on the wall of the colon. In the small intestine, the outer longitudinal layer of smooth muscle is a complete circumferential layer. In the colon, however, the longitudinal muscle is limited to three longitudinal strips called the taenia coli. The three taenia coli that are found on the ascending colon and caecum converge at the base of the appendix to form a continuous longitudinal layer on the appendix. Therefore, following any of the taenia will lead to the base of the appendix. (287)

25. What is the source of the blood supply to the appendix?
The appendix is supplied by the appendicular artery, which is a branch of the ileocolic artery, which arises from the superior mesenteric artery. The appendicular artery reaches the appendix by passing through the mesoappendix. This artery must be controlled when an appendectomy is performed.(287)

26. What are the three locations in the ureter at which a calculus is most likely to become impacted?
The ureter has three sites of narrowing at which a calculus may become impacted. The first is at the ureteropelvic junction at the top of the ureter, where the renal pelvis empties into the ureter. The second is where the ureter crosses the pelvic brim to pass from the abdomen into the pelvis. The third is at the ureterovesical junction, where the ureter enters the wall of the bladder. Each point of narrowing is smaller than the one above, so that the smallest diameter of the ureter is at the ureterovesical junction. Therefore, the ureterovesical junction is the most common site for impaction of a ureteral stone. (293–294)

27. What is the pathway of the urine after it leaves the distal end of the nephron?
When urine leaves the nephron, it enters a collecting tubule. Collecting tubules drain into the minor calyces of the kidney. Minor calyces drain into major calyces, and major calyces converge to form the renal pelvis. Urine leaves the renal pelvis and enters the ureter. It travels through the ureter to reach the urinary bladder and then empties from the bladder through the urethra. (292–293)

28. What is the anatomical basis for the prevention of reflux of urine from the bladder into the ureter?
The ureter has an oblique course through the bladder wall. Because of this oblique course, when the muscle of the bladder wall (detrusor muscle) contracts during micturition, it compresses the intramural portion of the ureter. This prevents the urine in the bladder from passing retrograde into the ureter. Failure of this mechanism results in vesicoureteral reflux. (293)

29. What is the source of the blood supply to the ureter?
The ureter receives its blood supply from multiple sources. The upper part of the ureter receives branches from the renal artery. As the ureter descends through the abdomen, it receives branches from the gonadal artery, the abdominal aorta, and the common iliac artery. In the pelvis, the blood supply of the ureter comes from branches of the internal iliac artery. (294)

30. What is the neural pathway for sensory innervation of the ureter that is responsible for carrying pain sensation?
The sensory nerve fibers that carry pain sensation from the ureter travel in parallel with the sympathetic innervation to the bladder. Because the preganglionic sympathetic nerve fibers involved in the innervation of the ureter arise from spinal cord levels T10 through L2, the pain sensory fibers enter the spinal cord through the dorsal roots of the T10 through L2 spinal nerves, and their cell bodies are in the corresponding dorsal root ganglia. (294–295)

31. What is the marginal artery (of Drummond)?
The marginal artery is formed by a series of anastomosing branches from the superior and inferior mesenteric arteries. From the superior mesenteric artery, the ileocolic artery, right colic artery, and middle colic artery contribute to the marginal artery. From the inferior mesenteric artery, the left colic artery and sigmoidal arteries contribute to the marginal artery. Each of the contributing arteries divides into proximal and distal branches as it approaches the colon. The distal branch of one artery anastomoses with the proximal branch of the next artery. Collectively, these anastomosing branches form a continuous blood vessel known as the marginal artery. (301)

32. Which parts of the colon have mesenteries, and which parts are retroperitoneal?
The transverse colon, sigmoid colon, and appendix have mesenteries; they are called, respectively, the transverse mesocolon, the sigmoid mesocolon, and the mesoappendix. The ascending colon, descending colon, and rectum are retroperitoneal. The caecum is variable. It may have a short mesentery, it may be retroperitoneal, or it may be partially peritoneal and partially retroperitoneal. (302)

33. Which abdominopelvic organs drain into the inferior vena cava, and which drain into the portal vein?
All primarily retroperitoneal organs drain into the inferior vena cava. All of the secondarily retroperitoneal organs and the peritoneal organs drain into the portal vein. (307)

34. How does the blood in the portal venous system reach the heart?
The blood in the portal system enters the liver at the porta hepatis. It then passes through the sinusoids of the liver to enter the central veins of the liver. The central veins drain into the hepatic veins. The hepatic veins drain into the inferior vena cava, which drains into the right atrium of the heart. (307)

35. What veins drain the rectum?
The rectum is drained by the superior, middle, and inferior rectal veins. The superior rectal vein is the terminal branch of the inferior mesenteric vein and is part of the portal venous system. The middle and inferior rectal veins are part of the caval venous system. The middle rectal vein is a branch of the internal iliac vein, and the inferior rectal vein is a branch of the internal pudendal vein, which is a branch of the internal iliac vein. (311)

36. What veins drain the esophagus?
The lower portion of the esophagus is drained by esophageal branches of the left gastric vein, which is a branch of the portal vein. The thoracic portion of the esophagus drains into the esophageal braches of the azygos vein. The azygos vein drains into the superior vena cava. (309–311)

UNIT V

Pelvis and Perineum

35

Prolapse of the Uterus

A 67-year-old woman presents to the outpatient department with the following concerns. She has noted a "heaviness" or pressure sensation in her pelvis over the past 2 months, which increases with prolonged standing. She often has backaches, particularly if she is on her feet all day. She also complains of urinary symptoms, such as frequency of urination and burning on urination, and has had three urinary tract infections in the past 6 months. She states that she has had increased vaginal discharge that has not changed in color or consistency. The patient has had four children, all via normal spontaneous vaginal delivery. Her last menstrual period was 15 years ago.

Examination

On general physical examination, the patient appears nervous and anxious. Her head, eyes, ears, nose, and throat (HEENT) examinations are normal, as are the heart and lung examinations. The abdominal examination reveals active bowel sounds, no distention or scars, and no organomegaly or masses.

Gynecological examination reveals mild vaginal atrophy in addition to a moderate downward bulging of the anterior vaginal wall that increases on straining. Reduction of the anterior vaginal wall with a speculum reveals urinary incontinence on straining. On examination in the erect position, the cervix of the uterus is found in the vagina close to the vestibule. It recedes somewhat when the patient is supine but does not assume its normal position. The cervix is elongated (Fig. 35.1).

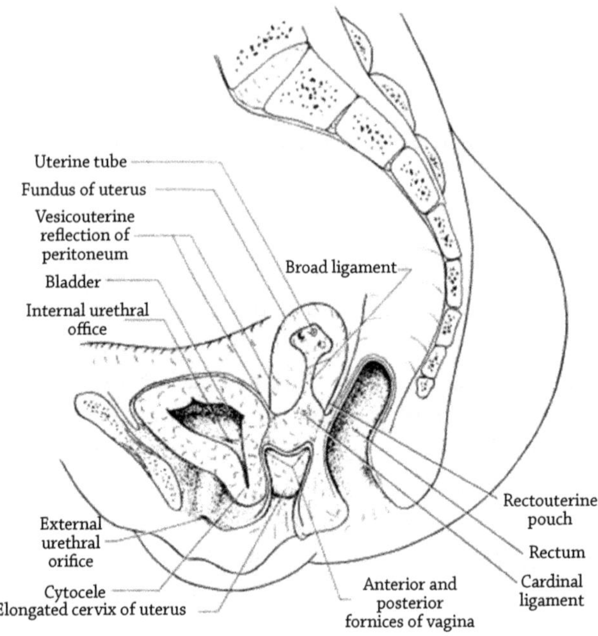

FIGURE 35.1

Prolapse of the uterus and cystocele. Notice the retroverted position of the partially descended uterus, the elongation of the cervix, and the bulging of the bladder into the anterior vaginal wall.

Diagnosis

The diagnoses are prolapse (descensus or downward displacement) of the uterus into the vagina and cystocele (bulging of the bladder into the anterior vaginal wall) with a hypermobile urethra.

Therapy and Further Course

The patient is fitted with a pessary as a temporary measure to help relieve her symptoms until surgical repair is accomplished. Because she is otherwise in good health, is active, and is relatively young, reconstructive surgery is recommended. Under general anesthesia, the patient is placed in the lithotomy position (supine, with legs flexed on the thighs and thighs flexed on the abdomen and abducted). Examination reveals that with traction the cervix descends to the level of the hymenal ring. Associated with the uterine prolapse is the cystocele, which also descends to the same level. There is marked loss of the urethrovesical angle, which is clinically referred to as rotational urethral descent or more commonly as a hypermobile urethra. The posterior vaginal wall in this patient has not collapsed, and there is no rectocele. The perineal body and vaginal axis are normal.

The surgery, done vaginally, consists mainly of vaginal hysterectomy and shortening of the uterosacral and cardinal ligament complexes, which will form the mainstays of support for the apex of the vagina after hysterectomy. After the uterus is removed, redundant peritoneum of the rectouterine pouch (of Douglas) is excised. After the hysterectomy, the anterior vaginal mucosa is incised in the midline to the urethral meatus. The anterior wall is dissected free from the posterior aspect of the bladder. The fascia of the bladder is imbricated (folded) in the midline to reduce the cystocele anteriorly. The urethrovesical angle is corrected, and resupport of the urethra is achieved by shortening of the pubovesical ligaments.

The following are the actual steps of these procedures. An elliptical incision is made through the anterior fornix, extending into the lateral fornices. By sharp dissection, a plane between the bladder and the cervix is developed within the intervening fascia. The peritoneal cavity is entered by cutting through the peritoneum forming the vesicouterine pouch. The rectouterine pouch is entered similarly by sharp dissection through the posterior fornix. The uterosacral and cardinal ligament complexes and the uterine artery are clamped, divided, and ligated with sutures. The ends of the uterosacral ligaments and cardinal ligaments are held separately for later use in the repair.

The uterus, the round ligaments, and the uterine (fallopian) tubes are extracted through the vagina. The ovarian ligaments are divided, and the ovaries are preserved. Although the patient is postmenopausal, there is no clinical rationale for removal of the ovaries with its associated additional risk of bleeding with division of the suspensory ligaments of the ovary. Then the rectouterine pouch is reentered to remove any excess peritoneum from the rectum so to prevent collapse of the rectum anteriorly (rectocele). The sutured uterosacral ligaments are brought across the rectum and attached to each other in the midline, which effectively shortens them and obliterates the rectouterine pouch.

Resuspension of the vaginal cuff is done by suturing the reconstructed uterosacral ligaments to the posterior wall of the vagina. Likewise, the ends of the cardinal ligaments are sewn into the lateral vaginal walls for additional support. A pursestring suture, laced through peritoneum, is placed high in the peritoneal cavity to gather peritoneum and eliminate the communication between the peritoneal cavity and the vagina. The vaginal wall and mucosa are then closed. At this point, the vagina should be of normal length and within normal limits of caliber. With the patient in the supine position, the vaginal axis should be angled slightly posteriorly. A normal urethrovesical angle should have been achieved.

Postoperatively, an indwelling transurethral catheter is used for 48 hours, and the patient is taught to perform self-catheterization. Only rarely is a patient able to void normally during the first few days after this type of repair. After 2 weeks, however, the most patients are voiding normally, and their preoperative urinary symptoms have resolved. Our patient is discharged from the hospital on the third day after surgery. Reexaminations after 3 and after 6 months show no recurrence of the prolapse.

Discussion

Although the cause of the discomfort resulting from prolapse of the uterus remains poorly understood, most gynecologists believe it is related to venous congestion and traction on the nerves and support structures of the pelvic floor caused by the pull of the prolapsed organ. Because of the dislodgment of the bladder and the change in the urethrovesical angle resulting from the cystocele, residual urine remains in the bladder after urination, leading to periodic infection of the stagnating urine and cystitis. Frequency and burning are typical signs of this disorder that result from urinary retention.

A pessary is a plastic or silicone device that is placed in the vagina to help support pelvic organs. In this patient, it was used as a temporary measure while awaiting surgery. It can also serve to provide an indication of whether surgical repair will provide relief of symptoms. In other patients, for whom surgery is either not indicated or not desired, a pessary can provide long-term nonsurgical support of prolapsed pelvic organs. A pessary does not provide a cure for organ prolapse, but it does provide relief of symptoms and can slow the progress of the prolapse.

Flexion and Version of the Uterus

The uterus is a highly mobile organ, subject to constant changes in position depending on the state of filling of the organs in its neighborhood, mainly the bladder and rectum. With these organs empty or almost empty, the most common position of the uterus is anteverted, denoting an anterior angle of somewhat more than 90 degrees between the long axes of the cervix and the vagina. In addition, the uterus is usually also anteflexed, denoting an anterior angle between the uterine body and the cervix. When the bladder fills, the uterus is readily elevated (retroflexed) or even retroverted by the upper surface of the bladder; filling of the rectum may increase the anteversion and anteflexion of the uterus (Fig. 35.2). In the normal anteverted uterus, the ostium of the cervix opens posteriorly into the vagina, whereas the cervical opening faces anteriorly if the uterus is retroverted.

In contrast to earlier beliefs, retroversion and retroflexion by themselves are of questionable clinical significance. Only if uterine supports are weakened does a retroverted and retroflexed position of the uterus tend to promote descent of the uterus, because it then lies in the extension of the longitudinal axis of the vagina (Fig. 35.1). Intra-abdominal pressure further accentuates the downward displacement of the cervix. Congestion and swelling gradually result in elongation of the cervix, as in this patient.

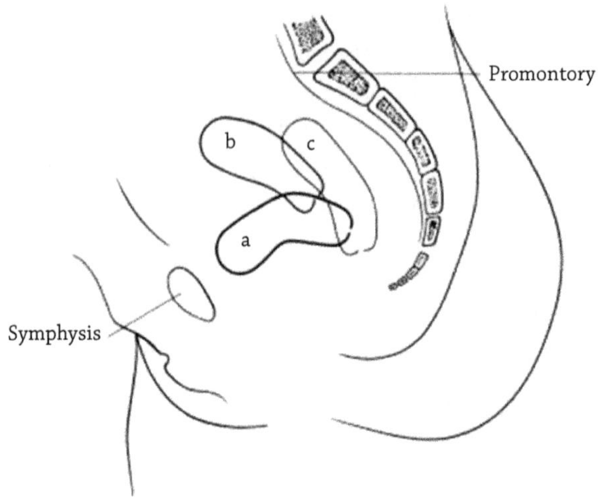

FIGURE 35.2

Variable positions of the uterus in the pelvis depending on the state of filling of the rectum and bladder. The positions of the uterus with bladder and rectum empty (a), with the bladder and rectum filled (b), and with a full bladder and empty rectum (c) are shown. (After Merkel.)

Uterine Support

Uterine prolapse, often combined with a cystocele (as in this patient), is one of the most frequently encountered gynecological disorders. Advancing age brings increased relaxation and loss of tonus of the pelvic diaphragm and the ligaments that constitute the support of the pelvic viscera. This fact is mainly responsible for the disorder. Tearing and overstretching of the supporting tissues during childbirth greatly enhance the chances for prolapse.

The pelvic diaphragm is a thin, conical muscle that is composed of the paired levator ani and coccygeus muscles and covered on both surfaces by deep fascia. Its muscular part is often partly replaced by connective tissue after having been stretched during childbirth. Its right and left halves are separated in front by a narrow gap, the urogenital hiatus, through which the vagina and urethra pass to the perineum. The importance of the pelvic diaphragm for support of the uterus is demonstrated by cases in which congenital paralysis of the pelvic diaphragm in malformations of the spinal cord leads to a prolapse of the uterus in the early years of childhood. This support of the uterus is mainly indirect, however, in that the uterus rests on organs that are maintained in position by the intact pelvic and urogenital diaphragms. These organs are the bladder, on which the normally anteverted and anteflexed uterus rests, and the ampulla of the rectum, which supports the cervix of the uterus and the vagina inferiorly and posteriorly.

Particularly controversial is the role of the cardinal (lateral or transverse cervical) ligaments. They are condensations of parametrial connective tissue (endopelvic fascia) in the base of the broad ligaments that surround the uterine vessels and its autonomic nerves. The cardinal ligaments extend from the lateral pelvic wall to the cervix and upper part of the vagina. The uterosacral ligaments are continuous with the cardinal ligaments but extend posteriorly toward the sacrum, where they fan out into condensations of pararectal tissue inserting into the connective tissue anterior to the sacrum. Although they do not directly attach to the sacrum, they contain some of the sensory nerves of the uterus and are shortened in most vaginal repairs for prolapse.

Finally, the fibrous connective tissue between the vagina and bladder and between the vagina and urethra provide additional support. Clinicians have given them the names vesicovaginal and urethrovaginal septa (or fasciae). They are a part of the pelvic visceral fascia and cover the walls of the bladder, vagina, and rectum.

Applied Anatomy of Prolapse Surgery

Care must be taken to avoid injury to the ureters during uterine surgery. During repair of a prolapsed uterus, the ureters are usually somewhat displaced from their normal position next to the lateral vaginal fornices. Great care must be exercised during division of the cardinal ligaments to prevent damage to the ureters. The ureters pass by the sides of the lateral fornices of the vagina at a distance of only 1 to 2 cm. Here they are located in the base of the broad ligaments. The uterine artery, which arises from the internal iliac artery, crosses superior to the ureter ("water runs under the bridge"), giving a small branch to it. The ureter should be identified and protected when ligating the uterine artery during surgical removal of the uterus. The vaginal artery, also a branch of the internal iliac artery or of the uterine artery, passes immediately inferior to the ureter and should also be identified and protected when the uterine artery is being ligated.

36

Vasectomy

A 37-year-old male geologist had a vasectomy, or excision of a segment of the ductus deferens (vas deferens, vas) 5 years ago for the purpose of sterilization after his first wife died. He has since remarried, and he and his second wife desire children. He consults a urologist to find out whether reunion of the deferent ducts can be done. The urologist recommends the operation but does not promise success.

Therapy and Further Course

With the patient under local anesthesia, an incision into the scrotum is made at the site of the previous operation. On identification and opening of the ductus deferens, copious clear fluid is noted. A sample of this fluid is sent to the pathology laboratory, which identifies the presence of motile sperm. Among patients who desire reversal of their vasectomy, the presence of motile sperm in the ductus deferens is highly predictive (94%) of the return of motile sperm to the ejaculate.

Both ends of the previously ligated ductus deferens are freed for 2 cm and brought to the surface. They are trimmed back to the point at which patency can be observed. Then an end-to-end anastomosis is established with all layers of the duct being properly approximated. The duct of the opposite side is repaired in the same manner. The incisions are closed, and a support is prescribed to immobilize the scrotal contents. Laboratory studies on two occasions within the next months prove the presence of live spermatozoa in the semen. Six months later, the patient reports that his wife is pregnant.

Discussion

Applied Anatomy of Vasectomy

This operation is performed with the use of local anesthesia. A skin incision is made on the front of the scrotum, just above the level of the head of the epididymis, and the ductus deferens is identified among the other constituents of the spermatic cord. In addition to the ductus deferens, the components of the spermatic cord are the artery and vein of the ductus deferens, which along with some fine nerves pass to the epididymis; the testicular artery, which is accompanied by testicular nerves; the pampiniform plexus of veins; lymph vessels; and the strandlike remnants of the processus vaginalis in the anterior part of the cord. All of these structures are embedded in areolar connective tissue that is continuous with the extraperitoneal connective tissue (Figs. 36.1 and 36.2).

The ductus deferens is directly continuous with the epididymis and lies in the posterior part of the spermatic cord; it is identified by its hard and cordlike feel when it is rolled between the thumb and index fingers. This firmness results from the presence of a thick muscular wall surrounding a narrow lumen. The muscular coat consists of outer and inner longitudinal fibers and a heavy circular middle layer; by peristaltic action it propels the semen into the prostatic urethra during ejaculation. The epididymis is a tightly coiled tube, located immediately posterior to the testis, in which sperm are stored before ejaculation. The pampiniform (tendril-like) plexus consists of 8 to 10 venous branches of the testicular vein. Most of these branches lie in front of the ductus deferens and surround the testicular artery. A few venous branches may be located posterior to the duct (Figs. 36.1 and 36.2).

To gain access to the duct for ligation, the coverings of the spermatic cord are separated. Although these fascial coverings are not easily identified individually, they consist of three layers: (1) the thin internal spermatic fascia, which is derived from the transversalis fascia; (2) the cremasteric muscle and fascia, which are derived from the internal oblique muscle and fascia; and (3) the external spermatic fascia, which is the continuation of the fascia of the

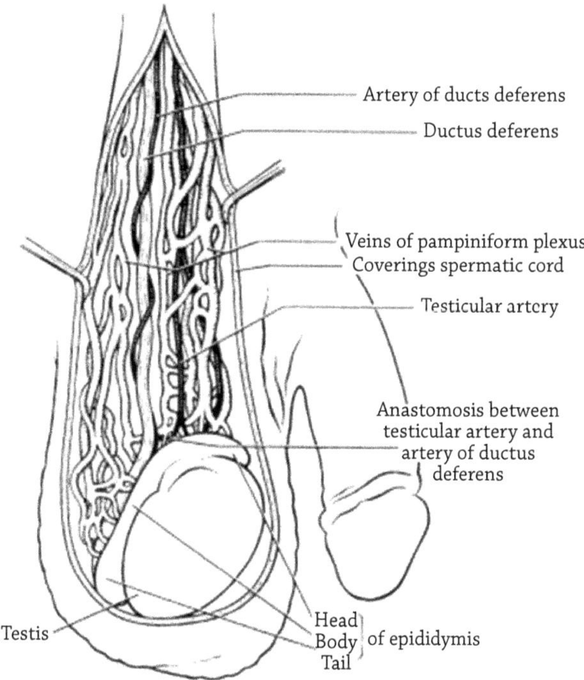

FIGURE 36.1

Dissection of the right spermatic cord. The coverings of the cord have been incised and the contents separated. Notice the veins of the pampiniform plexus in front and behind the ductus deferens.

external abdominal oblique muscle and aponeurosis extending over the cord. How the spermatic cord gains these fascial coverings as it passes through the inguinal canal is described in chapter 25.

After the duct has been stripped free of the areolar tissue in its neighborhood, it is grasped with forceps. The small artery of the ductus deferens is either pushed aside or ligated. This artery is usually a branch from one of the vesicle arteries, and it accompanies the ductus deferens from the pelvis through the inguinal canal to the testis. A small segment of the duct, 1.5 to 2 cm long, is removed, and both ends are ligated. The two ends are separated and cauterized to reduce

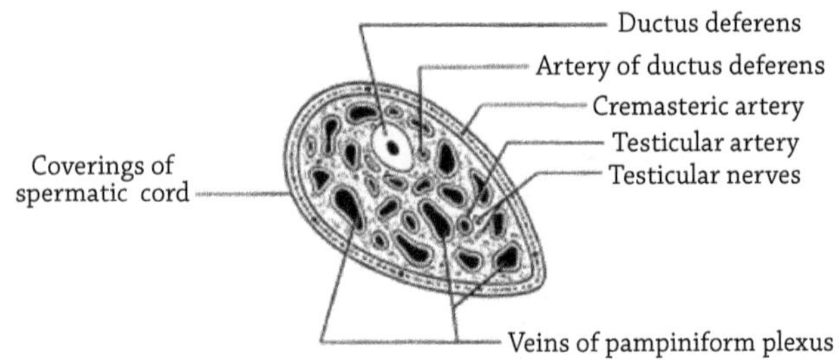

FIGURE 36.2

Cross section of the spermatic cord at the scrotal level shows ductus deferens, veins of pampiniform plexus, testicular artery, artery of ductus deferens, and cremasteric artery.

the possibility of recanalization of the duct. Then the wound is closed with sutures, and the operation is repeated on the other side.

Vasectomy typically does not affect the ability of the testes to produce sperm or androgens. Clinical and experimental evidence has shown that after vasectomy neither the seminiferous epithelium nor the interstitial cells degenerate. In most cases, potential for spermatogenesis is preserved after ligation; only the ejection of spermatozoa from the testes is prevented. This serves as the rationale for attempts at reunion and recanalization of the ductus deferens after previous surgical vasectomy (vasovasostomy). The preservation of spermatogenesis after ligation of the duct makes it feasible to reanastomose the ligated ends to restore the anatomical and functional integrity of the ducts. Restoration of sperm in the ejaculate may be achieved in 70% to 95% of patients when modern microsurgical techniques are used, depending on the length of time since the initial vasectomy (the longer the interval, the lower the success rate). Successful pregnancies are achieved in approximately 30% to 70% of cases, also depending on the length of time since vasectomy. Spontaneous reanastomosis of the ductus does occur in some cases after vasectomy, resulting in the patient retaining fertility.

Three arteries travel within the spermatic cord and provide the blood supply of the testis. They usually form an efficient anastomotic system, establishing testicular circulation. Therefore, if one of these arteries is damaged in the performance of the vasectomy, neither the contents of the cord nor the testis is under major risk of infarction. These arteries are the testicular artery, which arises directly from the abdominal aorta and is the most important blood supply to the testis; the artery of the ductus deferens, which arises from a vesicle artery and anastomoses with the testicular artery at the tail of the epididymis; and the cremasteric artery, a branch of the inferior epigastric artery. The cremasteric artery supplies the coverings of the spermatic cord and the scrotal sac. It enters into functioning anastomotic connections with the testicular artery and the artery of the ductus deferens in two-thirds of men.

Failure of Vasectomy

As mentioned earlier, spontaneous anastomosis of the ductus deferens may occur, depending in part on the surgical technique, defeating the purpose of the procedure. The regenerated adventitia of the two ends of the duct apparently serves as a splint guiding the separated fragments to reunite. In addition to spontaneous recanalization, other reasons could explain retention of fertility after vasectomy. Sperm may stay alive in the ductus deferens for 6 weeks or longer. During this period after vasectomy, the patient remains potentially fertile. Other reasons for failure of vasectomy are the presence of accessory ducts that bypass the ligated site and the surgeon's failure to identify correctly and remove a segment of the ductus deferens.

Other Consequences of Duct Ligation

Because the sperm from the testes contribute less than 5% of the volume of the ejaculate, vasectomy has only a minimal effect on the volume of semen that is ejaculated. Secretions from the seminal vesicles contribute approximately 60% of the volume of semen and are unaffected by vasectomy. The seminal vesicles are glands located posterior to the urinary bladder. Each gland has a short duct that joins with the ductus deferens to form an ejaculatory duct, which empties into the prostatic urethra. The fluid from the seminal vesicles is viscous and contains fructose, which provides an energy source for the sperm; prostaglandins, which contribute to the motility and viability of the sperm; and proteins, which cause slight coagulation reactions in the semen after ejaculation. The prostate contributes most of the remainder of the semen and is similarly unaffected. The prostate is a firm, dense organ located just inferior to the urinary bladder. Numerous short ducts from the prostate empty into the urethra. The prostatic secretion enhances the motility of the sperm. The volume of semen in a single ejaculation may vary from 1.5 to 6.0 mL. There are usually between 50 and 150 million sperm per milliliter of semen. Sperm counts lower than 10 to 20 million per milliliter usually are associated with fertility problems.

Erectile function is not affected by vasectomy. The ability of the male to have an erection is based largely on hormonal production (mainly by the testes) and blood supply to the erectile bodies of the penis. Atherosclerotic disease is a major cause of erectile dysfunction, and this factor is independent of whether a vasectomy has been performed. The interstitial cells (of Leydig) of the testes, which produce testosterone, remain unaffected by vasectomy. As an endocrine gland, the testis secretes this hormone into the bloodstream. Interruption of the ductus does not affect testosterone secretion, and erectile function is preserved.

37

Urethral Rupture

A 56-year-old man is brought to the emergency department by ambulance after having been in a severe motor vehicle accident. He is complaining of abdominal and pelvic pain. He is conscious and able to speak in complete sentences. He denies shortness of breath or chest pain. Intravenous fluids are administered while a thorough examination is performed.

Examination

The patient's heart rate is 110 bpm, and his blood pressure is 120/62 mm Hg. His respiration is shallow at a rate of 22 breaths/min. Different members of the health care team proceed to examine the various regions of his body to identify his injuries. It is noted that there is ecchymosis in the perineum and blood at the urethral meatus of the penis. The bladder is palpably full. Digital rectal examination reveals that the prostate is in a normal position. Because these findings are suggestive of a urethral injury, the decision is made not to place a Foley catheter in the patient. After completion of the secondary survey, a radiograph of the pelvis is obtained which reveals multiple fractures of the pelvic ring. A retrograde urethrogram is ordered. A small-bore urethral catheter is placed into the navicular fossa of the urethra, and contrast dye is gently injected into the urethra under fluoroscopic observation. It is seen that there is leakage of dye into the superficial perineal space, confirming a tear of the urethra (Fig. 37.1).

Diagnosis

The diagnosis is fracture of the pelvis with rupture of the urethra.

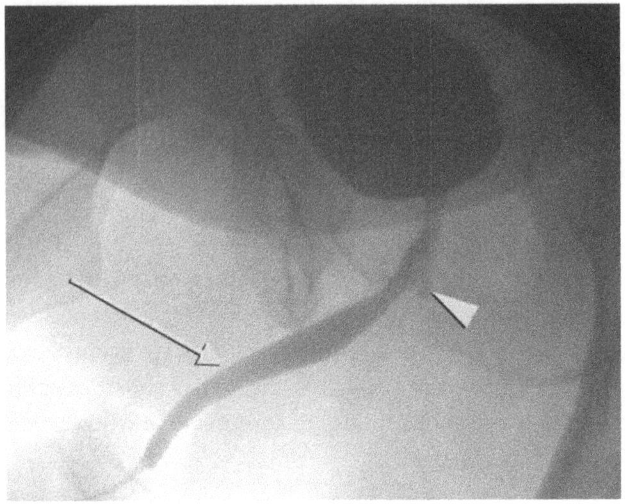

FIGURE 37.1

Urethrogram. The urethra (*arrow*) contains radiopaque dye. Notice the small leak of dye from the spongy urethra (*arrowhead*).

Therapy and Further Course

To provide drainage from the bladder, a suprapubic cystostomy tube is placed. A small infraumbilical incision is made to allow inspection of the bladder to determine whether any damage exists and to introduce a large-bore tube through the dome of the bladder to provide drainage. The decision is made to delay repair of the urethra until the patient has been stabilized and the pelvic fracture and the other, more emergent injuries are addressed. After 3 days, the patient is stable and the orthopedic surgeons have completed the surgical fixation of the pelvis. Additional imaging of the urethra is done by repeat retrograde urethrogram and by a cystogram with the dye introduced through the cystostomy tube. Evaluation of the images indicates that there is a partial tear of the urethra at the junction of the membranous urethra and the spongy urethra. Alignment of the urethra is accomplished by careful passage of a urethral catheter, which is left in place as a stent for 6 weeks to allow time for the urethra to heal. After 6 weeks, the catheter is removed and the cystostomy tube is left in place. After 10 more days, the patient is routinely passing urine though the urethra. The cystostomy tube is removed, and the bladder is closed.

Discussion

Although urethral rupture is fairly uncommon, it does occur in approximately 10% to 15% of pelvic fractures. Such injuries typically result from high-velocity impact such as a motor vehicle accident or a fall from great height. Because of the ring shape of the pelvis, pelvic fractures typically occur as multiple fractures, as in this patient. The shearing forces associated with these injuries put the urethra at risk of rupture.

Anatomy of the Urethra

Anatomically, the male urethra is divided into three parts: the prostatic urethra, which passes through the prostate; the membranous urethra, which passes through the urogenital diaphragm; and the spongy urethra, which passes through the bulb of the penis and the corpus spongiosum (Fig. 37.2). Clinicians divide the male urethra into two parts: the posterior urethra (which includes the prostatic urethra and the membranous urethra) and the anterior urethra (the spongy urethra). The external meatus of the urethra is its distal opening in the glans penis. The external meatus is the narrowest part of the urethra, which means that any catheter that can be introduced into the external meatus is small enough to traverse the full length of the urethra.

The navicular fossa (Fig. 37.2) is a fusiform dilatation of the spongy urethra that extends inward from the meatus for about 2.5 cm to the level of the corona of the glans penis. The distal end of the navicular fossa, near the external opening, is lined by stratified squamous epithelium; this is the part derived from the ectodermal glandular plate in the embryo. The remainder of the spongy portion is lined by epithelium of the stratified columnar type; this is the part derived from the endoderm of the urogenital sinus.

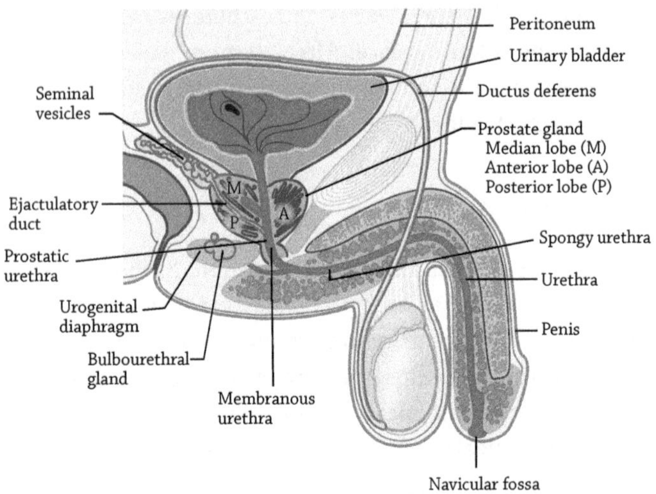

FIGURE 37.2

Sagittal section of the male bladder and urethra. (Courtesy of Kaplan Medical.)

The female urethra is much shorter than the male urethra (approximately 4 cm versus 20 cm). The female urethra emerges from the bladder, passes through the urogenital diaphragm, and opens into the vestibule, anterior to the vagina.

Parts of the Male Urethra

The *prostatic* urethra begins at the neck of the bladder (Figs. 37.2 and 37.3). At the neck, it is surrounded by circular smooth muscle, the internal urethral sphincter, which is sympathetically innervated. The internal urethral sphincter serves not only to retain urine within the bladder but also to prevent retrograde flow of seminal fluid from the prostatic urethra into the bladder during ejaculation. As the prostatic urethra continues through the prostate, it receives the right and left ejaculatory ducts and approximately 20 prostatic ducts. It is in the prostatic urethra that seminal fluid is introduced into the

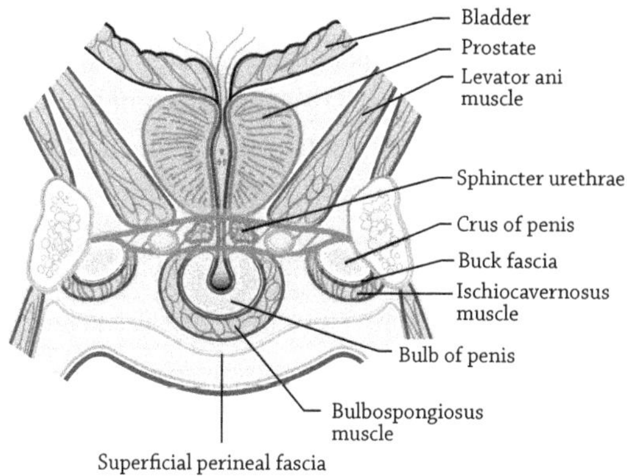

FIGURE 37.3

Frontal section through male urethra. (Courtesy of Kaplan Medical.)

urethra. The ejaculatory ducts are formed by the union of the ductus deferens (which carries sperm from the testis) and the duct of the seminal vesicle. The secretion of the seminal vesicle is high in fructose, which serves to maintain the viability and motility of the sperm. The multiple ducts of the prostate enter the prostatic urethra and carry the prostatic secretion, which, together with the seminal vesicle secretions, accounts for about 95% of the volume of semen.

The *membranous* urethra passes through the urogenital diaphragm, which is immediately below the prostate (Figs. 37.2 and 37.3). The urogenital diaphragm comprises two layers of fascia with a layer of skeletal muscle between them. The urogenital diaphragm stretches across the pelvic outlet from one ischiopubic ramus to the other. The skeletal muscle layer of the urogenital diaphragm is divided into two parts, the deep transverse perineal muscle and the sphincter urethrae muscle. The sphincter urethrae muscle surrounds the membranous urethra and serves as the external sphincter of the urethra. This sphincter is somatically innervated by branches of the pudendal nerve.

When the membranous urethra emerges from the urogenital diaphragm, it enters the bulb of the penis, which is attached to the fascia of the inferior surface of the diaphragm. Beginning at this point, the urethra is called the *spongy* urethra (Figs. 37.2 and 37.3). The bulb of the penis, which contains spongy erectile tissue, continues forward into the penis as the corpus spongiosum of the penis. The spongy urethra continues through the corpus spongiosum to reach the glans penis. There, it expands into the navicular fossa and then narrows again at the external urethral meatus.

The bulbourethral (Cowper's) glands are two small glands located posterior and to the right and left of the membranous urethra. They are housed within the muscle layer of the urogenital diaphragm. Each gland is drained by a duct that leaves the urogenital diaphragm, pierces the bulb of the penis, and terminates in the bulbous portion of the spongy urethra (Fig. 37.2). The bulbourethral glands have a mucoid secretion that makes up a small component of the seminal fluid.

The membranous urethra is bound within the muscle layer of the urogenital diaphragm, which is tightly attached to the bony pelvis; it is the most fixed part of the male urethra. In contrast, the bulb of the penis and its contained spongy urethra have no bony attachment; therefore, it is less stable. With severe shearing forces, such as occur in automobile accidents, the junction of the membranous urethra with the spongy urethra is prone to rupture, as it did in this patient. When such a rupture occurs, urine from within the urethra can escape into the superficial perineal space, the region surrounding the bulb of the penis.

Superficial Perineal Space

The superficial perineal space is the region bounded above by the urogenital diaphragm and below by the superficial perineal fascia (Colles' fascia) (Fig. 36.3). The superficial perineal fascia is tightly attached to the right and left ischiopubic rami, thus closing the lateral borders of the space. Posteriorly, the superficial perineal fascia is attached to the posterior edge of the urogenital diaphragm, thus closing the posterior border of the space. Therefore, urine that extravasates from the urethra into the superficial perineal space is limited with regard to where it can flow. It cannot escape posteriorly into the gluteal region, and it cannot escape laterally into the medial thigh. It can escape anteriorly, which would allow it to extravasate into the scrotum, into the penis, and onto the anterior abdominal wall.

Because the urine is in the superficial perineal space, which is immediately deep to the Colles' fascia, it will remain in that plane on the anterior abdominal wall, immediately deep to Scarpa's fascia, which is the same fascial layer. This accumulation of urine and blood in the superficial perineal space accounts for the butterfly-shaped perineal hematoma that is a classic sign of urethral rupture. The accumulation of urine and blood in the superficial perineal space also can account for a "high-riding" prostate that is observed in patients who have a complete urethral rupture. In that situation, the fluid accumulation pushes the prostate superiorly.

Surgical Repair of the Urethra

This patient was fortunate in that there was only a partial tear of the urethra and healing was possible without surgery by stenting the urethra with a catheter. When there is complete separation of the urethra, surgical repair is usually necessary. With the patient in the lithotomy position, a perineal incision is made. The bulbar portion of the spongy urethra is mobilized, and the prostatic urethra is identified at the apex of the prostate. Care is taken to remove all fibrotic scar tissue from the margins of the urethra, and the prostatic urethra is anastomosed to the spongy bulbar urethra. Although endoscopic repair of the urethra may be possible, there has been only limited success with this technique.

Prognosis

The rate of successful anastomoses of the urethra after rupture is very high. However, several complications can be anticipated. After urethral repair, patients are at risk for development of urethral strictures; these will require dilatation, which can usually be done endoscopically. Because the urogenital diaphragm with its contained external urethral sphincter is disrupted, patients are at risk for urinary incontinence. However, many patients are able to retain continence by action of the internal sphincter alone. Erectile dysfunction is also a significant risk in these patients, regardless of whether surgical repair of the urethra is required. It is likely that the injury itself is responsible for this outcome. Erectile dysfunction can be caused by injury to the cavernous nerves, arterial or venous injury, or direct injury to the erectile bodies.

38

Ectopic Tubal Pregnancy

A 27-year-old woman is brought to the emergency department by her husband and is complaining of lower abdominal pain. She reports that she has been having the pain intermittently for the past 2 weeks but that it has acutely worsened in the past 24 hours and is localized principally to the left side. She initially attributed the pain to an "upset stomach," perhaps related to "something I ate." However, the pain has persisted and has not responded to the over-the-counter medications that she had used successfully in the past for abdominal upset. The pain is constant and is reported to be about a 6 on a scale of 1 to 10, with 10 being most severe. She cannot identify any exacerbating or mitigating factors.

The patient reports that she has regular sexual activity with her husband. She had an intrauterine device placed several years ago for contraception. She reports that it has been about 7 weeks since her last menstrual period. Because she frequently has irregular menstrual periods, she did not pay any special attention to the length of time since her last period. However, for the past 2 or 3 weeks she has had some mild vaginal bleeding, which she thought might be related to her irregular period. Her medical history includes pelvic inflammatory disease secondary to *Chlamydia* infection when she was 17 years old. The infection resolved after treatment with antibiotics.

Examination

On physical examination, she localizes the abdominal pain to her left lower quadrant. Mild tenderness is elicited with deep palpation, but there is no percussion tenderness or guarding that would be suggestive of peritoneal irritation. A urine sample is obtained for assay of human chorionic gonadotropin (β-hCG) for pregnancy testing. Results show a hormone level indicative of pregnancy. Vaginal pelvic examination reveals a softened cervix and a slightly enlarged uterus. Both fullness and tenderness are noted in the left adnexa. Transvaginal ultrasound imaging is ordered and confirms the clinical diagnosis.

Diagnosis

Ectopic tubal pregnancy is diagnosed.

Therapy and Further Course

In discussion with the patient, it is explained that although she is pregnant, the conceptus has implanted ectopically in the left fallopian (uterine) tube. Therefore, she will be unable to carry the pregnancy, because there will be no room for the embryo to expand. The risk to her life due to a potential tubal rupture is explained, and the need to terminate the pregnancy is agreed upon. The options for medical and surgical treatment are explained. Because of the early stage of the pregnancy, the fact that there has not been a rupture of the uterine tube, and the recognition that the patient will be compliant with follow-up care and treatment, it is agreed that medical treatment will be pursued.

An intramuscular injection of methotrexate (50 mg/m^2) is administered. The patient returns 4 days and 7 days later for repeat assays of β-hCG. There is a 20% reduction in hormone level on day 7. Subsequent weekly assays of β-hCG continue to demonstrate decreasing levels until the hormone is undetectable at week 5. The patient is counseled regarding the risk of future ectopic pregnancies and advised to consult with her obstetrician about future attempts at pregnancy.

Discussion

It is estimated that approximately 2% of pregnancies are ectopic. An ectopic implantation is an implantation anywhere other than within the endometrium of the uterus (Fig. 38.1). Approximately

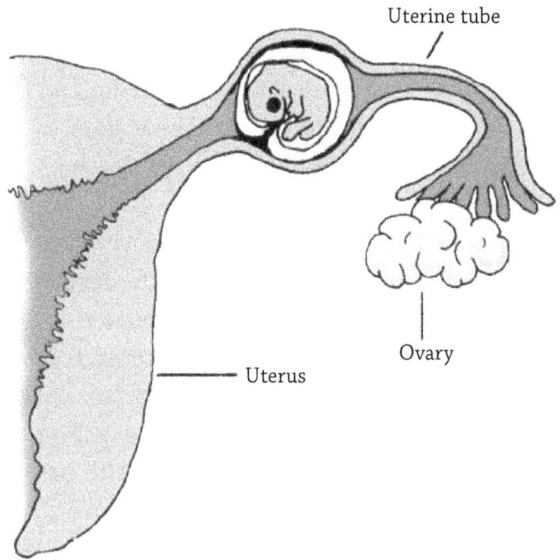

FIGURE 38.1

Ectopic pregnancy in the left uterine tube.

95% of all ectopic pregnancies are tubal pregnancies. Because the wall of the uterine tube does not have the capacity to expand in the way that the uterine wall does, tubal pregnancies, if undiagnosed and left untreated, pose a high risk of tubal rupture with significant hemorrhage and possible death. Because of the risk to the mother, tubal pregnancies are typically terminated.

Ovulation, Fertilization, and Implantation

Midway through the menstrual cycle, ovulation occurs. The cell released from the ovary is a secondary oocyte, which is arrested in metaphase of the second meiotic division. This cell is, for a brief time, in the peritoneal cavity. It is then usually swept into the uterine tubes by the action of the ciliated epithelium of the fimbria of the uterine tube. If the woman has been sexually active, there may be sperm in the uterine tube. Fertilization usually occurs in the ampulla (the wider portion) of the uterine tube. After penetration by a sperm, the secondary oocyte completes its second meiotic division to become an ovum. The nucleus of the ovum and the nucleus of the sperm fuse to produce a zygote. The zygote then begins a series of mitotic divisions, known as cleavage divisions, to increase the cell number of the developing embryo.

During the first 6 days after fertilization, as cleavage divisions proceed to eventually produce the blastocyst, the developing embryo is migrating down the uterine tube toward the uterus. Typically, by the sixth day, the blastocyst has entered the uterus. It is on the sixth day that implantation begins. Therefore, implantation normally occurs in the uterus. However, if the developing embryo is impeded in its progress along the uterine tube, by the sixth day it may still be in the tube and implantation may occur in the tube. A history of pelvic inflammatory disease, as in this patient, presents the possibility of scarring of the uterine tube, which could result in impaired transport of the developing embryo. Such a medical history is a significant risk factor for tubal implantation.

If the ovulated secondary oocyte fails to enter the uterine tube, it remains free in the peritoneal cavity. If it encounters sperm in the peritoneal cavity, it can be fertilized and development will proceed. When the sixth day of development is reached, implantation will begin. Implantation will occur on whatever surface the developing embryo is in contact with. Such an ectopic implantation is called an *abdominal pregnancy*. An abdominal pregnancy poses grave risk to the mother, because when the placenta later separates, the normal uterine muscle mechanism to stop the bleeding will not be present, and exsanguination could occur.

Anatomy of the Uterine Tube

The uterus is in the pelvic cavity within a fold of peritoneum that is elevated from the floor of the pelvis. This fold of peritoneum is a mesentery known as the *broad ligament*. Like other mesenteries, it carries within it the blood supply for the enclosed organ. In this case, the uterine arteries, branches of the internal iliac arteries in the lateral pelvic walls, reach the uterus by traveling within the base of the broad ligament. The broad ligament divides the pelvic portion of the peritoneal cavity into the rectouterine pouch, behind the broad ligament, and the vesicouterine pouch, in front of the broad ligament.

The uterine tube is suspended in the upper free edge of the broad ligament. A posteriorly directed extension of the posterior leaf of the broad ligament encloses the ovary. This extension of mesentery is called the *mesovarium*. The upper portion of the broad ligament, above the level of the mesovarium, is called the *mesosalpinx* because it suspends the uterine tube. The uterine tube receives its blood supply from arteries that travel in the mesosalpinx. These arteries are branches of the ovarian artery that reach the uterine tube from its distal end and branches of the uterine artery that reach the uterine tube from the proximal end. These arterial branches anastomose within the mesosalpinx and thereby establish a collateral pathway between the ovarian artery (a branch of the abdominal aorta) and the uterine artery (a branch of the internal iliac artery).

The uterine tube is approximately 10 cm long. It is traditionally divided into four parts. The most distal part is the infundibulum, a funnel-shaped portion designed for receiving the ovulated secondary oocyte. The infundibulum has finger-like extensions, the fimbria, which embrace the ovary and aid in moving the secondary oocyte into the uterine tube. The next portion is the ampulla, the wider portion of the tube, which has a relatively thin wall. It is in the ampulla that fertilization typically occurs. The next portion is the isthmus, which is narrower than the ampulla and has a thicker, more muscular wall. The last and most proximal portion is the uterine portion. This is the part of the uterine tube that traverses the uterine wall to enter the uterine cavity.

Medical Treatment

Medical treatment was chosen over surgical treatment in this case. Because it allows termination of a pregnancy without surgical disruption of the uterine tubes, and because this patient is young and desirous of getting pregnant in the future, medical treatment is the preferable option. This option is possible in this case because the embryo is still quite small and there is little risk that the uterine tube will rupture during the course of the treatment. Also, there is confidence that the patient will comply with the necessary follow-up visits to monitor the progress of the treatment.

Methotrexate is an antimetabolite that inhibits folic acid metabolism. It acts by blocking DNA and RNA synthesis. Therefore, its greatest effect is on cells that are rapidly dividing, such as the cells of the early embryo and the trophoblast cells of the placenta. As the trophoblast is reduced, the secretion of β-hCG is reduced; this hormone can be repeatedly assayed to monitor the effectiveness of the treatment. If there is not a significant decrease of β-hCG after 7 days, one or more additional injections of methotrexate may be given.

Surgical Treatment

An alternative option that is available to treat tubal pregnancy is surgical removal of the embryo and placenta. This can be accomplished by salpingostomy or salpingectomy, both of which can be done laparoscopically. In salpingostomy, the uterine tube is opened with a linear incision by needle cautery along the antimesenteric border of the uterine tube. The products of conception are removed by grasping them or flushing them from the tube. In salpingectomy, a portion of the uterine tube that contains the products of conception is resected. In both approaches, to ensure that no persistent trophoblastic tissue is left behind, β-hCG is measured in the days and weeks after the procedure.

Unit V

Review Questions

The number in parentheses is a reference to the page on which information about the question may be found.

1. What do the terms *anteverted* and *anteflexed* mean with regard to the position of the uterus?
Anteversion refers to the angle between the long axis of the vagina and the long axis of the cervical canal. Normally, this angle is approximately 90 degrees anteriorly, and this is referred to as anteversion. If the angle is significantly greater than 90 degrees, it is referred to as retroversion. Anteflexion refers to the angle between the uterine body and the cervical canal. Normally, the uterine body is angled anteriorly relative to the cervix such that it lies upon the bladder. This is referred to as anteversion. If the uterus is in line with the cervix, this is referred to as retroflexion. (331)

2. What is the pelvic diaphragm?
The pelvic diaphragm forms the floor of the pelvic cavity. It is composed of a layer of skeletal muscle between two layers of fascia. The skeletal muscle layer is comprises two muscles: the levator ani muscle and the coccygeus muscle. The pelvic diaphragm is suspended from the lateral pelvic walls by its attachment to the obturator internus fascia. The diaphragm is cone shaped and is responsible for supporting the pelvic organs. (332–333)

3. What is the transverse cervical ligament?
The transverse cervical (cardinal) ligament is a condensation of the parametrium, the connective tissue in the base of the broad ligament. The uterine artery and vein are contained within the transverse cervical

ligament as they travel from the internal iliac vessels on the lateral pelvic wall to the cervix of the uterus. (333)

4. What is the relationship between the ureter and the uterine artery?
The uterine artery crosses from lateral to medial through the base of the broad ligament as it extends from the internal iliac artery on the lateral pelvic wall to the cervix. The ureter crosses from posterior to anterior across the base of the broad ligament as it extends from the posterior pelvic wall to the bladder. The ureter passes slightly lateral to the cervix and under the uterine artery. (333–334)

5. What is the pathway for a sperm from the testis to the urethra?
When a sperm leaves the seminiferous tubule in the testis, it enters an efferent duct to reach the epididymis. It passes through the tightly coiled epididymis, which becomes the ductus deferens. The ductus deferens leaves the scrotum and travels within the spermatic cord to pass through the inguinal canal and enter the abdomen. As the ductus deferens approaches the prostate, it is joined by the duct of the seminal vesicle to form the ejaculatory duct. The sperm continues through the ejaculatory duct, which passes through the prostate and enters the prostatic portion of the urethra. (336–337)

6. Why does a vasectomy not significantly reduce the volume of semen?
A vasectomy interrupts the pathway for the transport of sperm from the testis. The sperm account for only about 5% of the volume of semen. Most of the semen comes from the seminal vesicles and the prostate. These secretions are not affected by a vasectomy. (339–340)

7. What arteries are found in the spermatic cord, and from what arteries do they branch?
Included in the spermatic cord are the testicular artery, the artery of the ductus deferens, and the cremasteric artery. The testicular artery is a direct branch of the abdominal aorta. The artery of the ductus deferens is a branch of the vesicle artery. The cremasteric artery is a branch of the inferior epigastric artery. (338–339)

8. What are the three anatomical parts of the male urethra?
The male urethra is divided into the prostatic urethra, the membranous urethra, and the spongy urethra. The prostatic urethra passes through the prostate. The membranous urethra passes through the urogenital diaphragm. The spongy urethra passes through the bulb of the penis and the corpus spongiosum of the penis. (343)

9. Which part of the male urethra has the smallest diameter?
The external meatus of the urethra has the smallest diameter. This is significant because any instrument that is able to enter the distal meatus of the urethra is small enough to traverse the entire length of the urethra and enter the bladder. (343)

10. What are the two sphincters of the urethra, and where are they located?
The internal urethral sphincter is at the neck of the bladder. It is composed of smooth muscle that is circularly arranged around the urethral orifice. This sphincter is sympathetically innervated. The external urethral sphincter is within the urogenital diaphragm. It is composed of skeletal muscle (the sphincter urethrae muscle) that is circularly arranged around the membranous urethra and is somatically innervated by branches of the pudendal nerve. (344–345)

11. What is the superficial perineal space?
The superficial perineal space is the compartment between the urogenital diaphragm and the superficial perineal fascia (Colles' fascia). The compartment is closed posteriorly by the fusion of the superficial perineal fascia to the urogenital diaphragm. It is closed laterally by the fusion of the superficial perineal fascia to the ischiopubic rami. Within the superficial perineal space are found the bulb of the penis and the crura of the penis. (346–347)

12. What cell is released from the ovary at ovulation?
The cell that is released from the ovary at ovulation is a secondary oocyte. This cell is in the second meiotic division and is arrested in metaphase. This second meiotic division will be completed if the secondary oocyte is

fertilized. On fertilization, when the second meiotic division is completed and the cell divides, one of the two resulting cells is the ovum and the other is the second polar body. (351)

13. When and where does implantation occur?
Implantation occurs on the sixth day after fertilization at the blastocyst stage of development. Normally, at this time the blastocyst is in the uterus, and it implants into the endometrium. If transport through the uterine tube is impeded, at the sixth day the blastocyst will still be in the uterine tube, and implantation will occur there, resulting in a tubal pregnancy. If the secondary oocyte does not enter the uterine tube and fertilization occurs in the peritoneal cavity at the sixth day of development, implantation will occur on a peritoneal surface, resulting in an abdominal pregnancy. (352)

14. What is the broad ligament, and what are its parts?
The broad ligament is the mesentery of the uterus. Extending from the posterior leaf of the broad ligament is the mesovarium, which suspends the ovary. The portion of the broad ligament above the mesovarium is the mesosalpinx. Enclosed within the edge of the mesosalpinx is the uterine tube. The largest part of the broad ligament, which extends laterally from the uterus, is the mesometrium. (352–353)

VI

Upper Limb

39

Fracture of the Clavicle

A 25-year-old skier fell on his left shoulder while negotiating the expert slopes. He immediately complained of severe pain in the area of his collarbone. All movements of his left arm are painful. He tries to avoid painful motion by holding his left arm close to his body and by supporting the left elbow with his right hand. He is transported by ski patrol to the base of the mountain and from there by his friends to the local emergency room.

Examination

In the emergency room, the patient is in good spirits but has considerable left shoulder pain. His vital signs are stable. On visual examination, his left shoulder is displaced inferiorly and anteriorly when support of the left arm is removed. There is a clear midshaft deformity of the left clavicle with overlying ecchymoses. His heart examination is normal. The breath sounds are clear and equal to auscultation bilaterally. The neurovascular examination of the left upper extremity is normal. There is marked tenderness and swelling at the fracture site. By passing the fingers along the border of the clavicle, the examiner can discern the projecting ends of the fragments. The sternal fragment is angulated upward (Fig. 39.1). Passive movement of the left shoulder is quite painful. A radiograph confirms the diagnosis of clavicular fracture at the expected site (midshaft) and shows depression of the outer fragment.

Diagnosis

The diagnosis is fracture of the clavicle.

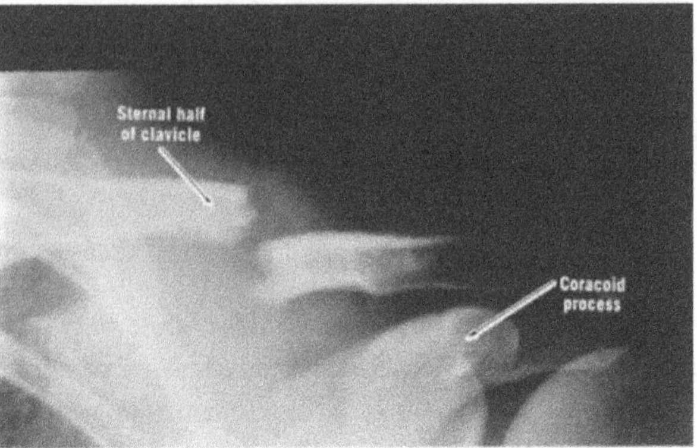

FIGURE 39.1

Radiograph of fractured clavicle shows typical displacement of the fragments. Notice that the sternal end is displaced upward, whereas the distal end sags because of gravity.

Therapy and Further Course

The fracture is reduced (closed reduction) by pulling the shoulder upward and backward, and correct alignment of the fragments is achieved via immobilization using a sling. Although a figure-of-eight bandage is also a treatment option, studies have not demonstrated an advantage to either method. Significant displacement of the bony fragments may require surgical fixation (open reduction) in specific cases. The sling is maintained for comfort and may be discontinued after 1 to 2 weeks as the pain diminishes. Passive range-of-motion exercises can then be performed as tolerated, with increased activity and strength exercises over 4 to 8 weeks.

Discussion

Clavicular fracture is one of the most common fractures. The clavicle is the only skeletal connection of the shoulder girdle to the trunk, and it serves as a strut to maintain the shoulder and arm at the proper distance from the chest. As such, it is exposed to any force that tends to thrust the arm medially against the chest, as exemplified in this patient, who fell on his shoulder. If unbroken, the clavicle maintains a constant distance between the acromion and the midline of the body; a decrease in this distance, compared with the normal side, is a rough indication of the amount of overriding of the fracture fragments.

Ligaments Anchoring the Clavicle

Forces applied to the clavicle, either directly, as in this case, or indirectly by force transmitted along the upper limb, can cause fracture or dislocation of the clavicle. Although the bony articulation at the sternoclavicular joint appears to be quite unstable and vulnerable to dislocation, this joint is actually extremely stable and almost never dislocates because of the strong ligaments at the joint. (Fig. 39.2). These are the costoclavicular ligament, the anterior and posterior sternoclavicular ligaments, and the articular disk, which is attached to the clavicle above and to the first costal cartilage below.

At the lateral end of the clavicle is the acromioclavicular joint, which binds the clavicle to the scapula. The coracoclavicular

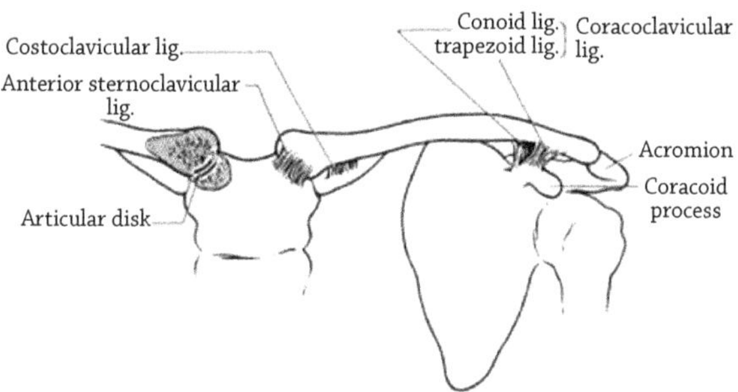

FIGURE 39.2

Ligaments of the clavicle. The disk, the sternoclavicular ligaments, and the costoclavicular ligament protect the integrity of the sternoclavicular joint and prevent dislocation. Notice that the disk is attached to the clavicle above and to the first rib below. Fractures most commonly occur between the costoclavicular and coracoclavicular ligaments. lig., ligament.

ligament with its two parts, the conoid and trapezoid ligaments, along with the acromioclavicular ligament, protects the integrity of the acromioclavicular joint and prevents the acromion from being driven under the clavicle. The ligaments of this joint are less strong than those of the sternoclavicular joints, and dislocations do occur here. A dislocation of the acromioclavicular joint is known as a *shoulder separation.*

Fractures of the clavicle typically occur between the attachments of the costoclavicular and the coracoclavicular ligaments, which anchor the clavicle at either end. These midshaft fractures are the most common type of clavicular fracture, occurring in 75% to 80% of cases. Most (>90%) heal with immobilization alone.

Clavicular Fracture at Birth

Fractures of the clavicle are particularly common in the newborn. In fact, they are more frequent than all other birth fractures combined. The clavicle may be fractured by the hand of the obstetrician in breech (buttocks) presentation, or it may break on its own during passage of the child through the birth canal by being pressed against the maternal symphysis pubis. Because the clavicle begins to ossify earlier than any other bone, with its primary ossification centers first appearing at about 6 weeks of development, it is fairly rigid at birth and subject to fracture.

Muscles Involved in Clavicular Fracture

Displacement of the fracture fragments in a clavicular fracture is rather characteristic and depends on the action of the muscles attached to the shoulder girdle and on the weight of the arm. The pull of the clavicular portion of the sternocleidomastoid muscle is responsible for the upward tilt of the medial fragment (Fig. 39.1). The weight of the arm and the pull of deltoid muscle, which attaches to the lateral third of the clavicle, displaces the lateral fragment downward. In our patient, these factors cause the left arm to hang lower than the right, as evidenced on the physical examination.

The pectoralis major muscle and the latissimus dorsi connect the trunk to the arm and adduct the arm toward the thorax, causing a decrease in the distance between the acromion and the midline and therefore an overlapping of the fracture fragments. Because the medial rotators of the arm (pectoralis major, subscapularis, teres major, and latissimus dorsi) are stronger than the lateral rotators (infraspinatus and teres minor), and because the bracing action of the clavicle is nullified by the fracture, the arm is also medially rotated. This medial rotation of the arm also explains why the medial end of the lateral fragment commonly points posteriorly.

Despite the superficial location of the clavicle and the frequent presence of bony fragments at the site of fracture, piercing of the skin by osseous spicules is rare. The subcutaneous location of the platysma, which allows the skin to move freely over the clavicle, protects the skin and usually prevents fragments from piercing it, thus precluding the occurrence of an open fracture with its danger of secondary infection at the fracture site. More important is the protective action of the subclavius muscle, a muscle that lies deep to the clavicle and attaches it to the first rib. This muscle guards the underlying subclavian vessels and the brachial plexus against injuries from bony fragments of a clavicular fracture. These important structures, which pass over the first rib and under the clavicle on their way into the axilla, can be injured by posteriorly displaced fragments, as can the apex of the lung. Although injuries to these structures are uncommon, examination of the lungs and neurovascular examination of the extremities should always be performed.

Chapter 40

Thoracic Outlet Syndrome

A 39-year-old woman who is otherwise healthy has suffered for the past year with right-sided shoulder pain. She describes the pain as deep, aching, and persistent and rates it as 5 out of 10 in severity (10 being the worst). She notes that the pain is made worse with certain activities, particularly swimming, and persists even with rest, although it lessens in intensity. The pain is increased by downward traction, such as carrying heavy objects. Recently, after the patient took on additional work, the pain worsened. It now radiates down the medial side of the arm and forearm into the hand. Her pain increases toward the end of the day and at night. Sometimes the fingers on the ulnar side of the hand tingle and feel numb. The right arm seems weaker than the left.

Examination

Examination of the neck reveals no evidence of cervical spine pathology. Examination of the right shoulder demonstrates good range of motion and is negative for evidence of joint pathology. There is some tenderness and resistance in the right supraclavicular area, but nothing definite can be palpated. Both pulling downward on the arm and lateral flexion of the neck to the left increases the pain, and pulling down on the arm specifically causes a loss of the radial pulse. There is obvious wasting of the right thenar eminence. On testing, the opponens pollicis and abductor pollicis brevis seem to be particularly involved.

Diagnosis

The diagnosis is thoracic outlet syndrome, possibly caused by a cervical rib. This diagnosis is based on the resistance in the right supraclavicular fossa and on the presence of subjective symptoms and objective neurological signs pointing to involvement of the lower trunk of the brachial plexus; both sensory and motor fibers are affected. Radiological studies confirm the diagnosis and show an accessory rib on the right side that articulates with the seventh cervical vertebra, pointing forward and downward and ending bluntly.

Therapy and Further Course

After a trial of conservative therapy (physical therapy and antiinflammatory medication) followed by local injection of the anterior scalene with botulinum toxin (Botox), which provides only temporary symptomatic relief, surgery is recommended. At operation, the cervical rib is found to be continued anteriorly as a fibrous band attached to the first rib. The brachial plexus is elevated, as is the subclavian artery, both of which pass over the cervical rib. The inferior trunk of the plexus appears rather taut and is stretched over the accessory rib (Fig. 40.1). The cervical rib is excised.

After removal of the cervical rib, the symptoms gradually disappear during the next few months. Strength seems to return to the hand, and the wasting of the thenar eminence also gradually diminishes.

Discussion

The sensory disturbances in this case do not correspond to the cutaneous distribution of any one peripheral nerve but involve an area that is supplied by at least three named nerves. The medial brachial and antebrachial cutaneous nerves and the ulnar nerve supply the involved area with sensory fibers. In addition, the motor deficit in the thenar eminence concerns two muscles supplied by the median nerve. The involvement of fibers distributed through four peripheral nerves makes a peripheral nerve lesion highly improbable.

Localization of Neural Lesion

A lesion involving sensory and motor nerve fibers, proximal to the level at which the brachial plexus is formed, would explain all the

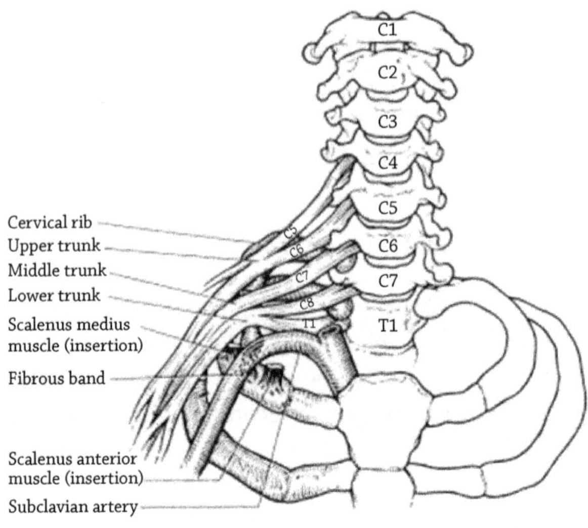

FIGURE 40.1

The cervical rib on the right side is continued as a fibrous band that attaches to the first rib. The brachial plexus and subclavian artery are elevated, and the lower trunk of brachial plexus seems particularly taut and stretched by the cervical rib.

sensory and motor defects in this case. Reference to a dermatome chart (Fig. 40.2) indicates that the C8 and T1 spinal nerve segments correspond to the region of the sensory symptoms. The opponens pollicis and the abductor pollicis brevis most commonly receive their main motor supply via the median nerve from segments C8 and T1. These are the same segments that display the sensory defects.

It is most likely that the lesion is located outside the spinal cord, distal to the point where sensory and motor fibers combine to form the mixed spinal nerve, because both types of fibers are involved. The lesion is likely beyond the point of division of the mixed spinal nerve into ventral and dorsal rami, because there is no sign of neurological deficiency in the back, the area of distribution of the dorsal rami of the C8 and T1 spinal nerves.

The observation at surgery that the inferior truck of the brachial plexus was being stretched by the cervical rib is consistent

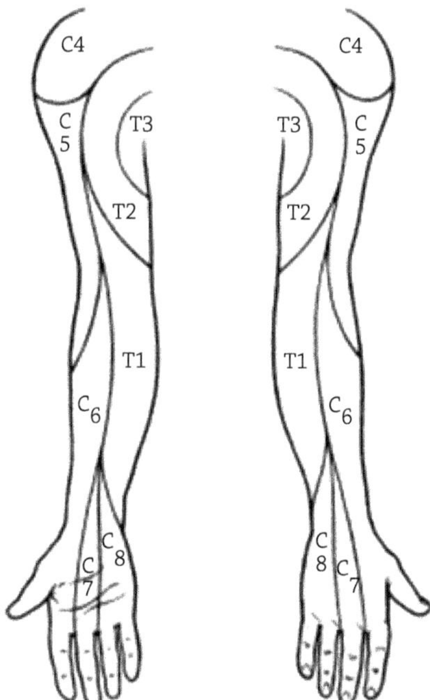

FIGURE 40.2

Dermatome chart of anterior and posterior aspects of upper extremity. Notice particularly the representation of segments C8 and T1 on the medial side of the arm, forearm, and hand. (From Foerster.)

with all of the signs and symptoms in this patient. Clinical examination shows that the opponens pollicis and the abductor pollicis brevis are particularly involved. How would the action of these muscles be tested? Keep in mind that it is the function of the abductor pollicis brevis to pull the thumb away from the palm in a plane at right angles to the palm. It is the function of the opponens pollicis to advance the thumb across the palm in an arc, rotating it simultaneously, so that at the end of the motion the palmar surfaces of the thumb and little finger are in opposition to each other. Consequently, these muscles may be tested for integrity of function by asking the patient to execute these motions against resistance.

Further clinical study in this patient reveals that certainly not all motor fibers coming from C8 and T1 are affected. The muscles of the hypothenar eminence seem to have escaped, a common occurrence in nerve lesions. This is probably explained on the basis of the location of nerve fibers within the trunk.

The brachial plexus and the subclavian artery pass through the neck in the scalene triangle. The anterior and posterior boundaries of this triangle are the anterior and middle scalene muscles, respectively. The inferior boundary is the first rib. Anything that causes a decrease in the size of this triangle can result in compression of its contents. It is noteworthy that the subclavian vein passes anterior to the anterior scalene muscle; therefore, it is not in the scalene triangle and is not compressed in thoracic outlet syndrome. Because it is the inferior boundary of the triangle that is elevated by the cervical rib in this case, the most inferior structures in the triangle are those that are being compressed. The inferior trunk and the subclavian artery are the most inferior structures in the triangle.

Why do the symptoms become noticeable later in life, although the underlying condition is congenital? With progressing age, the tone and strength of the muscles suspending the shoulder decrease, and there is less muscular resistance to the downward pull of the arm. A conservative alternative to the radical surgical removal of the cervical rib includes physical therapy to strengthen the muscles suspending the shoulder, thereby decreasing the stretching of the compressed neurovascular bundle and enlarging the space within the scalene triangle. The injection of botulinum toxin into the anterior scalene muscle is aimed at paralyzing that muscle and thus enlarging the triangle. Surgical section of the anterior scalene muscle (scalene myotomy) where it inserts into the scalene tubercle of the first rib has the same effect. Similarly, surgical resection of the cervical rib enlarges the space in the scalene triangle and relieves the compression on the lower trunk of the brachial plexus and the subclavian artery.

41

Subclavian Steal Syndrome

A 69-year-old retired postal worker is seen in the outpatient department after a syncopal (fainting) episode and is later admitted to the hospital. He reports that for the past year he has experienced transitory periods of dizziness accompanied by vertigo and nausea. These episodes have been accompanied by blurring of vision and usually last from only a few seconds to a few minutes. In the past month, they have occurred more frequently and have interfered with his daily activities. Yesterday evening, he experienced a brief fainting spell while seated. On further questioning, he reports occasional pain and numbness in the left arm that increases with use and subsides with rest. The arm fatigues easily. He denies any history of chest pain, palpitations, or shortness of breath. His past medical history is significant for hypertension (high blood pressure), hypercholesterolemia, and tobacco use. He reports no history of coronary artery disease.

Examination

On examination of this well-nourished, not acutely ill patient, a marked difference in blood pressure between right and left arm is noted. The pressure is 180/95 mm Hg on the right and 93/70 mm Hg on the left. The carotid pulsations are normal, and there are no carotid bruits. The lungs are clear to auscultation bilaterally without wheezes or rales. The cardiac examination reveals a normal point of maximum impulse (PMI), regular rate and rhythm, normal S_1 and S_2 heart sounds, and no murmurs or gallops. The examination of the upper extremities demonstrates diminished pulsation in the left brachial artery, accompanied by a systolic bruit. The brachial and radial pulses are diminished on the left compared with the right. On exercise of the left upper extremity, the patient complains of numbness and

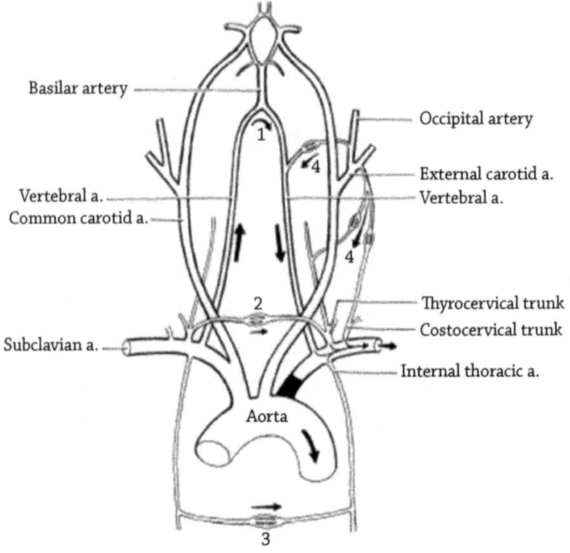

FIGURE 41.1

Various arterial pathways involved in proximal occlusion of the left subclavian artery. Collateral routes include branches of the two subclavian arteries such as the vertebral arteries (1), the inferior thyroid arteries (2), the internal thoracic arteries (3), and branches of the ipsilateral external carotid and subclavian arteries (4) distal to the occlusion. a., artery.

tingling in the arm, lightheadedness, and vertigo. Magnetic resonance angiography of the aortic arch and its branches demonstrates severe narrowing (80% stenosis) of the left subclavian artery proximal to the origin of its vertebral branch (Fig. 41.1). Doppler ultrasonographic studies reveal retrograde flow in the left vertebral artery, with the flow directed toward the subclavian artery.

Diagnosis

The diagnosis is subclavian steal syndrome on the left side, probably due to atherosclerotic plaques in the subclavian artery proximal to the origin of the vertebral artery.

Therapy and Further Course

Because spontaneous relief cannot be expected and there is no effective medical therapy, surgical repair is proposed. The surgeon recommends percutaneous transluminal angioplasty with placement of a stent.

Access to the arterial system is gained through the femoral artery at the groin. At the start of the procedure, contrast dye is injected for angiography of the aorta and the subclavian and vertebral arteries to determine whether any other lesions exist. The angiography confirms stenosis of the subclavian artery with a 1.5 cm lesion proximal to the emergence of the vertebral artery. The artery is dilated, and a stent is placed. One year after the operation, the patient is asymptomatic with normal blood pressure and pulses in both arms.

Discussion

Since the first reports of subclavian steal in 1960 and 1961, this syndrome has now become well recognized in some patients with occlusive disease of the subclavian artery. Familiarity with the anatomical course, distribution, and anastomoses of the subclavian and vertebral arteries is necessary for understanding of subclavian steal syndrome (Fig. 41.1).

Mechanics of Subclavian Steal

The term *subclavian steal* implies that blood is being "stolen" from another region to supply the upper limb. The presence of stenosis of the subclavian artery causes a great decrease in pressure between the prestenotic portion of the artery and its distal patent part. If the stenosis is proximal to the emergence of the vertebral artery, the reduced pressure in the subclavian artery will cause blood from the vertebral artery to flow in a retrograde direction into the subclavian artery. In this case, this blood is coming from the contralateral right vertebral artery by way of the basilar artery. This blood would normally pass into the basilar artery on the inferior surface of the pons and supply the brain stem, cerebellum, and occipital lobe of the brain. Instead, the blood is “stolen” and courses down the left vertebral artery in a retrograde direction to supply the patent poststenotic portion of the left subclavian artery.

Anatomy of the Subclavian Artery

The term *subclavian artery* refers to the artery's location deep to the clavicle. The subclavian artery supplies blood via its branches to areas as far cranially as the cerebral hemispheres and as far inferiorly as the anterior portion of the thorax, including the breast and the anterior abdominal wall. Its blood courses distally to the fingers and medially to structures such as the vertebral column and the thyroid gland. Students and physicians alike often incorrectly think of the artery as being responsible for the blood supply to the upper limb only.

Subclavian steal resulting from atherosclerotic plaques occurs much more commonly on the left side (>70%), which can be partially explained by the difference in origin and length of the right and left arteries. The right subclavian artery arises from the brachiocephalic trunk of the aorta, behind the right sternoclavicular joint, and arches upward and laterally, often above the level of the clavicle. By contrast, the left subclavian artery arises considerably lower, directly from the arch of the aorta, and ascends through the superior mediastinum into the supraclavicular fossa. This difference in origin between the right and left subclavian arteries makes the left vessel 3 to 4 cm longer than the right.

Anatomy of the Vertebral Artery

The main function of the vertebral artery, which is the first, largest, and most important branch of the subclavian artery, is to supply the brain and spinal cord. It has been estimated that the vertebral arteries supply the brain with about 25% to 30% of its arterial blood. After it courses through the transverse foramina of the upper six cervical vertebrae and the dura of the spinal canal, the vertebral artery passes through the foramen magnum and joins its counterpart from the opposite side to form the basilar artery. Just before the formation of the basilar artery, it gives off its largest branch, the posterior inferior cerebellar artery; in addition, the vertebral artery sends off the anterior and posterior spinal arteries to the spinal cord.

Arterial Anastomoses

If there is stenosis (narrowing) or occlusion (blockage) of the first part of the subclavian artery, blood can be carried by various alternative pathways. The retrograde flow in the ipsilateral vertebral artery may be supplemented by extracranial anastomoses from the contralateral vertebral artery and from the ipsilateral occipital artery (Fig. 41.1). Anastomoses also occur between other branches of the ipsilateral external carotid artery and the thyrocervical and costocervical trunks of the subclavian artery. The ipsilateral internal thoracic (mammary) artery also assists in supplying blood to the poststenotic left subclavian artery. The internal thoracic artery is now commonly used for coronary artery grafts, and stenosis of the subclavian artery proximal to the emergence of the internal thoracic artery may result in coronary-subclavian steal syndrome, leading to symptoms of cardiac ischemia in patients who have had such a graft performed.

Explanation of Objective Signs and Subjective Symptoms

Several of the patient's symptoms, such as the episodes of fainting, dizziness, vertigo, nausea, and blurred vision, can be explained by ischemia of the central nervous system. In this case, the combination of eye symptoms and general signs (e.g., fainting, vertigo) was caused by temporary depletion of blood from the posterior cerebral cortex and the brain stem.

One must keep in mind that the classic distribution of blood vessels in the central nervous system does not always hold true; variations are fairly common. One variation that would preclude the function of the left vertebral artery as a conduit for additional blood supply to the left upper limb would be its origin directly from the aorta, which occurs in 5% of individuals.

The differences in blood pressure between right and left upper limbs, the auscultatory phenomena over the left brachial artery, the decrease in pulse volume on the left, and the subjective symptoms of tingling and numbness in the left arm in this patient were cause by the narrowing of the first part of the subclavian artery. The extent of the blood pressure differential between right and left is an indication of the amount of narrowing. The diagnosis of subclavian steal was supported in this patient by the simultaneous appearance of neurological signs of cerebral ischemia and vascular insufficiency of the extremity when the left arm was exercised. Exercising of the left arm increases the demand for oxygen by the muscles of the left upper limb, thereby increasing blood flow to the limb.

42

Supracondylar Fracture of the Humerus

A 9-year-old boy is brought to the emergency department by his mother. She reports that approximately 45 minutes earlier he had been playing on the jungle gym in a playground and fell to the ground on his outstretched left hand. He immediately complained of pain in the region of his elbow, and the elbow began to swell. The mother also thinks that the arm appears "deformed." At home, the patient would not move his forearm or hand because of the pain, so his mother brought him to the hospital. He has no significant medical or surgical history and is up to date on all age-appropriate vaccinations.

Examination

On presentation in the emergency department, the patient is in significant pain. His initial vital signs are stable. After discussion with the parents, intravenous access is obtained in the right upper limb, and mild narcotic analgesia is provided before physical examination. On inspection, there is an S-shaped supracondylar deformity, but there is no apparent tenting of the skin or break in the skin over the fracture. The left hand is slightly pale compared with the right and exhibits delayed capillary refill. There is no palpable radial or ulnar pulse on the left side. He is able to move all of his fingers, and he can touch the tips of his index finger and thumb together. He is also able to extend his thumb and to fully abduct all his fingers. Examination of sensation reveals some hypesthesia on the palmar aspect of his left hand in the region of the lateral palm and the lateral 3½ fingers. Radiography of the left elbow region confirms a fracture of the supracondylar region of the left humerus with posterior displacement of the distal fragment (Fig. 42.1).

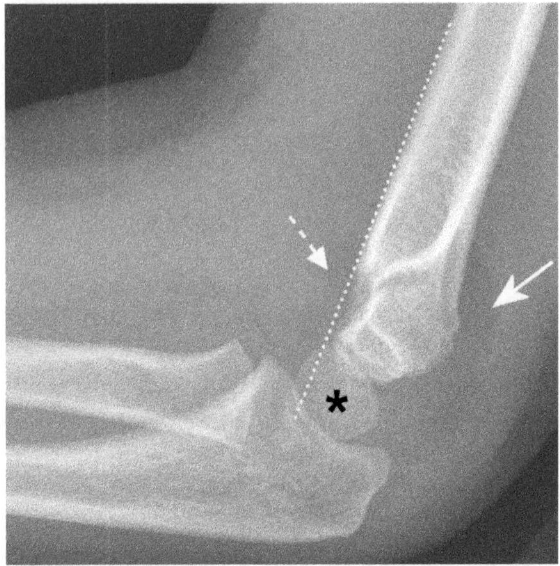

FIGURE 42.1

Radiograph of supracondylar fracture of the humerus. Notice the posterior displacement of the distal fragment. The anterior humeral line (*dotted line*) does not pass through the middle of the capitellum epiphysis(*), as it should, because of posterior displacement of the distal humerus fracture fragment. Solid arrow and dotted arrow indicate effusion in region of the injury.

Diagnosis

The diagnosis is supracondylar fracture of the humerus with compression of the brachial artery and median nerve.

Therapy and Further Course

The patient is transported to the operating room and sedated. Reduction of the fracture is performed and the hand quickly regains its warmth, normal color, and radial and ulnar pulses. The fracture is set and pinned. On completion of the procedure, it is determined that the circulation to the hand remains good but there is persistent diminished sensation on the palmar aspect of the hand. Normal sensation is regained after 2 weeks. On follow-up visits, the sensory and motor examinations of the limb are normal and the vascular supply to the forearm and hand are normal.

Discussion

Supracondylar fractures are the most common elbow fractures in children. The mechanism of injury is typically a fall on the outstretched hand, as in this case. These fractures are less common in adults. In children, the bone strength in this region is less than the strength of the ligaments. Therefore, stresses that tend to deform the elbow are more likely to fracture the bone than to tear the ligaments. Because of the direction of force that caused the fracture, the distal fragment of the fracture is usually displaced posteriorly. Passing across the anterior side of the elbow are the brachial artery and the median nerve. The displacement of the distal fragment of the humerus causes the brachial artery and median nerve to be stretched across the fracture site, resulting in compression of these structures. Because the brachialis muscle lies between the humerus and the brachial artery and median nerve, laceration of the artery and nerve by the fractured end of the bone is unlikely. The brachial artery and median nerve in the cubital fossa can be located by their position relative to the biceps brachii tendon. The artery is immediately medial to the tendon, and the nerve is medial to the artery.

Location of Pulse in Ulnar and Radial Arteries

Both ulnar and radial pulsations were absent in this patient. It is essential for the clinician to know where these pulses can be palpated. Remember, a pulse is best felt in areas where the artery is superficial and is resting on a firm structure such as a bone or a ligament. This is the case for both arteries in the region of the distal forearm and wrist. The ulnar artery lies superficial to the flexor retinaculum on the radial side of the pisiform bone. The pulse can be palpated at this location by compressing it against the retinaculum. It is also possible to palpate the ulnar pulse a bit more proximally in the distal forearm. The ulnar artery lies along the lateral border of the flexor carpi ulnaris tendon, and the pisiform is a sesamoid bone within this tendon. The tendon can be traced proximately from the pisiform, and the ulnar artery pulse can then be palpated at the lateral border of the tendon by compressing it against the ulna. The pulse of the radial artery is felt on the lateral side of the distal forearm, lateral to the tendon of the flexor carpi radialis, by compressing it against the radius.

Collateral Circulation Around the Elbow

The absence of both radial and ulnar pulses suggests occlusion of the brachial artery proximal to its bifurcation. This is consistent with an occlusion at the site of the fracture proximal to the elbow. Two arteries provide the source of collateral circulation around the elbow. The brachial artery, the major artery of the arm, is the distal continuation of the axillary artery (Fig. 42.2). The name of the artery changes from axillary to brachial as the artery passes the inferior border of the teres major, which is the inferior border of the posterior wall of the axilla. In the distal arm, the brachial artery gives rise to the superior and inferior ulnar collateral arteries. These cross the elbow and anastomose with the anterior and posterior ulnar recurrent arteries, which are branches of the ulnar artery.

Immediately after the brachial artery enters the arm from the axilla, it gives rise to the profunda brachii (deep brachial) artery. This artery accompanies the radial nerve in the musculospiral groove and thus passes from the medial side of the humerus to the lateral side by spiraling around the back of the humerus. The profunda brachii artery divides into the radial collateral artery and the middle collateral artery. The radial collateral artery anastomoses with the radial recurrent artery, a branch of the radial artery (Fig. 42.2). The middle collateral artery anastomoses with the interosseous recurrent artery, a branch of the posterior interosseous artery, which ultimately is a branch of the ulnar artery.

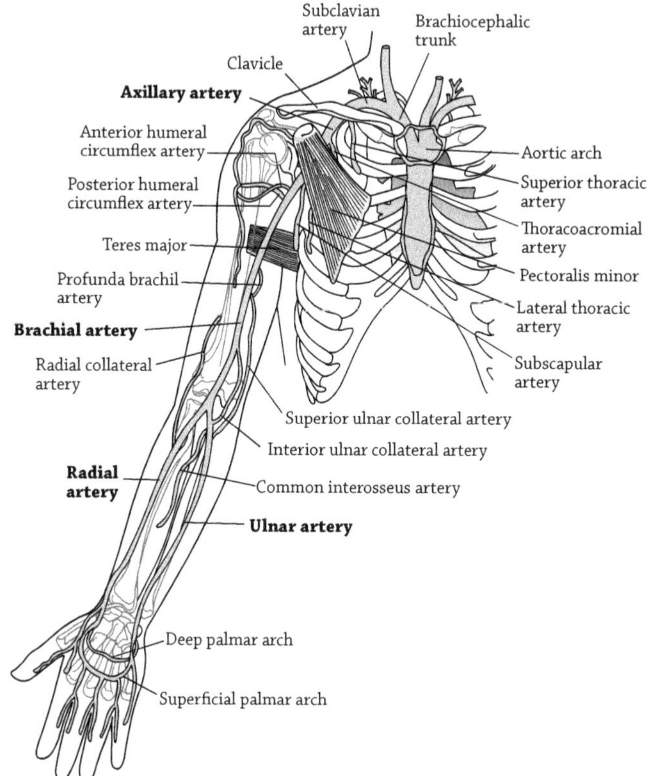

FIGURE 42.2

Arterial supply to the upper limb.

Although these collateral pathways are effective in maintaining the blood supply distal to the elbow during the kinking and bending of the brachial artery with movements of the elbow, they are not adequate when the brachial artery is completely occluded. For this reason, our patient had signs of vascular compromise distal to the elbow. If this condition had not been corrected promptly, the muscles of the forearm would have suffered ischemic damage, which could lead to severe disability of the hand (see later discussion).

The Median Nerve

The displaced fracture in this patient is causing stretch or compression of the median nerve as it crosses in front of the fracture site. The median nerve forms in the axilla from branches of the lateral and medial cords of the brachial plexus. The nerve then passes through the arm without providing any innervation in this region. In the forearm, the median nerve provides innervation to all of the muscles of the anterior compartment except for the flexor carpi ulnaris and the ulnar half of the flexor digitorum profundus. The forearm muscles innervated by the median nerve are responsible for pronation of the forearm, flexion of the wrist, and flexion of the digits.

After the median nerve enters the hand by passing through the carpal tunnel, it innervates the thenar muscles and the first and second lumbrical muscles. It also provides sensory innervation to the skin of the palmar surfaces of the lateral 3½ digits and the corresponding region of the palm of the hand. This patient has sensory symptoms in the region of the hand innervated by the median nerve but does not display any motor weakness in the muscles innervated by this nerve, as evidenced by his ability to make the "okay sign" (touching the tips of his index finger and thumb). The okay sign tests the flexor digitorum profundus to the index finger and flexor pollicis longus, both of which are innervated by the anterior interosseous nerve, a branch of the median nerve. It also tests the opponens pollicis, which is innervated by the recurrent branch of the median nerve.

It is common for nerve compression to cause sensory symptoms before any motor deficits are seen. In this patient, if the compression of the median nerve is not relieved, motor weakness is likely to ensue. Because the patient can extend his thumb and abduct his fingers, we know that his radial nerve is intact (extend thumb) and that his ulnar nerve is intact (abduct fingers).

Volkmann Ischemic Contracture

It is fortunate that the patient's mother brought him to the emergency department as soon after the injury as she did. This allowed the reduction of the fracture and restoration of the blood supply to the forearm and hand in a timely manner. In as little as 4 hours, the absence of blood supply can result in irreversible necrosis of muscle tissue. Such tissue injury results in edema, which further compromises blood supply because of the increased pressure within the anterior compartment. In time, the necrotic muscle becomes fibrotic and contracted and is replaced by scar. This leads to wrist and finger flexion contractures, which make the hand functionless. This condition is known as Volkmann ischemic contracture and was first described by Dr. Richard von Volkmann in 1881.

43

Peripheral Venous Access

A 47-year-old woman with a past surgical history of an appendectomy at age 15 presents to the emergency room with a 6-hour history of generalized abdominal pain accompanied by multiple episodes of nausea and vomiting. The pain is periumbilical and is crampy in nature. The severity of the pain varies from 5 to 8 on a scale of 10 (10 being worst). She reports no radiation and no prior episodes of this nature. She has not had a recent bowel movement and states that she is not passing flatus. She reports no fever or chills. She has no significant past medical history, has no allergies, and takes no medications. She is a nonsmoker.

Examination

The patient appears uncomfortable. She is afebrile, and her heart rate is 110 bpm. Her blood pressure is 140/80 mm Hg supine and 110/50 mm Hg seated. Her mucous membranes are dry. Her neck veins are flat. Examination of the lungs reveals clear and equal breath sounds bilaterally. The heart examination detects a regular rhythm, but the patient is tachycardic. Normal S_1 and S_2 heart sounds are auscultated, and there are no murmurs or gallops. Her abdomen is distended. There is a well-healed transverse scar in the right lower quadrant, consistent with a surgical history of appendectomy, without evidence of hernias. The bowel sounds are hyperactive with frequent rushes and succussion splashes (sloshing). On palpation, there is diffuse mild tenderness without peritoneal signs. No masses are palpable. The rectal examination is normal, and there is no stool in the rectal vault. An abdominal radiograph is obtained and demonstrates multiple dilated loops of small bowel with a small amount of air in the right and left colon.

Diagnosis

The diagnosis is partial small bowel obstruction, most likely resulting from postsurgical adhesions.

Therapy and Further Course

A nasogastric tube is immediately placed to drain the stomach and to prevent the further accumulation of fluid and air in the intestine. This management strategy in itself often provides enough intervention to relieve the obstruction without the need for further action. A second, important consideration is obtaining intravenous access. A bowel obstruction can result in a significant sequestration of fluid within the lumen of the intestine, resulting in serious intravascular volume depletion. In addition, the patient is likely to have lost additional fluid due to the multiple episodes of vomiting. Intravascular volume loss is evident in this patient, who is tachycardic, demonstrates postural changes in blood pressure, and has dry mucous membranes. Should she require operative intervention to relieve the obstruction, it is essential that her intravascular volume status be restored before the surgery. To accomplish this, intravenous access allows the delivery of crystalloid or colloid solutions, blood products, or medications directly into the bloodstream. In the case of fluids, the goal of therapy is to correct the patient's existing losses, replace any ongoing losses (e.g., enteric contents lost through the nasogastric tube), and provide the patient with maintenance fluid to prevent further dehydration.

In general, to obtain intravenous access, the most peripheral site on the arm is chosen. If access is emergent, usually the median cubital vein is targeted in the antecubital fossa. However, this is not an ideal site for longer-term access, because as the patient flexes the elbow, the patency of the indwelling catheter can be compromised. Typically, a more distal target, such as the cephalic vein in the forearm, is selected. All necessary equipment should be prepared before visiting the patient's bedside, including intravenous fluid, tubing, tape, gauze, tourniquet, alcohol swabs, and an intravenous catheter of appropriate size. Importantly, one should always use gloves and other protective equipment. The tourniquet is placed above the patient's antecubital fossa (usually, the patient prefers the nondominant arm to be used, unless there is a contraindication) with the forearm in a dependent position. The tourniquet should be tied in such a way that it can be released with one hand. The patient's forearm and hand are then carefully inspected on the palmar and dorsal sides to identify the best target vein—usually one that is large, easily visualized, and compressible. The tourniquet should then be released while the intravenous set and equipment are prepared.

Once everything is ready, gloves are worn and the tourniquet is reset. The area is palpated and cleansed with alcohol swabs. While it dries, the intravenous catheter is grasped in the dominant hand and is held between the thumb and index finger, bevel side up. The non-dominant hand is used to retract the skin gently distally and thereby prevent the vein from rolling. The needle is inserted slightly lateral to the vein wall and at a 45-degree angle. A small "pop" is often felt as the needle enters the vein, and typically a flash of blood is visualized in the hub of the catheter. With the end of the needle held steady, the catheter is advanced over the needle into the vein until the hub is flush with the skin. The tourniquet can then be released. After a gauze pad is placed under the catheter hub, the needle is removed and replaced with intravenous tubing that allows fluid infusion. The area is dried, and the catheter is secured with a transparent dressing and tape.

Discussion

Veins can be divided into two groups: superficial veins and deep veins. Superficial veins are those found in the superficial fascia (i.e., between the skin and the deep fascia). Deep veins are those found deep to the deep fascia. With some exceptions, deep veins accompany arteries. Superficial veins are not accompanied by arteries. Examples of superficial veins include the cephalic and basilic veins in the upper limb, the long saphenous and short saphenous veins in the lower limb, the external jugular and anterior jugular veins in the neck, and the thoracoepigastric veins in the abdominal wall. All superficial veins drain into deep veins.

Upper Limb

In the upper limb, the major superficial veins are the cephalic vein and the basilic vein (Fig. 43.1). The cephalic vein is on the lateral side of the limb and drains into the axillary vein. The cephalic vein arises from the lateral side of the dorsal venous network in the superficial fascia of the hand. Although the precise course of the cephalic vein is variable, as it reaches the proximal portion of the limb, it enters the deltopectoral groove. It continues into the deltopectoral triangle and then pierces the clavipectoral fascia to enter the axilla and drain into the axillary vein. The basilic vein arises from the medial side of the dorsal venous network of the hand and ascends on the anteromedial side of the forearm in the superficial fascia. After passing the elbow, the basilic vein pierces the deep fascia of the arm and continues deep to the deep fascia through the arm. At the proximal arm, the basilic vein joins with the brachial vein to form the axillary vein.

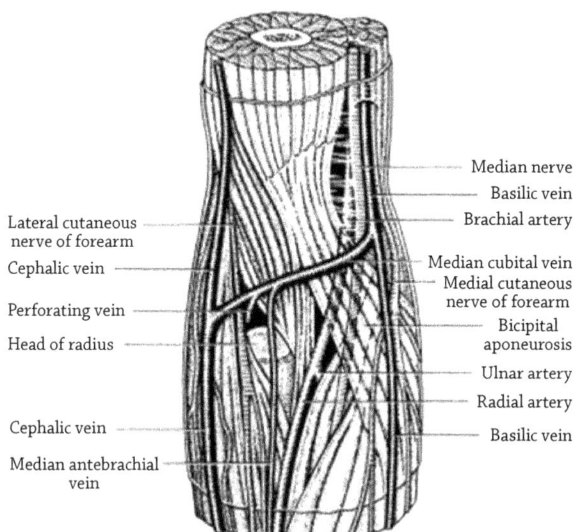

FIGURE 43.1

Superficial veins of the elbow and forearm. Note the relationship of the basilic vein to the median nerve and the brachial artery.

There are multiple communications between the superficial and deep veins by way of penetrating veins that pierce the deep fascia of the arm and forearm. There is a prominent communication between the cephalic vein and the basilic vein in the cubital fossa. This is the median cubital vein, which crosses obliquely across the cubital fossa (Fig. 43.1). Because of the visibility of this vein and ease of access, the median cubital vein or the cephalic vein near the median cubital vein is often used for venipuncture to obtain a sample of venous blood or for intravenous infusion. If the median cubital vein is used, it should be approached lateral to the biceps brachii tendon. The brachial artery and median nerve are located on the medial side of the biceps brachii, just deep to the bicipital aponeurosis (Fig. 43.1). Staying lateral to the tendon avoids an accidental penetration of the brachial artery. However, it should also be kept in mind that, as a possible variation, a superficial radial artery may arise from the brachial artery proximal to the elbow and passes superficial to the bicipital aponeurosis. As mentioned earlier, for longer-term peripheral venous access, the distal cephalic vein is often used.

Lower Limb

In the lower limb, the major superficial veins are the long saphenous (or great saphenous) vein and the short saphenous vein (Fig. 43.2). The long saphenous vein is homologous to the cephalic vein, and the short saphenous vein is homologous to the basilic vein. However, the long saphenous vein is on the medial side of the lower limb, whereas the cephalic vein is on the lateral side of the upper limb, and vice-versa for the basilic and short saphenous veins. This reflects the rotation of the limbs that occurs during embryonic development: The lower limb rotates medially, and the upper limb rotates laterally. Both saphenous veins arise from the dorsal venous plexus of the foot, which forms the dorsal venous arch. The long saphenous vein arises from the medial side of this arch, ascends on the anteromedial side of the limb, and then passes through the saphenous hiatus of the fascia lata to enter the femoral triangle and drain into the femoral vein. The short saphenous vein arises from the lateral side of the

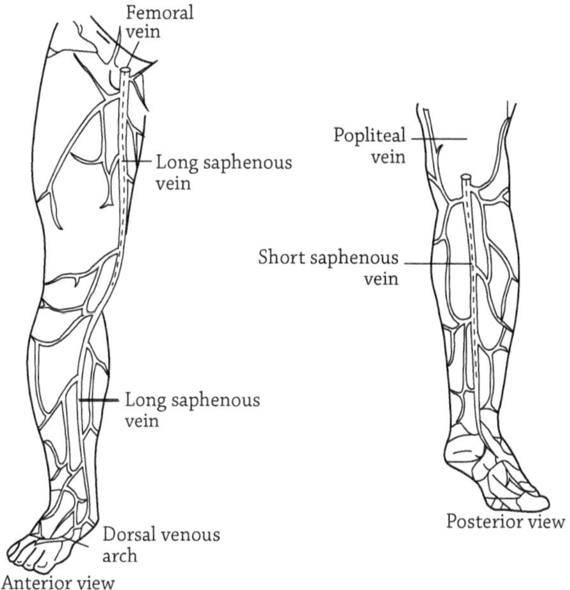

FIGURE 43.2

Superficial veins of the lower limb. Notice the long saphenous vein entering the femoral vein and the short saphenous vein entering the popliteal vein.

dorsal venous arch of the foot, ascends on the posterolateral side of the leg, and then pierces the crural fascia to enter the popliteal fossa and drain into the popliteal vein.

There are multiple communications between the superficial and deep veins by way of penetrating veins that pierce the deep fascia of the leg and thigh. Because of the effect of hydrostatic pressure, the valves found in the saphenous veins are particularly important. These valves are designed to reduce the effect of hydrostatic pressure in the erect posture. The valves in the superficial veins allow flow toward the heart and prevent backflow that gravity would tend to cause. The penetrating veins have valves that allow flow from the superficial veins toward the deep veins. The deep veins have the advantage of the musculovenous pump to help propel blood toward the heart. When the muscles of the limb contract, they compress the veins and help to propel blood. Because the superficial veins lack this mechanism, the tendency for blood to pool in these veins is greater. Over time, the valves in the superficial veins may fail, and this contributes to the development of varicose veins in the lower limb.

Neck

The superficial veins of the neck are the external jugular vein and the anterior jugular vein (Fig. 43.3). The external jugular vein arises

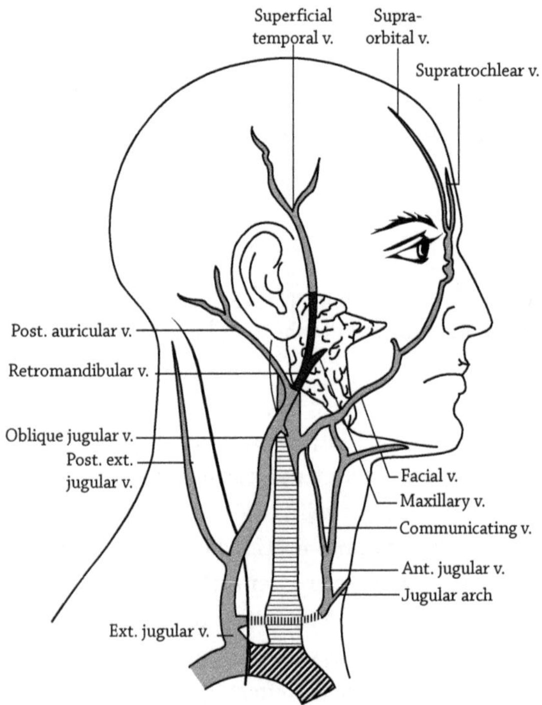

FIGURE 43.3

Superficial veins of the neck. Notice the external jugular vein entering the subclavian vein and the anterior jugular vein entering the external jugular vein. Ant., anterior; ext., external; post., posterior; v., vein.

from the union of the posterior auricular vein and a branch from the retromandibular vein. The external jugular vein descends in the superficial fascia of the neck on the superficial surface of the sternocleidomastoid muscle. It then pierces the investing fascia of the neck to enter the posterior triangle and drains into the subclavian vein. The anterior jugular vein is variable in its course. It usually forms from the union of small veins in the submental region and descends in the superficial fascia. It usually drains into the external jugular vein, or it may drain directly into the subclavian vein. Often, there is a jugular venous arch in the suprasternal space that unites the right and left anterior jugular veins (Fig. 43.3). Because of the superficial position of the external jugular vein, it is a useful indicator of elevated central venous pressure (e.g., in heart failure). When central venous pressure rises, the external jugular vein becomes engorged with blood and is visible on the side of the neck. Assessment of the external jugular vein is usually included as part of a physical examination.

Abdominal Wall

In the superficial fascia of the anterior abdominal wall are found the thoracoepigastric veins. These veins drain inferiorly into the femoral vein by way of the superficial epigastric vein and the superficial circumflex iliac vein. They anastomose superiorly with tributaries of the axillary vein. The thoracoepigastric veins can serve as an anastomotic communication between the superior vena cava and the inferior vena cava. These veins may enlarge and may become prominent on the anterior abdominal wall if there is obstruction to flow in either the superior or the inferior vena cava. Because there are also anastomotic connections with the paraumbilical veins from the portal venous system, enlargement of the thoracoepigastric veins can also occur with portal hypertension.

44

Scaphoid Fracture

A 28-year-old man was playing racquetball when he tripped over the foot of his partner and fell to the ground. He broke his fall with his outstretched right hand and immediately experienced pain in the region of his right wrist. He ended the game and went home. He told his wife about the incident and told her that he thought that he might have sprained his wrist. He iced the wrist and took some ibuprofen to reduce the moderate pain. As the evening progressed, he noticed some swelling in his wrist and some bruising at the base of his right thumb. The ibuprofen was somewhat effective in reducing the pain, but movement of the thumb or movement of the wrist increased the pain, as did gripping an object. When the pain did not subside by the next day, he called his primary care physician's office and went to see him the following day.

Examination

Examination of the patient's hand reveals minimal swelling and ecchymosis on the lateral side of the wrist in the region of the base of the thumb. He reports that the pain in his wrist is a 6 on a scale of 1 to 10, with 10 being most painful. The physician elicits tenderness in the anatomical snuff box (Fig. 44.1). Tenderness is also elicited when the physician extends the patient's wrist with one hand and presses with the other hand on the lateral side of the wrist at the level of the proximal wrist crease. The physician compresses the proximal phalanx of the thumb longitudinally along the long axis of the first metacarpal, and this too elicits tenderness in the wrist. The patient is sent for radiography of his wrist and is referred to an orthopedic surgeon. The radiologist reports that no fracture can be seen in the wrist, hand, or forearm.

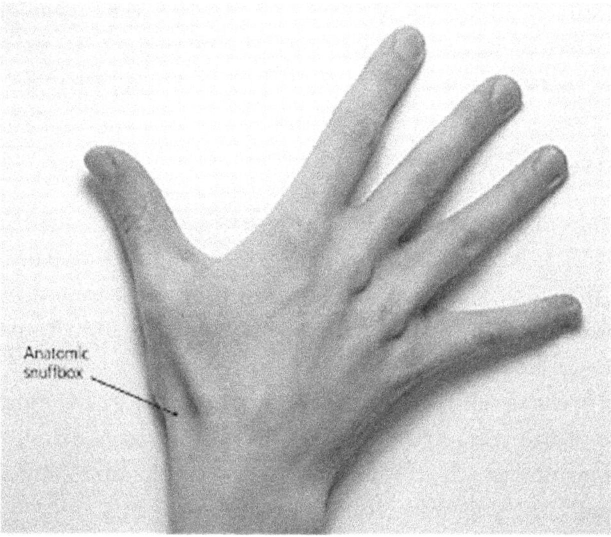

FIGURE 44.1

The anatomical snuff box is located between the tendons of the extensor pollicis longus and the extensor pollicis brevis. The scaphoid is in the floor of the snuff box.

Diagnosis

A tentative diagnosis of fracture of the scaphoid is made.

Therapy and Further Course

Based on the presumptive diagnosis of scaphoid fracture, a short arm thumb spica cast is applied to keep the wrist in radial deviation and 10 degrees of flexion. The forearm, wrist, and thumb are included in the cast. The remaining fingers are left mobile. The patient is instructed to try to keep his hand at or above the level of his heart as much as possible to minimize edema. The patient is scheduled for another radiograph of the wrist in 2 weeks.

The subsequent radiograph demonstrates a nondisplaced fracture of the midscaphoid. The patient is told that the wrist will remain casted for an additional 10 weeks. After 10 weeks, radiography reveals that the fracture is well healed. The patient is referred to physical therapy to restore mobility of the wrist and thumb.

Discussion

The scaphoid is the most radial of the proximal row of carpal bones (Fig. 44.2). It is the most frequently fractured of the carpals. From lateral to medial, the proximal row comprises the scaphoid, lunate, and triquetrum. The distal row comprises the trapezium, trapezoid, capitate, and hamate bones. The pisiform bone is a sesamoid bone located in the tendon of the flexor digitorum ulnaris on the anterior surface of the triquetrum. The scaphoid articulates distally with the trapezium, which articulates distally with the first metacarpal. Proximally, the scaphoid articulates with the radius.

Mechanism of Injury

The articulation between the carpus and the forearm is primarily between the scaphoid and lunate and the radius (Fig. 44.2). The ulna plays very

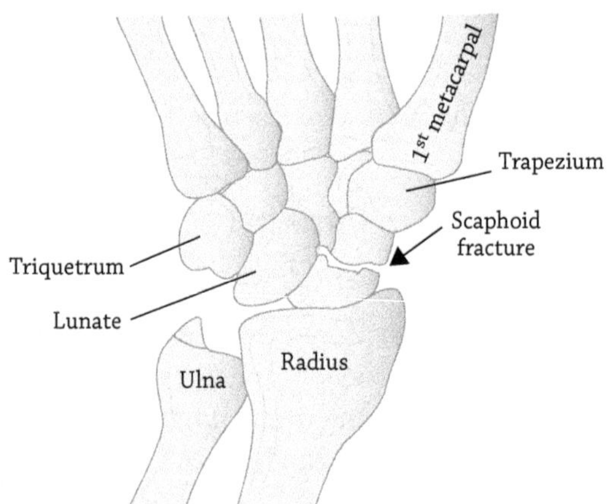

FIGURE 44.2

Fracture of the scaphoid.

little role in this articulation, and therefore the more medial carpal bones have little role. When this patient fell on his outstretched hand, the force of the ground against the hand was transmitted up along the upper limb. The transmission of force is from the hand to the radius, from the radius to the ulna, from the ulna to the humerus, and from the humerus to the shoulder girdle. The transmission from the hand to the radius is primarily across the radioscaphoid joint and the radiolunate joint; the transmission from the radius to the ulna is across the interosseous membrane; the transmission from the ulna to the humerus is across the humeroulnar joint of the elbow; and the transmission from the humerus to the shoulder girdle is across the glenohumeral joint.

Based on this pathway, it is clear why the common injuries resulting from a fall on an outstretched hand (FOOSH injuries) are scaphoid fractures, lunate dislocations, radial fractures, elbow dislocations, humeral fractures, shoulder dislocations, and shoulder separations. In the distal part of the upper limb, the scaphoid or distal radius may fracture or the lunate may dislocate. Scaphoid fractures account for 70% of carpal fractures. Although the other carpal bones do fracture, those fractures are typically caused by direct trauma rather than a FOOSH injury. Fractures of the scaphoid occur most commonly in young adults, whereas distal radial fractures (Colles' fractures) occur more frequently in children and older adults because the radius is weaker in these age groups. Lunate injuries may occur as a FOOSH injury, but this is typically an anterior dislocation with the lunate displaced into the carpal tunnel and possibly causing compression of the median nerve.

Diagnosis of a Scaphoid Fracture

Because of the many ligaments that tightly hold the carpal bones together, scaphoid fractures are commonly nondisplaced fractures. Because of the lack of displacement, identification of a fracture line on standard radiographs is often difficult or impossible. In this patient, initial radiographs did not identify the fracture. However, because of the bone resorption that occurs during the early phase of fracture healing, commonly a fracture line can be identified radiographically 10 to 14 days after the injury, as was the case in this patient. For this reason, the presumptive diagnosis of scaphoid fracture is typically made based on physical findings. If, after 2 weeks, radiography does not reveal a fracture but there remains a high suspicion of fracture, a magnetic resonance imaging study may be necessary to make the diagnosis.

The scaphoid is located in the floor of the anatomical snuff box (Fig. 44.1). The anatomical snuff box is the triangular recess found on the dorsum of the hand near the base of the thumb, between the tendons of the extensor pollicis longus and the extensor pollicis brevis. Tenderness in the floor of the snuff box is a classic finding in scaphoid fractures. However, although this is a very sensitive test, it is not a specific test, and there are many false positives. There are many causes of pain and tenderness in this region other than scaphoid fracture. The use of additional tests on physical examination can increase the specificity. The tubercle of the scaphoid can be palpated on the radial side of the dorsum of the wrist at the level of the proximal wrist crease when the wrist is extended. Elicitation of tenderness by this maneuver is additional evidence suggestive of scaphoid fracture. Because the first metacarpal articulates with the trapezium, which then articulates with the scaphoid, axial compression of the first metacarpal causes compression of the scaphoid and will elicit tenderness if there is a fracture. These three findings in our patient were highly suggestive of a scaphoid fracture even though there was no radiological evidence at that time. For this reason, the wrist and thumb were immobilized with a spica cast, and radiography of the wrist was repeated after 2 weeks to confirm that there was a fracture.

Blood Supply to the Scaphoid

The scaphoid receives its blood supply from branches of the radial artery, which enter the distal end of the scaphoid. The proximal end of the scaphoid receives its blood supply by way of branches that traverse within the scaphoid. When there is a fracture of the scaphoid, the proximal end of the scaphoid is at risk of being deprived of its blood supply and may be subjected to avascular necrosis. For this reason, it is important to immobilize the scaphoid as soon after the fracture as possible, to try to minimize the disruption of the blood supply to the proximal scaphoid. Therefore, suspected scaphoid fractures are immobilized until a definitive radiological diagnosis made.

Bone healing is very dependent on blood supply. The quality of healing is related to the quality of the blood supply. For this reason, the location of the fracture within the scaphoid is an important determinant of the likelihood of its healing and how long it will take to heal. Approximately 10% of scaphoid fractures occur in the distal third (where the blood supply is the best), and, if they are not displaced, almost all of these will heal in 6 to 8 weeks. Most scaphoid fractures occur in the central "waist" region of the bone, and 80% to 90% of these will heal in 8 to 12 weeks if nondisplaced. Approximately 20% of scaphoid fractures occur in the proximal third (where the blood supply is the poorest); only 60% to 70% of these will heal if nondisplaced, and some may require more than 20 weeks for union to occur.

When healing fails to occur, it is often necessary to surgically repair the fracture with the use of screws. Displaced fracture of the scaphoid increases the risk of avascular necrosis of the proximal pole, and surgical repair is usually indicated. If avascular necrosis occurs, the use of a vascularized bone graft may be necessary. Left untreated, avascular necrosis can lead to arthritis of the wrist with chronic pain and limitation of movement.

45

Carpal Tunnel Syndrome

A 55-year-old computer analyst who is right-hand dominant consults her physician, complaining of tingling and burning pain over the palmar aspect of her thumb, index, and middle fingers and the lateral side of the ring finger of her right hand. The symptoms began gradually over the last 2 years and lately have become more intense. They are most marked during the night, and they often awaken her from her sleep. She complains that when she gets up in the morning her fingers feel puffy and stiff, but her symptoms gradually subside during the morning. If she overworks, particularly if she does extensive keyboarding, the pain and discomfort increase again. Recently, she has experienced difficulties in holding tableware, resulting in frequent breakage. Also, she can hardly keep her grasp on a pencil. At the same time, she notices that the movements of her right thumb are not as strong as before. This change is accompanied by some wasting in the outer half of the ball (thenar eminence) of this thumb. For the last few weeks, she has also had occasional burning in the corresponding area of the thumb and fingers of her left hand.

Examination

On inspection of the patient's right hand, flattening of the outer half of the thenar eminence is noticed. On testing, there is loss of power and limitation of range of motion on abduction and opposition of the thumb. Diminished sensation (hypesthesia and hypalgesia) over the palmar aspect of the thumb, index, and middle fingers and the lateral aspect of the ring finger of the right hand is demonstrated by impaired appreciation of light touch and pin pricks and decreased differentiation between sharp and blunt stimuli. Sensation over the lateral aspect of the palm, including the thenar eminence, is unaffected. Pressure and tapping over the lateral portion of the flexor retinaculum cause tingling and a sensation of "pins and needles" in the involved fingers (Tinel's sign). On study of the motor functions of the muscles of the right forearm and fingers, no interference with active motion of the elbow, wrist, or fingers is observed (except for the described deficiencies in the motion of the thumb). Extreme flexion of the wrist, performed by flexing the wrists with the fingers hanging down and compressing the backs of the hands together (Phalen's test), reproduces the typical pain in the lateral 3½ digits of her hand.

Diagnosis

Carpal tunnel syndrome is diagnosed and is confirmed by electrodiagnostic testing.

Therapy and Further Course

Conservative treatment with immobilization of the wrist during the night by splinting and physical therapy with heat, massage, and mild exercises are tried for several weeks but have no effect. Antiinflammatory treatment with hydrocortisone injections also does not lead to any improvement. Therefore, surgical treatment consisting of division of the flexor retinaculum is agreed on.

With the patient under local anesthesia and a tourniquet around the upper arm to obtain a bloodless surgical field, the flexor retinaculum is divided with attention to and avoidance of the superficial palmar vascular arch and the motor or recurrent branch of the median nerve. At operation, the synovial sheath of the flexor tendons beneath the flexor retinaculum appears swollen, with the median nerve somewhat flattened and compressed in the narrowest part of the carpal tunnel. This decompression operation results in a dramatic disappearance of her pain and other subjective symptoms and gradual cessation of the deficiencies in the next few months. Motor recovery also occurs, although somewhat later. Because the patient is right-handed and can now use her dominant hand without hindrance, the symptoms on the left side also gradually subside.

Discussion

Sensory Deficiencies

This patient presents the subjective symptoms of paresthesias (tingling and numbness) and pain in the lateral 3½ digits of her right hand as well as the objective signs of sensory loss, including loss of pain perception on stimulation over approximately the same cutaneous area. The apparent contradictory finding of spontaneous pain and interference with pain perception in approximately the same area should be understood. The former is an irritative phenomenon caused by stimulation of certain sensory nerve fibers; the latter is an indication of damage and loss of function of certain other sensory fibers. This combination occurs frequently in neurological disorders. In carpal tunnel syndrome, the larger, myelinated fibers that supply voluntary muscle and those that carry tactile discrimination impulses are more affected than the smaller, unmyelinated fibers that transmit pain.

Motor Deficits

There is a loss of motor function of the abductor pollicis brevis and opponens pollicis combined with wasting at the site of these two muscles in the lateral part of the ball of the right thumb. Because it is the function of the abductor pollicis brevis to pull the thumb away from the palm in a plane at right angles to it, the patient is asked to point her thumb toward the ceiling against resistance while her forearm is supine and the dorsum of her hand is resting on a table. The opponens pollicis pulls the thumb across the hand in an arch, rotating it at the same time so that at the end of the motion the palmar surfaces of the thumb and little finger are in opposition to each other. Testing is done by having the patient execute this motion against the resistance of the examiner's outstretched finger.

Site of the Lesion

Where, then, is the site of the lesion that causes the combined sensory and motor deficits? We can exclude systemic diseases of the central nervous system, such as multiple sclerosis, which cause more widespread impairments than are present in this case. We can likewise rule out involvement of a spinal nerve before its division into ventral and dorsal rami at the site of the intervertebral foramen, because there is no indication of sensory or motor deficiencies on the posterior aspect of the trunk supplied by dorsal rami.

By contrast, it might be tempting in this case to place the lesion in one or more ventral rami in the neck, where they form the roots and trunks of the brachial plexus. What roots or trunks of the brachial plexus would have to be involved? A dermatome chart would place the sensory deficiencies in the ventral rami of C6 and C7, which form part of the upper and all of the middle trunk of the brachial plexus. However, the muscles affected in this patient, the abductor pollicis brevis and the opponens pollicis, receive their motor supply from segments C8 and T1 by way of the median nerve. A widespread lesion involving practically all the roots of the brachial plexus from C6 to T1 would be required to accommodate all the deficits in this case. In view of the limited extent of the neurological defect, this seems very unlikely. Consequently, it must be assumed that the lesion is more peripheral than the brachial plexus.

The median nerve supplies the two affected muscles and provides sensory innervations to the skin of the lateral 3½ digits on their palmar aspects.

Level of Median Nerve Involvement

To identify the level of the median nerve where the lesion has occurred, we must locate a site where the lesion would cause the described impairments but leave the other important motor and sensory functions of the median nerve intact.

Although the median nerve does not innervate any muscles in the arm, in the forearm it supplies the pronators of the forearm, the flexors of the wrist (with the exception of the flexor carpi ulnaris), and the long flexors of the fingers (with the exception of the medial half of the flexor digitorum profundus). Because the muscles of the forearm supplied by the median nerve display normal function in this patient, the lesion must be located distal to the origin of the branches to these muscles but proximal to the origin of the motor nerve to the opponens pollicis and the abductor pollicis brevis. This motor nerve is often called the recurrent branch of the median nerve; it leaves the lateral side of the median nerve as the latter emerges distally from beneath the flexor retinaculum (Fig. 45.1). It runs superficial to or through the substance of the flexor pollicis brevis to supply the two involved muscles of the thumb. The same nerve also supplies the superficial portion of the flexor pollicis brevis, but loss of function of the flexor pollicis brevis cannot be demonstrated by ordinary clinical testing. The other muscles of the hand that are innervated by the median nerve are the lateral two lumbrical muscles. These receive their nerve supply from the terminal portion of the median nerve but via the first two common palmar digital branches, which are otherwise sensory nerves.

The action of other muscles, such as the interossei, which are supplied by the ulnar nerve, obscures the deficiency of the lumbrical muscles. By contrast, clinical experience indicates that the abducting action of the abductor pollicis longus, innervated by the radial nerve, is not usually strong enough to compensate for the paralyzed abductor pollicis brevis.

Can we derive similar localizing indications from the sensory deficiencies in this case? Sensation over the lateral aspect of the palm and the thenar eminence is unaffected. This region of skin receives its sensory innervations from the palmar cutaneous branch, which arises from the median nerve just proximal to the upper margin of the flexor retinaculum (Fig. 45.1). By contrast, the terminal sensory branches of the median nerve supply the skin of the lateral 3½ digits that display the sensory loss. Therefore, we can pinpoint the lesion in that portion of the median nerve located distal to the origin of the unaffected palmar cutaneous branch but above its terminal division into the three common palmar digital branches.

In summary, this lesion of the median nerve must be located where the nerve runs through the carpal tunnel. This common site for median nerve involvement has been known to clinicians since the early 1950s as the site of carpal tunnel syndrome.

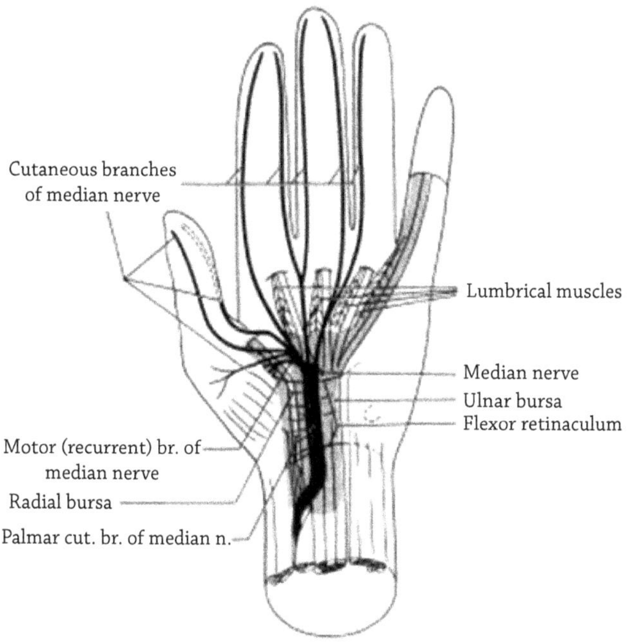

FIGURE 45.1

The median nerve in the carpal tunnel and its distribution in the palm of the hand. br., branch; cut., cutaneous; n., nerve.

Definition and Contents of the Carpal Tunnel

The carpal tunnel is a fibro-osseous canal, the trough of which is formed by the palmar concavity of the carpal bones; its roof consists of the flexor retinaculum—a rigid, inelastic ligament that attaches to the scaphoid and trapezium on the lateral side and to the pisiform and hook of the hamate on the medial side. The distal of the two creases on the palmar aspect of the wrist marks the proximal margin of the flexor retinaculum. The distal margin is at the level of the abducted and extended thumb. The retinaculum is 2 to 3 cm long and almost as wide. A rectangular postage stamp of this size, laid with its narrower edge on the distal crease, would outline the area occupied by the retinaculum.

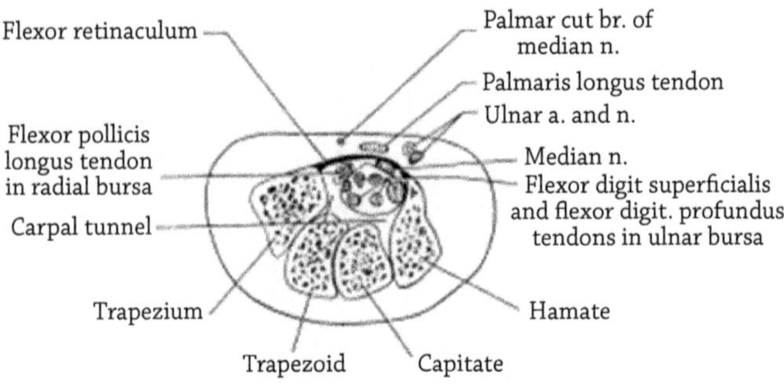

FIGURE 45.2

Proximal view of the left carpal tunnel shows structures in the tunnel and those superficial to the flexor retinaculum. a., artery; br., branch; cut., cutaneous; digit., digitorum; n., nerve.

The contents of the carpal tunnel, or carpal canal, are the tendon of the flexor pollicis longus in its synovial sheath (also called the radial bursa), the tendons of the flexor digitorum superficialis and the flexor digitorum profundus in their common synovial sheath (the so-called ulnar bursa), and the median nerve (Figs. 45.1 and 45.2). The latter, with which we are concerned in this case, lies superficial to the two most lateral tendon slips of the flexor digitorum superficialis and against the deep surface of the flexor retinaculum. Although the median nerve innervates the muscles whose tendons are contained within the carpal canal, it does so in the forearm, well proximal to the carpal tunnel.

Reasons for Compression of Median Nerve

The carpel tunnel, being occupied by the structures listed and covered by a rigid ligament, appears crowded as it is. Therefore, it is not surprising that any space-occupying alteration within the canal, such as a chronic thickening of the synovial sheath of the common flexor tendons, leads to compression of the median nerve. This would explain the clinical signs and symptoms of irritation and impairment of the median nerve described in our case.

The thickening of the synovial sac of the common flexor tendon sheath, a tenosynovitis, is probably caused in this patient by occupational strain and repetitive movement of these tendons during keyboarding. It is not surprising that the symptoms are aggravated by motions that increase the pressure within the tunnel, such as hyperflexion and hyperextension. Hormonal disturbances, such as myxedema or acromegaly, that lead to fluid accumulation and deposition of additional connective tissue in the carpal tunnel also compress the median nerve. Fluid retention, which often accompanies pregnancy, may have the same effect, and it is probably the hormonal changes of menopause that account for the high frequency of carpal tunnel syndrome in perimenopausal women. Increase in clinical symptoms during the night can be explained on the basis of venous stasis during rest and flexion of the relaxed wrist while sleeping. For this reason, use of a splint to maintain the wrist in a slightly extended position during sleep often offers relief to a patient with carpal tunnel syndrome.

Some authors have explained the median nerve deficiency not by direct compression of the nerve itself but rather by interference with its blood supply as a result of pressure on the vasa nervorum. Others ascribe the nerve symptoms to increase in endoneural and perineural connective tissue within the nerve, such as might occur in older age groups or through possible scarring and shrinkage of the endoneural supporting tissue. Often more than one mechanism is responsible.

Surgically Endangered Structures Superficial to the Flexor Retinaculum

Structures that pass superficial to the flexor retinaculum must be protected during surgical approach to the retinaculum. The ulnar artery and the superficial branch of the radial artery both pass superficial to the flexor retinaculum. These arteries join in the hand to form the superficial palmar arch. The palmar branch of the median nerve arises from the median nerve before that nerve passes into the carpal tunnel. The palmar branch then passes superficial to the flexor retinaculum. Because the palmar branch is not in the carpal tunnel, and because it provides sensory innervations to the skin of the palm in the lateral portion of the hand, this region does not display sensory disturbance in our patient. The superficial branch of the ulnar nerve also passes superficial to the flexor retinaculum to enter the medial portion of the hand and provide sensory innervations to the skin of the palm and medial 1½ digits. The recurrent motor branch of the median nerve arises from the median nerve distal to the flexor retinaculum and then turns proximally to pass superficial to the retinaculum and innervate the thenar muscles. Care must be taken to avoid injury to this important nerve.

Other Nerve Entrapments

There are other areas where, because of their anatomical configurations, nerves can become entrapped. The cause is usually compression of a nerve where it runs through an inelastic fibrous ring or a rigid fibro-osseous tunnel. The compression may result from a local condition (e.g., callus formation after fracture), bony deformity, rheumatoid arthritis, osteoarthritis, bursitis, or synovitis with swelling. Systemic diseases such as hypothyroidism, acromegaly, or collagen disorders may also cause nerve compression by fluid accumulation and deposition of connective tissue in an already crowded space.

In addition to the carpal tunnel, compression may occur where the median nerve passes between the two heads of the pronator teres and dips under a fibrous band that connects the two heads of the flexor digitorum superficialis. The ulnar nerve may become entrapped at the wrist in a trough where it passes between the pisiform and the hook of hamate. The ulnar nerve may also be compressed in the ulnar groove behind the medial epicondyle. Other entrapment neuropathies, as these conditions are called, occur in the posterior interosseous branch of the radial nerve as it passes through the supinator muscle, in the suprascapular nerve as it passes between the transverse ligament and the scapular notch, in the common and superficial fibular nerves, and in the tibial nerve beneath the flexor retinaculum in the so-called tarsal tunnel.

Unit VI

Review Questions

The number in parentheses is a reference to the page on which information about the question may be found.

1. What are the two articulations of the clavicle?
The clavicle articulates medially at the sternoclavicular joint and laterally at the acromioclavicular joint. The sternoclavicular joint is extremely stable because of its strong anterior and posterior sternoclavicular ligaments and the costoclavicular ligament. The acromioclavicular is much less stable and frequently dislocates (shoulder separation). The intrinsic ligament of this joint is the acromioclavicular ligament. This joint is also stabilized by the coracoclavicular ligament, which binds the clavicle to the coracoid process. (363)

2. What muscles attach to the clavicle?
The clavicle serves as a bony attachment for the subclavius muscle, the sternocleidomastoid muscle, the pectoralis major muscle, and the deltoid muscle. The upward pull of the sternocleidomastoid muscle on the medial portion of the clavicle and the downward pull of the deltoid muscle on the lateral portion of the clavicle account, in part, for the displacement that is typically seen with a clavicular fracture. (364–365)

3. What is the scalene triangle, and what passes through it?
The scalene triangle is formed by the anterior scalene muscle, the middle scalene muscle ,and the first rib. The roots of the brachial plexus and the subclavian artery pass through the triangle. Narrowing of this triangle can cause compression of the artery and nerves found within it. (370)

4. What muscles receive their innervation from motor nerve fibers in the inferior trunk of the brachial plexus?
The inferior trunk of the brachial plexus contains nerve fibers from spinal levels C8 and T1. These motor fibers innervate muscles in the distal limb (i.e., hand muscles). Intrinsic hand muscles include the thenar muscles, the hypothenar muscles, the interosseous muscles, the adductor pollicis muscle, and the lumbrical muscles. (368)

5. What regions of skin receive their sensory innervation from sensory nerve fibers in the inferior trunk of the brachial plexus?
The inferior trunk of the brachial plexus contains nerve fibers from spinal levels C8 and T1. These sensory nerve fibers provide innervation to the C8 and T1 dermatomes. The C8 dermatome is on the medial side of the hand and the medial side of the distal forearm. The T1 dermatome is on the medial side of the proximal forearm and the medial side of the arm. (368)

6. What is the origin of the vertebral artery, and what regions does it supply?
The vertebral artery is the first branch of the subclavian artery. It ascends through the neck, passing through the transverse foramina of the upper six cervical vertebrae, then passes through the foramen magnum and meets with its contralateral counterpart to form the basilar artery. The vertebral artery supplies the brain stem, the cerebellum, and the occipital lobe of the brain. (374)

7. What is the origin of the subclavian artery?
The left subclavian artery is a direct branch of the aortic arch. The right subclavian artery is a branch of the brachiocephalic trunk, which is a branch of the aortic arch. Both subclavian arteries leave the thorax by passing over the first rib and under the clavicle to enter the root of the neck. They then pass downward to enter the axilla. While in the neck, the subclavian gives rise to several branches, including the vertebral artery, the internal thoracic artery, the thyrocervical trunk, and the costocervical trunk. (374)

8. What are the locations of the brachial artery and median nerve in the region of the elbow?
As the brachial artery and median nerve cross the anterior side of the elbow, they are located immediately medial to the tendon of the biceps brachii tendon. The brachial artery is medial to the tendon, and the median nerve is medial to the artery. The artery and nerve then pass deep to the bicipital aponeurosis. (379)

9. Where can the radial pulse and ulnar pulse be palpated?
The pulse of the radial artery can be palpated immediately proximal to the wrist on the ventral side of the forearm, just lateral to the flexor carpi radialis tendon. The artery can be compressed against the radius at this location. The pulse of the ulnar artery can be palpated on the ventral side of the carpus, immediately lateral to the pisiform bone; at that location it can be compressed against the flexor retinaculum. The ulnar pulse can also be palpated in the distal forearm, on the lateral side of the flexor carpi ulnaris tendon. At that location it can be compressed against the ulna. (379–380)

10. What arteries provide collateral pathways for arterial circulation around the elbow?
There are collateral pathways between the brachial artery and the ulnar artery by way of the superior and inferior ulnar collateral arteries, which are branches of the brachial artery, and the anterior and posterior ulnar recurrent arteries, which are branches of the ulnar artery. There is collateral pathway between the profunda brachii artery and the radial artery by way of the radial collateral artery, which is a branch of the profunda brachiii artery, and the radial recurrent artery, which is a branch of the radial artery. There is a collateral pathway between the profunda brachii artery and the ulnar artery by way of the middle collateral artery, which is a branch of the profunda brachii artery, and the interosseous recurrent artery, which is a branch of the posterior interosseous artery, which is a branch of the common interosseous artery, which is a branch of the ulnar artery. (380)

11. What is the distribution of motor innervation of the median nerve?
The median nerve provides motor innervation to all of the muscles of the anterior compartment of the forearm except the flexor carpi ulnaris and the medial half of the flexor digitorum profundus, which are innervated by the ulnar nerve. In the hand, the median nerve innervates all of the thenar muscles as well as the two most radial lumbrical muscles. (382)

12. What are the two major superficial veins in the upper limb, and into what deep veins do they drain?
The two major superficial veins are the cephalic vein and the basilic vein. The cephalic vein drains into the axillary vein. The basilic vein joins with the brachial vein to form the axillary vein. (387)

13. What are the two major superficial veins in the lower limb, and into what deep veins do they drain?
The two major superficial veins are the long saphenous and the short saphenous veins. The long saphenous vein drains into the femoral vein. The short saphenous vein drains into the popliteal vein. (388–389)

14. In the antecubital fossa, what is the relationship between the median cubital vein and the brachial artery?
The median cubital vein is in the superficial fascial. It crosses the antecubital fossa and connects the cephalic vein to the basilic vein. It lies superficial to the bicipital aponeurosis. The brachial artery lies deep to the bicipital aponeurosis on the medial side of the biceps brachii tendon. For this reason, when blood is drawn from the median cubital vein, it should be done on the lateral side of the biceps brachii tendon. (388)

15. Dilation of the thoracoepigastric veins indicates that blood is being shunted through these veins between other veins. From what other veins is this blood being shunting?
The thoracoepigastric veins communicate with branches of the superior vena cava, the inferior vena cava, and the portal vein. If either vena cava is obstructed, blood can be shunted into the other vena cava through

these veins. If there is an obstruction of flow through the portal vein or the liver, blood can be shunted from the portal system into the caval system through these veins. (391)

16. What are the carpal bones?
The carpal bones are found in two rows. The proximal row, from lateral to medial, comprises the scaphoid, the lunate, and the triquetrum. The distal row, from lateral to medial, comprises the trapezium, the trapezoid, the capitate, and the hamate. Another bone, included with the carpal bones, is the pisiform, which is a sesamoid bone within the tendon of the flexor digitorum ulnaris that articulates on the anterior surface of the triquetrum. (394)

17. What is the source of blood supply for the scaphoid?
The scaphoid receives its blood supply from branches of the radial artery. These branches all enter the distal end of the scaphoid. The proximal end of the scaphoid receives its blood supply from branches that traverse through the scaphoid from the distal end to the proximal end. If there is a fracture in the midregion of the scaphoid, the blood supply to the proximal end is compromised and necrosis may occur. (396–397)

18. How is force transmitted from the hand to the proximal upper limb?
Force that is applied to the hand is transmitted to the radius across the scaphoid and lunate bones, which form the raiocarpal joint with the radius. The force is transmitted from the radius to the ulna across the interosseous membrane. From the ulna, the force is transmitted to the humerus across the humeroulnar joint at the elbow. It is then transmitted from the humerus to the shoulder girdle across the glenohumeral joint at the shoulder. (395)

19. What is the carpal tunnel, and what passes through it?
The carpal tunnel is the space bounded by the carpal bones and the flexor retinaculum. The carpal bones form the posterior, lateral, and medial walls of the tunnel; the flexor retinaculum forms the anterior wall. Passing through the tunnel are the tendons of the flexor digitorum

superficialis, flexor digitorum profundus, and the flexor pollicis longus, which are covered by their synovial tendon sheaths, and the median nerve. (403–404)

20. Which muscles in the hand receive their motor innervation from the recurrent branch of the median nerve?
The recurrent branch arises from the median nerve after it has passed through the carpal tunnel. The recurrent branch innervates the muscles of the thenar compartment: abductor pollicis brevis, flexor pollicis brevis, and opponens pollicis. It does not provide any cutaneous sensory innervation. (402)

21. What region of the hand receives its cutaneous sensory innervation from the median nerve?
Before it passes through the carpal tunnel, the median nerve gives rise to a palmar cutaneous branch. This branch provides sensory innervation to the skin of the lateral portion of the proximal palm. After passing through the carpal tunnel, the median nerve divides into digital branches that provide sensory innervation to the skin of the palmar surfaces of the lateral 3½ digits as well as the corresponding region of the distal palm. (402)

UNIT VII

Lower Limb

46

Intragluteal Injection

A 39-year-old carpenter, who is a recovering alcoholic, is being supported in outpatient rehabilitation by intragluteal injection of naltrexone, an opioid antagonist, every 4 weeks. Immediately after the last injection into his right buttock, he complained of numbness, tingling, and burning in his right leg down to his toes. The next day, he developed a footdrop and was hospitalized.

Examination

On examination at the hospital, inspection of the right gluteal region shows an injection mark approximately over the course of the right sciatic nerve slightly above the gluteal fold. The sensory loss involves the outer side of the right calf and the dorsum of the right foot. On the motor side, there is an inability to dorsiflex the ankle or to evert the foot, with noticeable footdrop. There is also difficulty in extending the toes. When walking, the patient drags the front and the outer margin of his right foot.

Diagnosis

The diagnosis is sciatic nerve injury after intramuscular injections.

Therapy and Further Course

The patient is given deep heat followed by electrical stimulation of the involved muscles and reeducation exercises by the department of physical medicine and rehabilitation. After 4 months, he has essentially regained the motor functions of his right leg but still shows some sensory deficits.

Discussion

At the level of the gluteal fold, the sciatic nerve passes approximately midway between the greater trochanter and the ischial tuberosity. Of the two components of the sciatic nerve, the tibial nerve and the common fibular (peroneal) nerve, the common fibular seems to be exclusively involved in this case. The greater susceptibility of the common fibular nerve in injuries of the sciatic nerve is a characteristic feature that has often been observed. It is explained by the fact that the common fibular component is located more superficially. In addition, the more lateral location of this nerve makes it more vulnerable to injuries by intramuscular injection, which should be directed into the upper lateral quadrant of the gluteal region.

The sciatic nerve usually enters the gluteal region by passing through the greater sciatic foramen inferior to the piriformis muscle. In 15% of cases, however, the common fibular division of the sciatic nerve passes above or through the piriformis muscle instead of below it, increasing the danger to this division.

Neurological Deficiencies

The sensory deficit over the lateral portion of the calf is accounted for by the lateral sural cutaneous nerve (a branch of the common fibular nerve) and the superficial fibular nerve, which provide this area with sensory fibers. The sensory deficit on the dorsum of the foot is accounted for by cutaneous branches of the superficial fibular nerve, which transmit sensory impulses from the dorsum of the foot. The nerve responsible for dorsiflexion of the foot and extension of the toes is the deep fibular nerve, which innervates the dorsiflexors of the foot and the extensors of the toes in the anterior compartment of the leg. The nerve that innervates the main evertors of the foot (the fibularis longus and fibularis brevis muscles) is the superficial fibular nerve. Because the neurological deficits in this patient involve functions of the superficial and deep fibular nerves, the nerve that is injured is most likely the common fibular nerve.

Applied Anatomy of Intragluteal Injections

The gluteal region is a common site for intramuscular injection of drugs. Intramuscular rather than intravenous injections are given when prolonged action is preferred to immediate effect. Intramuscular injections are also more easily administered and are often better tolerated. In addition, oily preparations cannot be injected directly into the bloodstream but can be given intramuscularly. Irritant drugs are excluded from the otherwise simpler subcutaneous application, where they may cause sloughing or abscess formation. The rich blood supply of the superior and inferior gluteal arteries to the large gluteal musculature makes this area a favorable site of parenteral (nongastrointestinal) administration of drugs.

How can the inadvertent application of drugs into the subcutaneous tissue or the even more dangerous penetration of the drugs into the gluteal vessels be avoided? Keep in mind that the subcutaneous adipose layer over the gluteal area varies greatly in thickness and may reach a depth of 6.5 cm, particularly in women. The injection needle must penetrate beyond this layer if painful indurations and abscesses are to be avoided. Intravenous application into one of the gluteal veins should be guarded against by slightly withdrawing the plunger of the syringe and inspecting the syringe for blood. If an oily suspension were to be injected into one of the thin-walled gluteal veins, such an embolus would traverse the gluteal vein into the internal and common iliac veins, and then into the inferior vena cava, the right atrium and right ventricle, and the pulmonary artery to be arrested in the pulmonary circulation.

If, as stipulated, the injection is made into the upper outer quadrant of the gluteal region, it will be given into either the gluteus maximus or the gluteus medius, depending on whether the solution is injected into the lower inner portion or the upper outer portion of this quadrant (Fig. 46.1). To avoid injury to the sciatic nerve, the needle should not be directed downward and medially.

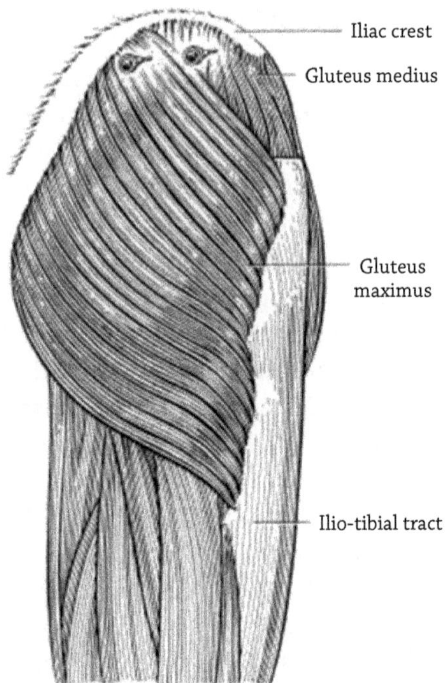

FIGURE 46.1

Superficial aspect of the musculature of the gluteal region. Two needles for intramuscular injection are shown in place in the upper outer quadrant of the gluteus maximus and gluteus medius.

Injury to Superior and Inferior Gluteal Nerves

Two other motor nerves, the superior and inferior gluteal nerves, are occasionally damaged by intragluteal injection. Both of these nerves exit the pelvis through the greater sciatic foramen, most of which is occupied by the piriformis muscle. The superior gluteal nerve and vessels exit through the foramen immediately superior to the piriformis, whereas the inferior gluteal nerve and vessels exit immediately inferior to the piriformis. The superior gluteal nerve innervates the gluteus medius and minimus and runs in the plane between these two muscles (Fig. 46.2). Because of the deep location

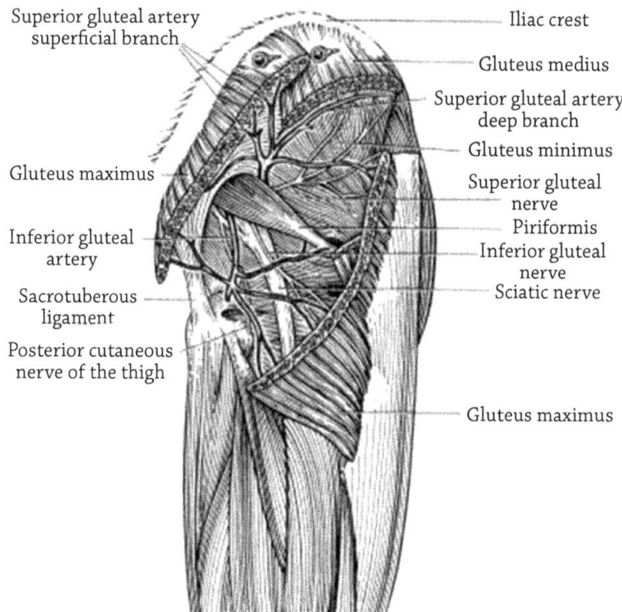

FIGURE 46.2

Anatomy of the gluteal area, with needles shown in place, after partial section of the gluteus maximus and medius. Shown are the sciatic nerve and the superior and inferior gluteal arteries and nerves. Notice that both gluteal arteries, but only the inferior gluteal nerve, supply the gluteus maximus. The superior gluteal nerve lies on the deep aspect of the gluteus medius, between it and the gluteus minimus, and supplies both of those muscles.

of this nerve and because it branches near its exit from the pelvis, this nerve is rarely injured in intragluteal injection, even though it is in the upper outer quadrant where the injection is done. In contrast, the superior gluteal vessels have more superficial branches in the plane between the gluteus maximus and gluteus medius, and these vessels may be injured by intramuscular injection in this region.

The inferior gluteal nerve may likewise be damaged in improperly located injections. This nerve is the only innervation for the gluteus maximus muscle. This muscle receives its blood supply from branches of both the inferior and the superior gluteal vessels, and these branches may also be injured in intragluteal injections (Fig. 46.2).

Other Locations of Intramuscular Injections

Other muscle sites that have been recommended for intramuscular injections are the vastus lateralis of the quadriceps femoris, the deltoid, and the more anterior aspects of the gluteus medius and gluteus minimus, inferior and posterior to the anterior superior spine of the ilium.

47

Femoral Neck Fracture

A 72-year-old widow who lives with her oldest son is found on the floor of her bedroom, unable to rise. She tells her son that she slipped on a rug and fell to the floor. She complains of severe pain in her right hip and is unable to stand. Because no physician is immediately available, an ambulance is called, and she is taken to the hospital on a stretcher. On arrival, she is given intravenous morphine to reduce her pain and is made more comfortable by immobilization of her limb with pillows and sandbags and by gentle longitudinal traction. She has no significant past medical or surgical history and takes no medications.

Examination

The patient is a frail, elderly woman in mild distress. Her vital signs are stable, with a blood pressure of 139/80 mm Hg and a heart rate of 89 bpm. A primary survey and secondary survey are performed to assess her injuries. Head, neck, chest, and abdominal examinations are unremarkable. Musculoskeletal examination reveals that her right leg is externally rotated and shortened. This is confirmed by measuring the distance between the anterior superior iliac spine and the distal tip of the medial malleolus of the tibia and comparing the result with that obtained in the left leg. There is shortening of her right leg by 4 cm. The greater trochanter on the right side appears higher and more prominent than on the left. No abrasions or hematomas are evident. On palpation, there is tenderness in the femoral triangle in front of the right hip joint. She is in significant pain, despite the morphine, and is unable to lift her right heel from the stretcher. No numbness or paresthesias are detected. Her extremities are warm and well perfused. The femoral, popliteal, dorsalis pedis, and posterior tibial arteries are palpable and are equal (2+) bilaterally.

Diagnosis

A presumptive diagnosis of fracture through the femoral neck (commonly referred to as hip fracture) is made. As with any suspected femoral neck fracture, anteroposterior and lateral radiographs are taken. Close comparison with the contralateral hip radiographs is important. This procedure confirms the diagnosis and demonstrates the fracture just below the head of the femur (subcapital). The neck of the femur is anteriorly angulated, and the angle between the head and neck of the femur and the shaft of the femur is decreased (varus deformity). The neck and shaft are externally rotated, and the fragments overlap with the neck and shaft, having moved superiorly against the head (Fig. 47.1). The pelvic skeleton and femur show marked demineralization (osteoporosis).

Therapy and Further Course

In this aged patient, who is frail, there are substantial risks associated with attempts at closed reduction of this fracture and the attendant extended periods of immobilization and limited mobility. These risks include bed sores, pneumonia, deep venous thrombosis, and pulmonary embolism with possible fatal outcome. In addition, because the head of the femur, when separated from its neck, has a poor blood supply left in the subcapital location of the fracture (10–30% of cases), nonunion of the fragments and late necrosis may develop. These complications frequently lead to secondary degenerative osteoarthritis, resulting in a painful and disabled hip. Finally, the degree of displacement of the bony fragments provides an additional contraindication to nonoperative management.

Therefore, in view of the poor prognosis of conservative treatment in this patient, surgery with removal of the femoral head and total hip prosthetic replacement is recommended. Recent

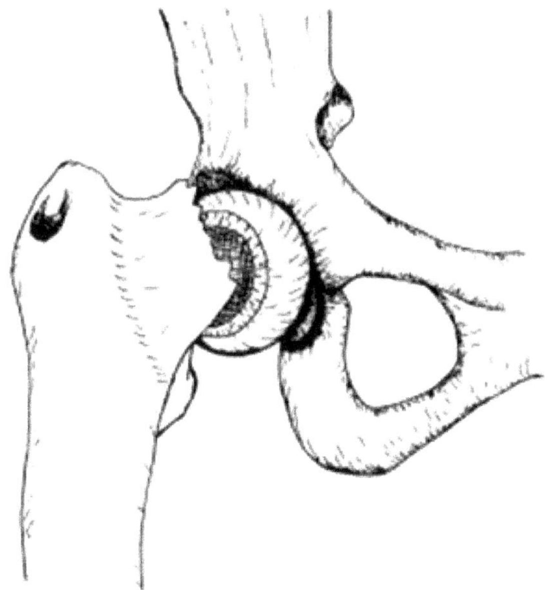

FIGURE 47.1

Intracapsular subcapital fracture through the neck of the femur. The neck of the femur points forward, and the neck and shaft are externally rotated. Notice the decrease in the angle between the head and the shaft of the femur (varus deformity).

data support this decision and indicate that total hip replacement in elderly patients with good cognitive function and a more independent lifestyle is associated with improved quality of life and lower morbidity compared with open reduction and external fixation of the fracture.

With the patient under spinal anesthesia, the hip is approached by an inferolateral skin and fascial incision through the lower part of the buttock. The iliotibial tract is identified, and the gluteus maximus is split in the direction of its fibers by blunt dissection. A 5-cm vertical incision is made to separate the gluteus maximus from its insertion into the iliotibial tract and give better access to the posterior aspect of the hip joint. The upper and lower portions of this muscle are separated and retracted, exposing the sciatic nerve and the lateral rotators of the hip. The latter are divided close to their insertion into the greater trochanter. After removal of the overlying fat, the capsule is incised and partly reflected. The head of the femur is dislodged out of the acetabulum and removed, and the ligament of the head is ligated and excised. The neck of the femur is sawed across, and the stem of a properly fitted titanium prosthesis is inserted into the marrow cavity almost halfway down the femoral shaft to anchor the head. The stem of the prosthesis is fenestrated (has windows), and bits of cancellous bone, removed from the upper end of the femur, are placed in these windows as bone grafts. It is expected that these bone chips will become dense new osseous tissue, locking the prosthesis in place and lending strength and stability to the femoral shaft for its weight-bearing function. Care is taken to preserve the normal forward angle of the neck and head. A tight fit of the prosthesis is obtained after the artificial head is moved into place. The acetabulum is enlarged to accommodate a replacement plastic acetabular cup, which is put into place.

The operation lasts 3 hours, and the patient is able to sit up in bed and eat on the afternoon of the day of surgery. Physical therapy is started on the next day. Two days after the surgery, the patient is walking with the help of a walker, and she leaves the hospital after 5 days. She is cautioned to use a walker, and only partial weight bearing is permitted for about 6 weeks. She is also warned not to expose her leg to too much strain and to avoid heavy weight gain.

On reexamination after 1 year, the patient reports that she can do her own housework and can walk with no limp or pain. She has practically normal function of her hip.

Discussion

Anatomy of Intracapsular and Extracapsular Fractures of the Neck of the Femur

Femoral neck fracture is a very common clinical condition in elderly patients, particularly women. Approximately 350,000 hip fractures occur annually in the United States in people older than 65 years of age, and 75% of these patients are women. Approximately 20% of hip fracture patients die within 1 year after the fracture, often as a result of complications cited earlier. With the aging population, it is estimated that there will be more than 500,000 hip fractures annually by the year 2040. The use of hip fixation and hip replacement procedures and concomitant early ambulation are expected to reduce the morbidity and mortality associated with hip fractures.

As described earlier, the rotational strain in slipping has caused a fracture with complete separation of the fragments. The fracture line is located just below the head of the femur, at the highest point of the neck (subcapital), and is therefore completely intracapsular. The fibrous joint capsule, lined by synovial membrane, arises from the margins of the acetabulum of the hip bone and extends, sleevelike, downward and laterally around the neck of the femur to attach near the intertrochanteric line anteriorly and near the middle of the neck posteriorly, a fingerbreadth above the posteriorly located intertrochanteric crest. From the attachments of the capsule, the synovial membrane is reflected onto the neck and up to the margin of the articular cartilage, which, as in all synovial joints, is not covered by synovial membrane.

Because the more lateral or distal portions of the posterior aspect of the femoral neck are outside the capsule, more distal neck fractures, in contrast to the injury in this case, may be partly intracapsular and partly extracapsular. Intertrochanteric fractures are always extracapsular.

Anatomy of Displacement of the Fragments

Typically in patients with femoral neck fractures, as in this case, the leg is externally rotated by the pull of the lateral rotators and the weight of the leg and foot. The lateral rotators of the hip are the piriformis, the obturator internus and obturator externus, the superior and inferior gemelli, the quadratus femoris, and the gluteus maximus. The external rotators are much more powerful than the internal rotators, which explains the position of the leg.

How do we explain the shortening of the extremity in this case? The force of the injury itself may drive the distal fragment superiorly, but in general it is muscle pull that leads to this result. The muscles whose pull causes shortening of the leg include the powerful gluteal muscles, the hamstrings, and the adductors, as well as the iliopsoas and other flexors of the thigh that arise from the pelvis or lumbar vertebral column above the fracture line and insert into the distal fragment. Their pull results in upward displacement of the lower fragment and shortening of the leg.

Angles of Inclination and Declination

Muscle pull also leads to a change in the angle of the femoral head and neck with the shaft. Normally this angle, called the *angle of inclination*, is about 125 degrees in adults; it is larger in children. As so often occurs in hip fractures, the radiograph in this case reveals that the angle is reduced, resulting in what is called a *coxa vara* (Fig. 47.1). By contrast, a fracture through the neck may occasionally take place with abduction of the thigh at the time of injury. If this happens, the neck will be driven in the abducted position into the head, where it will remain firmly impacted, increasing the angle of inclination and resulting in the so-called valgus position. Such a fracture has a better prognosis; there is no shortening of the leg and little pain.

Blood Supply of the Shaft, Neck, and Head of the Femur

A problem that has direct bearing on the course and handling of the fracture in this patient is the blood supply to the proximal portion of the femur (Fig. 47.2). The femur, like other long bones, is well supplied with blood vessels. These are derived from the following three sources.

1. The nutrient arteries, which enter the bone through the nutrient foramina, take an oblique course through the cortex of the bone until they reach the marrow cavity, where they divide into ascending and descending branches. The nutrient artery is largely concerned with supply of the bone marrow and the inner two-thirds

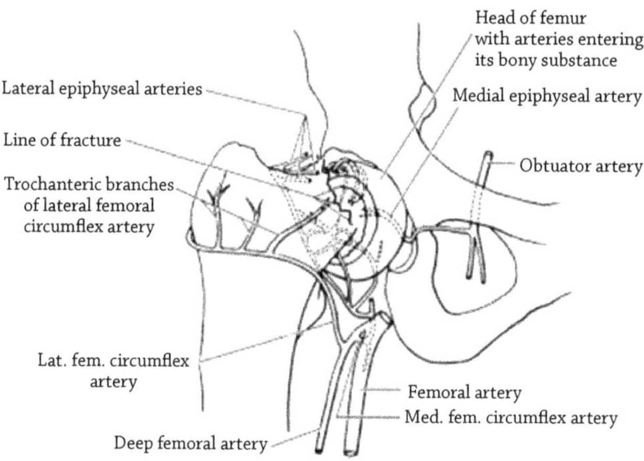

FIGURE 47.2

Blood supply of the head and neck of the femur. Notice that the main artery to the head is the medial femoral circumflex, through its lateral epiphyseal arteries, and that the lateral femoral circumflex artery contributes to the blood supply of the neck. The medial epiphyseal artery, a branch of the obturator artery, may or may not anastomose with the medial femoral circumflex artery. In this illustration, notice also that most of the important arteries to the head have been torn by the fracture.

of the cortex. In the femur, there are two nutrient foramina, and the nutrient arteries passing into them are derived from the perforating branches of the deep femoral artery.

2. The periosteal vessels form a communicating network that surrounds the bone. The number of periosteal vessels increases from the middle of the diaphysis toward the metaphyses, which are richly supplied with periosteal blood vessels. Fine branches of the periosteal network enter the outer third of the cortical bone and anastomose with vessels derived from the nutrient artery in the inner portion of the cortex. The two systems of nutrient and periosteal blood vessels may partially substitute for each other if the circulation in one or the other system is interrupted.

3. The main arteries of supply to the head of the femur come from the medial femoral circumflex, which is most commonly a branch of

the deep femoral artery. The posterior branches of the medial femoral circumflex artery represent the most important blood supply to the head. These vessels arise from a posterior branch of the medial femoral circumflex, which takes origin behind the femoral neck. They pierce the fibrous capsule of the hip joint and run upward and medially along the posterior aspects of the neck. There they course beneath the synovial membrane surrounding the neck to enter the head through bony foramina near the epiphyseal line.

It should be noted that the acetabular branch of the obturator artery sends a branch to the femoral head, which is carried through the ligament of the head of the femur (ligamentum teres capitis femoris). This is called the *foveolar artery*. Its extent and patency are variable, and its contribution to the blood supply of the head is usually not significant.

Necrosis of the Femoral Head in Subcapital Fractures

From the foregoing, it is clear that a subcapital fracture, such as in this case, leads to tearing of the important branches of the medial femoral circumflex artery beneath the synovial membrane and therefore to interruption of the main blood supply to the femoral head. On the other hand, trochanteric fractures outside the capsule have a much better chance to allow sufficient nourishment of the bone. The blood supply to the head of the femur via the foveal artery may be its only source of blood after fracture of the neck. This artery does not anastomose with the branches of the medial femoral circumflex artery in 20% of cases, and necrosis of the distal four-fifths of the head and the proximal neck is likely to occur in such cases. This type of necrosis is caused by isolation of the head and neck from its blood supply and is aseptic, in contrast to septic necrosis due to bacterial infection.

An interesting radiographic feature of aseptic necrosis of the head is a change in radiodensity in the fracture area, which becomes noticeable several weeks or months after the fracture has been sustained. The area surrounding the neck and shaft becomes increasingly translucent as a result of bone resorption from disuse and inflammation, whereas the dead head itself, cut of from its blood supply, preserves its normal bone density.

In the past, attempts were frequently made to immobilize the fragments by a plaster cast or by nailing in the hope that they would unite and vessels would grow across the fracture line. This effort often fails, particularly in subcapital fractures in elderly patients, and the previously described necrosis of the head results. To avoid this complication in this case, the head was excised and replaced by a prosthesis. Other bones in which fractures frequently lead to devascularization and the risk of necrosis of one fragment are the scaphoid and the talus.

Osteoporosis and Its Underlying Anatomy

The radiograph of the pelvis of this patient called attention to marked osteoporosis, which is common in the elderly, particularly in women. Osteoporosis is a bone disease in which there is a thinning of bone tissue and a reduction of bone mineral density. Although the cause of this disease is certainly multifactorial, it is clear that a reduction in estrogen secretion in women is a significant causal factor. It is estimated that 55% of Americans older than 50 years of age suffer from osteoporosis, and 80% of these individuals are women. A substantial percentage of these people will suffer fractures, primarily of weight-bearing bones such as the femoral neck or the vertebral body. For many years, hormone replacement therapy was recommended for postmenopausal women as a preventive measure. This no longer is recommended because, although estrogen replacement does reduce the risk of fractures, it increases the risk of cardiovascular disease and breast cancer. Currently, bisphosphonates are the major pharmacological treatment for osteoporosis.

Surgical Anatomy of the Operation

To gain access to the hip from a posterior approach, the fibers of the gluteus maximus are split by blunt dissection. These fibers run from above, laterally and downward. The muscle passes over the lateral surface of the greater trochanter of the femur and inserts into the iliotibial tract of the fascia latae and the gluteal tuberosity of the femur. A bursa interposed between the greater trochanter and the gluteus maximus reduces friction. Deep to the gluteus maximus are a series of muscles that are lateral rotators of the hip. From superior to inferior, they are the piriformis, the superior gemellus, the tendon of the obturator internus, the inferior gemellus, and the quadratus femoris. These muscles, with the exception of the quadratus femoris, are typically divided in this surgical procedure.

Sensory Nerve Supply of the Hip Joint and Hilton's Law

A brief comment on the sensory nerve supply of the hip joint is indicated, because it is responsible for the pain suffered by patients with hip fractures and explains the muscle spasms. Hilton's law is quite applicable to the hip joint; that is, a joint receives its proprioceptive and pain innervation from the same nerves that supply the muscles crossing the joint and distribute to the skin over these muscles and their insertions. This law also explains the reflex spasm of the overlying muscles in disease of the joint and the referral of joint pain to the adjacent skin. In the hip joint, the sensory nerve supply is derived from the femoral, obturator, and sciatic nerves.

"Unhappy Triad" of the Knee Joint

A 20-year-old student, while playing intramural football, suffered a severe twisting injury to his right knee. He was running hard, and while his foot was planted in the turf, another player ran into him, causing his trunk to twist. He lost his balance, felt a "pop" in his knee, and fell to the ground. In excruciating pain, he was taken to the health center on a stretcher.

Examination

The patient is seen later the same day by an orthopedist. His pain is intense, and his knee has begun to swell. He prefers to hold it in slight flexion. Abduction of the leg on the femur (valgus stress) aggravates the pain. There is tenderness when pressure is applied along the tibial attachment of the tibial (medial) collateral ligament but not at its femoral attachment. The clinical evaluation indicates that the ligament is sprained (overstretched). The Lachman test, a sensitive test for acute rupture of the anterior cruciate ligament (ACL), is performed. With the knee in 20 degrees of flexion and the leg externally rotated (which relaxes the iliotibial tract), the inner aspect of the calf is grasped by the examiner's right hand and traction is applied anteriorly while the left hand grasps and stabilizes the outer aspect of the distal thigh. There is excessive anterior displacement of the tibia compared with the contralateral leg, indicating a lax or absent ACL. Similarly, when the knee is then flexed to a right angle and an attempt is made to pull the tibia forward, there is a noticeable increase in anterior mobility (positive anterior drawer sign) compared with the uninjured knee. There is also marked restriction to passive extension of the knee joint.

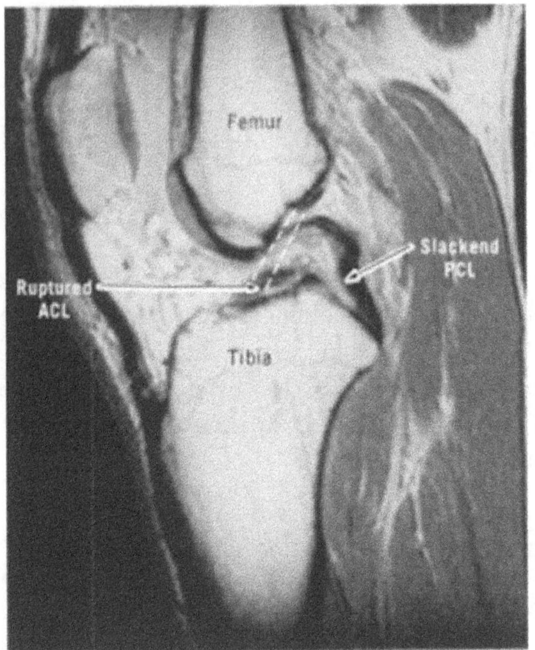

FIGURE 48.1

Sagittal magnetic resonance image through the knee joint shows a ruptured anterior cruciate ligament (ACL). The dashed line indicates the location of an uninjured ACL. The posterior cruciate ligament (PCL) is slackened and bent acutely because the tibia has translocated anteriorly.

A magnetic resonance image confirms a clinical diagnosis that the ACL is torn from its femoral attachment. It also demonstrates that the rim of the medial meniscus is torn, causing the central portion to displace into the joint (bucket-handle tear) (Fig. 48.1).

Diagnosis

The diagnoses are effusion (fluid collection) in the synovial cavity of the knee joint, rupture of the ACL at its femoral attachment, a bucket-handle tear of the medial meniscus, and a sprain of the lower portion of the tibial collateral ligament.

Therapy and Further Course

Injuries to the knee that disrupt its synovial lining frequently cause the knee to swell. This explains the swelling seen in this patient: The well-vascularized synovial membrane that attaches to the ACL and the outer margins of the medial meniscus was torn, causing effusion and hemorrhage. Restricted range of motion, also associated with swelling, explains why the patient prefers to hold his knee in slight flexion. In consultation with the patient, arthroscopic surgery for reconstruction of the ACL using a tendon graft is decided on but will not be performed until knee motion improves to normal, which may take as long as 6 weeks. Reconstruction of the ACL with graft material is indicated because a torn ACL does not heal well, even if the torn ends of the ligament are surgically repaired.

The decision to repair the torn medial meniscus will be made only after intraarticular assessment of the exact location and severity of the injury with the arthroscope. If it is repairable, the arthroscopic surgery will be performed in two stages: First the meniscus will be repaired, after which the ACL will be replaced by a graft. If the medial meniscus cannot be repaired, it will be partially excised by removal of the unstable flaps. The sprain of the tibial collateral ligament will heal without surgical treatment.

Six weeks later, in preparation for the arthroscopic surgery, the patient is placed in the supine position. An epidural block for the lumbar and sacral nerves is given, and a cephalosporin antibiotic (cefazolin) is given intravenously. A tourniquet is placed on the proximal thigh to reduce bleeding during surgery. The joint is injected with a mixture of Xylocaine and Marcaine (anesthetic agents) as well as epinephrine, a vasoconstrictor that will further reduce bleeding and will increase the duration of action of the anesthetic agents.

After anesthesia is induced, the surgery begins with small skin incisions on each side of the patellar tendon to create anteromedial and anterolateral portals, openings through which arthroscopic instruments are inserted into the joint cavity. The arthroscope, which is equipped with a light source and camera, is inserted into the joint through the anterolateral portal, and irrigation is carried out through a cannula inserted into the anteromedial portal.

Diagnostic Arthroscopy

During diagnostic arthroscopy, the ACL and the medial and lateral menisci are carefully inspected visually and probed with a nerve hook (a curved, round probe) to expose tears. To ensure the best possible visualization of a tear, the surgical assistant maneuvers the injured limb into various positions and degrees of varus, valgus, or rotational stress.

Inspection shows a large, displaced bucket-handle tear of the medial meniscus in the outer vascular zone of the meniscus, 3 mm from its periphery. The tear is about 2.5 cm long, and it curves from the posteromedial aspect of the meniscus to the posterior horn or root of the meniscus. Because the tear occurred in the vascular ("red") zone, it is deemed repairable by suturing the torn edges together. Tears of the thinly tapered inner part ("white" zone) are not repairable because this part is avascular. In those cases, the damaged tissue is unstable, and it is usually excised arthroscopically. The arthroscopic examination also reveals that the ACL is completely torn (avulsed) from its femoral attachment on the lateral wall of the intercondylar notch.

Repair of the Medial Meniscus

The surgeon chooses the "inside-out" technique of meniscal repair. A 3-cm skin incision, extending inward to the fibrous capsule, is made just behind the tibial collateral ligament. The sartorius muscle and the saphenous branch of the femoral nerve are retracted posteriorly out of harm's way. This incision exposes the posteromedial part of the fibrous capsule, which lies superficial to the torn medial meniscus.

In this inside-out technique of meniscal repair, the surgeon, working inside the joint, guides sutures attached to 8-inch-long, flexible needles through the meniscus and pushes them outward through the fibrous capsule of the knee, where the surgical assistant can grasp them so they can be tensioned and tied after the ACL reconstruction.

Reconstruction of the Anterior Cruciate Ligament

Before the surgery, a discussion was had with the patient about whether to use an allograft or an autograft to repair the ACL. An autograft would involve use of the patient's own tissue, typically a portion of the patellar ligament or hamstring tendon. An allograft would involve use of a cadaveric ligament. In general, an autograft provides a stronger graft but requires a longer surgical procedure and leads to a more painful recovery. Although in earlier times, allografts raised concern about transmission of disease, improved methods of sterilization have obviated these concerns. However, the sterilization procedure somewhat weakens the ligament. Because this patient does not participate in high-intensity sports (his participation in the intramural game during which he was injured was a rare event) and does not plan such activities in the future, it is decided to use a cadaver allograft. The cadaver tendon graft has a bony plug at each end with which to anchor the graft to the patient's bone.

The ACL is reconstructed in several stages:

1. Debriding (removing nonviable tissue) from the lateral side of the intercondylar notch at the femoral attachment of the ACL
2. Drilling of the tibial tunnel
3. Drilling of the femoral tunnel
4. Implanting the graft and fixing it into the femoral and tibial tunnels

5. Closing the incisions and making a postoperative evaluation.

Working through the anteromedial portal, the part of the ACL that remains attached to the anterior intercondylar area of the tibia and the site from which it was torn from the lateral wall of the intercondylar notch (the medial surface of the lateral condyle of the femur) are debrided with a motorized burr (resector). The resector is removed, and a small curved osteotome is then inserted through the portal to contour the lateral wall of the intercondylar notch in preparation for drilling of the femoral tunnel (Fig. 48.2), so as to make adequate room for the graft. Debris is removed by irrigation and suction.

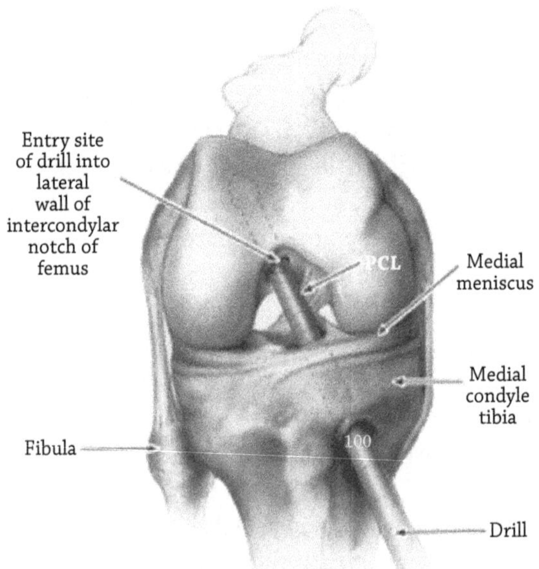

FIGURE 48.2

Schematic diagram shows the three-dimensional relationships of the drill passing through the right tibia upward through the joint space and the overlying tibia. (Reproduced with permission, Raven Press.)

The next step is drilling of the tibial tunnel. The angle of the tibial tunnel should align to the slope of the femoral tunnel when the knee is in 70 degrees of flexion, which allows the femoral tunnel to be drilled through the tibial tunnel.

The knee is now ready for graft implantation. An eyelet pin, which was threaded with sutures through the bony plug of the graft, is passed through the tibial and femoral tunnels and out the anterolateral thigh. This procedure positions the graft within the joint so that one bony plug lies in the femoral tunnel and the other in the tibial tunnel. Screws are inserted through the bony plugs into the femur and tibia for fixation. After the graft has been fixed, the knee is brought through a full range of motion to test the new graft.

Rehabilitation

The initial stage of postoperative rehabilitation is directed at minimizing swelling and reducing discomfort. This is done by icing of the knee, elevation of the knee, use of analgesic medication, and the use of crutches when the patient must ambulate. This stage is followed by range-of-motion exercises to gradually increase the range of motion of the knee. Then, strengthening exercises are used to restore the strength of the quadriceps femoris and the other muscles that cross and help to stabilize the knee.

Discussion

Anatomy of the Knee Joint

The knee joint has a complex structure. It includes two articulations, one between the femur and the tibia and the other between the patella and the femur. The fibula does not participate in the knee joint and is not a weight-bearing bone. The knee joint is enclosed by a fibrous capsule and is reinforced by both capsular ligaments and extracapsular ligaments. The knee also has a pair of intracapsular ligaments. The capsular ligaments, thickenings of the fibrous capsule that provide added stability to the joint, are the patellar ligament anteriorly and the oblique popliteal and arcuate popliteal ligaments posteriorly. The extracapsular ligaments are the tibial and fibular collateral ligaments, which are found on the medial and lateral sides of the joint, respectively. The intracapsular ligaments are the ACL and the posterior cruciate ligament (PCL). The extracapsular and intracapsular ligaments are discussed in more detail later.

The joint also contains two wedge-shaped cartilages, the medial and lateral menisci, which are interposed between the femoral condyles and the tibial condyles (Fig. 48.3). Also contributing to the stability of the knee joint are the strong muscles that cross this joint. As in other synovial joints, the inner surface of the fibrous capsule is lined by a synovial membrane. This membrane reflects from the fibrous capsule and attaches to the nonarticular surfaces within the joint. The synovial membrane attaches to the edges of the menisci and reflects around the cruciate ligaments. As such, although the menisci and the cruciate ligaments are within the fibrous capsule, they are outside of the synovial cavity.

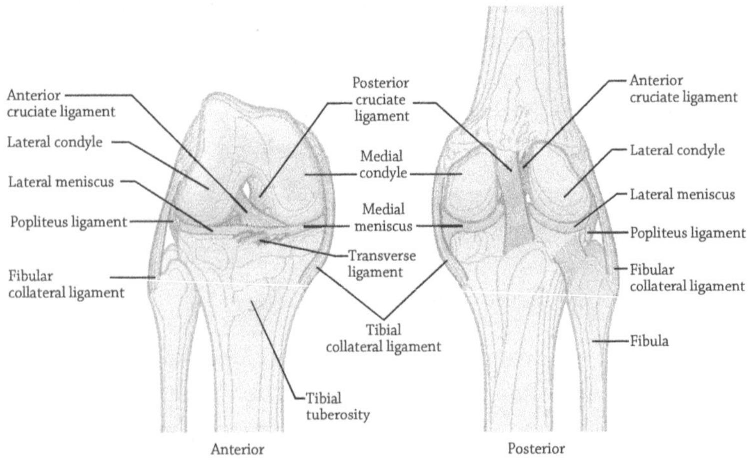

FIGURE 48.3

Supporting structures of the knee. (Courtesy of Kaplan Medical.)

The injury suffered by the patient in this case is a common one that has been designated the "unhappy triad" of the knee. The triad is classically described as consisting of injuries to the ACL, the medial meniscus, and the tibial collateral ligament. More recently, with the increased use of magnetic resonance imaging in the diagnosis of knee injuries, it has been observed that injury to the lateral meniscus, with or without injury to the medial meniscus, is often a component of this injury. The joint swelling in this case reflects damage to the interior of the joint, particularly the synovial lining. Joint swelling typically accompanies all types of intraarticular knee joint injuries.

There are many causes for ACL injury. A direct blow to the lateral side of the knee (creating valgus stress), as occurs in tackling, is not required. The considerable inertia of the body in rotating the femur medially over a planted foot and stable tibia is a frequent cause of ACL injuries, and excessive lateral rotation can also cause this injury. This injury can occur in a runner who is making a quick turn if the heel does not lift off the surface to spin with the runner's body, or in a skier whose ski becomes caught and cannot rotate freely with the skier's body. In summary, this injury can be caused by a variety of rather common misfortunes, all having to do with the inability of the knee joint to withstand the forces to which it is subjected.

Movements of the Knee Joint

Although the knee may initially appear to be a hinge joint, its movements are much more complex and include rolling, gliding, and rotation. In full extension, the matching articular areas of the femur and tibia are most congruent, and the strong stabilizing ligaments—ACL, PCL, tibial collateral, and fibular collateral—are taut. The knee is said to be "locked" when fully extended, and it is most stable in that position. The joint occupies this position during quiet standing. Movement from the locked position, as when assuming the sitting position or at the beginning of a stride, begins with flexion and a few degrees of lateral rotation of the femur on the tibia. These movements unlock the knee. The rotational component is caused by contraction of the popliteus muscle. Rotation at the knee is possible when the knee is flexed because in this position the collateral ligaments are slack. You can readily demonstrate this on yourself while sitting in a chair by keeping your heel on the floor and lifting your forefoot off the surface. While moving your foot from side to side, you can palpate the rotation of the tibia on the femur by placing your hands on the lateral and medial sides of the upper tibia. If you repeat this test while standing with your knee in full extension (locked), rotation will take place at the hip joint because the collateral ligaments of the knee are taut.

In summary, the unhappy triad injury in this case was caused by excessive medial rotation of the femur on a relatively stable tibia while the joint was partially flexed. It occurred during the moment when the body weight was borne by the stance limb.

The matching surfaces of the tibia and femur contribute little to this mobile joint's stability. Moreover, the contact area between the two bones decreases during flexion, leading to even greater instability. The main contributors to the strength and stability of the joint are the very strong muscles and tendons that cross the joint and the numerous ligaments (intraarticular, capsular, and extracapsular) that act as stabilizing elements. In addition, the menisci deepen the articular surfaces of the tibial condyles and accommodate the joint to variations in contact between femur and tibia. The fibrous capsule itself contributes greatly to maintaining the integrity of the joint.

Tibial Collateral Ligament

In this case, the tibial collateral ligament is injured to a lesser extent than the ACL or the medial meniscus. Medial rotation and adduction of the femur with the knee partially flexed caused this injury; the injury occurred when the foot was on the ground, thereby making the tibia relatively stable in reference to the femur. This motion, and the consequent separation of the medial tibial and femoral condyles, put more stress on the ligament than it could withstand. The tibial collateral ligament attaches the femur to the tibia. It attaches proximally to the medial epicondyle of the femur and distally to the medial condyle of the tibia, about 5 cm below the joint line. Its deeper fibers attach to the outer aspect of the medial meniscus. This explains the frequent coexisting injuries to both structures (see later discussion). Three tendons cross the tibial collateral ligament: the sartorius, gracilis, and semitendinosus tendons. They have a common insertion on the proximal portion of the tibia.

Anterior Cruciate Ligament

The second ligament injured in this case was the ACL, which is torn off its proximal attachment. The cruciate ligaments lie inside the fibrous capsule but outside the synovial cavity of the joint; the synovial membrane is reflected around them anteriorly and on their sides. The ACL is attached superiorly to the lateral surface of the intercondylar notch and is directed downward in a medial and anterior direction; it inserts on the anterior intercondylar area of the tibia. The PCL, which crosses the ACL posteriorly, also attaches to the intercondylar area of the tibia, but behind the ACL. The cruciate ligaments cross each other like the limbs of an X, hence the name (from the Latin *crux*, for "cross"). Both cruciate ligaments exert a stabilizing effect on all motions of the knee joint. They also limit anterior and posterior mobility of the tibia on the femur when the knee joint is in flexion. The ACL limits excessive anterior mobility, and the PCL limits excessive posterior mobility of the tibia on the femur.

The ACL is evaluated clinically with the knee flexed. The Lachman test is done with the knee in 15 to 30 degrees of flexion, and the anterior drawer test is done with the knee at 90 degrees of flexion. With the knee in the flexed position, the collateral ligaments are slackened, thus allowing movement of the tibia if a cruciate ligament is torn. The Lachman test is done with the leg externally rotated at the knee, which slackens the iliotibial band, to eliminate the stabilizing effect of this band. The iliotibial band is a lateral thickening of the fascia lata, the deep fascia of the thigh. The iliotibial band crosses the knee to attach to the tibia and thus contributes to the stability of the knee. Increased anterior mobility of the tibia with either test indicates injury to the ACL.

Medial Meniscus

The final injury is tearing of the medial meniscus. Both menisci are wedge-shaped, being thicker at their peripheral margins. In contrast to its lateral counterpart, the medial meniscus forms a three-quarter segment of a larger circle; that is, it is more C-shaped than the lateral meniscus, which displays a sharper curve and approximates a more complete, smaller circle. The anterior and posterior horns (ends) of the medial meniscus are attached to the anterior and posterior intercondylar areas of the tibia. A part of the fibrous capsule termed the *coronary ligament* attaches the menisci to the underlying tibia. The medial meniscus, in contrast to the lateral meniscus, is firmly anchored on its peripheral margin to the deep portion of the tibial collateral ligament, making it less mobile than its lateral counterpart. The same force that caused the stretching injury to the tibial collateral ligament and the rupture of the ACL displaced the medial meniscus more deeply into the joint, where crushing and shearing forces produced the bucket-handle tear.

The medial meniscus is injured more commonly than the lateral. This difference is partially explained by the firm anchorage of the medial meniscus to the collateral ligament. The lateral meniscus is not attached to the extracapsular fibular collateral ligament, which gives it increased freedom of movement and presumably allows it greater escape from damage. If the injury to the medial meniscus is left unrepaired, the patient is likely to suffer intermittent locking or buckling of the knee.

49

Intermittent Claudication

A 57-year-old man has been seeing his primary care physician for the past 4 years with concerns about recurrent leg pain. He is employed as a security guard, and his job requires a considerable amount of walking. Four years ago, he noticed that when he walked more than 5 or 6 blocks, he experienced a burning or aching pain in his right calf. If he stopped walking and rested, the pain would subside within a few minutes. At that time, his medical history included hypertension, which was well controlled on medication, and hypercholesterolemia, which was being treated with a statin medication. He was moderately overweight with a body mass index (BMI) of 28.3. He had a 40 pack-year history of cigarette smoking but has since been able to stop smoking. His family medical history includes the death of his father at age 60 after a myocardial infarction and the death of his mother at age 67 from a stroke.

The patient was started on daily low-dose aspirin (81 mg) for anticoagulation and pentoxifylline to decrease blood viscosity, and he began an exercise program of treadmill walking. He was instructed to walk until it became painful, rest until the pain subsided, and then walk again, continuing this regimen for 1 hour daily. After a period of 2 months, he reported an improvement in his tolerance to walking, and he continued on this regimen while being monitored by his physician.

On his current visit, the patient reports that the calf pain has recently worsened and that he can only walk a short distance (about 100 yards) before the onset of pain. It is now interfering with his ability to do his job, and he fears that he is at risk of being terminated. He reports that his reduced physical activity due to leg pain has led to an increase in his weight. He denies having calf pain at rest, and he reports no buttock or thigh pain. He has no difficulty maintaining an erection during intercourse.

Examination

The patient continues to be overweight, with a BMI of 29.7. Examination of the patient's extremities reveals that he has hair loss on the right leg below the knee. The skin of his right leg is shiny and tight, and there is a thickening of the toenails of his right foot. On vascular examination, there is a palpable abdominal aortic pulse of normal caliber. No abdominal or femoral bruits are auscultated. Bilateral femoral pulses are palpable immediately below the inguinal ligaments, but the pulse on the right side is noticeably weaker. The right popliteal pulse is barely palpable compared with the left. The posterior tibial and dorsalis pedis pulses on the right are not palpable, but those on the left are normal. His blood pressure measured in the right brachial artery is 134/92 mm Hg. Blood pressure measured at his right ankle in the dorsalis pedis artery, which is detected with a hand-held Doppler ultrasound device, is 76/58 mm Hg. With a systolic brachial pressure of 134 and a systolic ankle pressure of 76, his ankle-brachial index is 0.57, indicative of moderate obstruction in the arterial supply to the lower limb.

Diagnosis

The diagnosis is intermittent claudication in the right lower limb due to peripheral artery disease.

Therapy and Further Course

Because medical therapy has been used for the past 4 years but the disease has now progressed to the point that it is substantially interfering with the patient's lifestyle, he is referred to a vascular surgeon for evaluation. After a physical examination that confirms the previous finding of peripheral artery disease in the right lower limb, a careful evaluation of the carotid arteries by auscultation and Doppler ultrasound is done. These vessels appear normal with no indication of obstruction. The findings of a thorough cardiac examination are also normal. Imaging of the abdominal aorta, iliac arteries, and femoral arteries with digital subtraction angiography is ordered. Imaging reveals normal patency of the aorta and its bifurcation as well as the common iliac arteries. However, there is a 7-cm-long atherosclerotic lesion in the right external iliac artery that is causing a moderate narrowing of the artery and a 17-cm-long atherosclerotic lesion in the distal superficial femoral artery[1] that is causing a significant narrowing of the artery and reduced filling of the popliteal artery and its branches. Distal to the popliteal artery, flow appears normal with minimal evidence of arterial disease.

The need for revascularization of the right lower limb is discussed with the patient. The options of surgical bypass grafting and percutaneous transluminal angioplasty are described. Because of the size and number of lesions, it is decided that a surgical bypass graft is the better option because of the greater likelihood of a good long-term outcome.

At the time of surgery, the patient is prepared for an iliofemoral bypass with a synthetic graft. A retroperitoneal approach is made to the right common iliac artery. An oblique incision extending from near the tip of the right eleventh rib to 3 cm below the umbilicus is made. The external and internal oblique muscles are divided. The transversus abdominus muscle is split parallel to its fibers. The surgeon enters the preperitoneal plane and retracts the peritoneum medially. The ureter is mobilized away from the common iliac artery, and the external and internal iliac artery

1. The nomenclature commonly used by surgeons for the arteries of the thigh is different from that used by anatomists. Surgeons refer to the continuation of the external iliac artery as the *common femoral artery*, which then divides into the *superficial and deep femoral arteries*. Anatomists refer to the continuation of the external iliac artery as the femoral artery, which gives rise to the deep femoral artery. Surgeons say that the popliteal artery is the continuation of the superficial femoral artery, whereas in anatomical terminology the popliteal artery is the continuation of the femoral artery. Surgical nomenclature is used in this case study.

origins are mobilized. The common iliac artery is mobilized to its origin at the aortic bifurcation. A longitudinal incision is then made in the groin to expose the common femoral artery. A tunnel is created behind the inguinal ligament, anterior to the external iliac artery and the common femoral artery. The right common iliac artery is clamped, and a prosthetic bypass vessel is grafted into the artery. The prosthesis is passed through the tunnel and, at its other end, is grafted into the common femoral artery proximal to the origin of the profunda femoris (deep femoral) artery.

The patient is then prepared for the more distal bypass using an autologous venous graft. Proximal and distal vascular control is obtained. The great saphenous vein is harvested by making a longitudinal incision along the course of the vein. Tributaries of the vein are ligated and divided. A segment of vein is then removed, reversed, and flushed with heparinized saline. The vein is then stored in this flush solution until it is needed for the graft. The superficial femoral artery, proximal to the site of the atherosclerotic lesion in the femoral triangle, is mobilized. Access to the popliteal artery distal to the lesion is gained by making an incision on the medial side of the distal thigh with the knee in a slightly flexed position. The sartorius muscle is identified and retracted laterally. The deep fascia in the region of the adductor canal is dissected free, and the popliteal artery, posterior to the femur, is mobilized.

The saphenous vein is reversed, and the former distal end of the vein is grafted into the superficial femoral artery in the femoral triangle; the vein is then tunneled through the superficial fascia on the medial side of the thigh to reach the popliteal artery. The former proximal end of the vein is grafted into the popliteal artery. Arterial circulation is reestablished, and the grafts are checked for leaks. All incisions are closed. The patient is released to a rehabilitation facility 2 days after operation. Ambulation is increased over the next 5 days, and he is then released to home. He is referred for dietary counseling to reduce his lipids and to reduce his weight. On a follow-up visit, the patient reports that he is now able to walk unlimited distances without any pain in his lower limbs.

Discussion

The abdominal aorta bifurcates into the two common iliac arteries immediately anterior to the fourth lumbar vertebra. The common iliac artery continues to the pelvic brim, where it divides into the internal and external iliac arteries. The internal iliac artery passes over the pelvic brim to enter the pelvis, where it supplies the pelvic viscera, the pelvic wall, the gluteal region, and the perineum. The external iliac artery continues along the pelvic brim and then passes deep to the inguinal ligament to enter the thigh. At this point, its name is changed to *common femoral artery* (Fig. 49.1). This artery is contained within the femoral sheath, along with the femoral vein and lymphatic vessels. The artery continues into the femoral triangle and soon gives rise to the profunda femoris (deep femoral) artery. The profunda femoris gives rise to branches that are predominantly responsible for supplying the anterior, medial, and posterior compartments of the thigh. The superficial femoral artery continues within the femoral triangle, and at the inferior apex of the triangle, the artery enters the adductor (Hunter's) canal, the fascial plane between the sartorius anteriorly and the adductor longus and adductor magnus posteriorly. As the artery continues along the anterior surface of the adductor magnus tendon, it reaches the adductor hiatus, a gap within the tendon. The artery passes through the adductor hiatus to reach the popliteal fossa, on the posterior side of the femur. At this point, the name of the artery changes to *popliteal artery* (Fig. 49.1).

The popliteal artery crosses the knee joint and then divides into the anterior and posterior tibial arteries. The anterior tibial artery passes over the top of the interosseous membrane to enter the anterior compartment of the leg. The posterior tibial artery remains in the posterior compartment of the leg and it gives rise to the fibular (peroneal) artery. The anterior tibial artery supplies the anterior compartment, and the posterior tibial and fibular arteries supply the

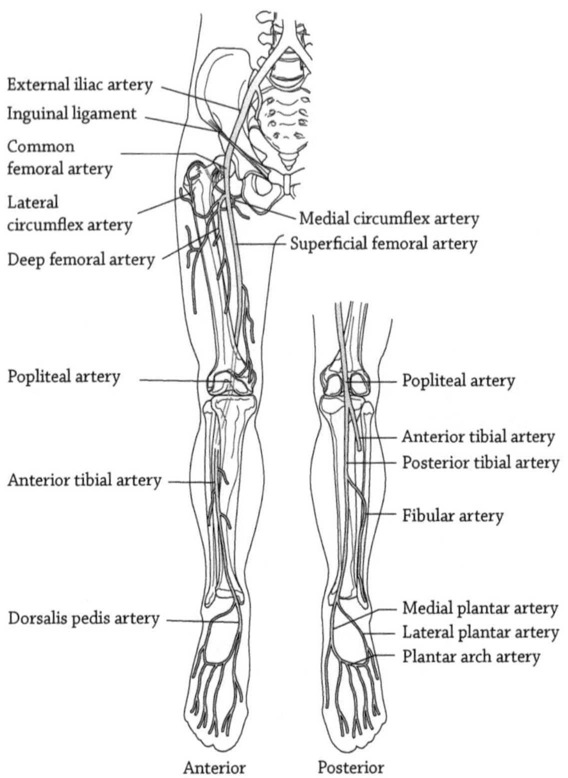

FIGURE 49.1

Arterial supply to the lower limb.

posterior and lateral compartments of the leg. The anterior tibial artery continues onto the dorsum of the foot as the *dorsalis pedis artery* (Fig. 49.1). The posterior tibial artery passes behind the medial malleolus to enter the plantar compartment of the foot.

In summary, the profunda femoris artery is chiefly responsible for the blood supply proximal to the knee, whereas the superficial femoral artery (through its continuation as the popliteal artery) is chiefly responsible for the supply distal to the knee. For this reason, this patient, who had a significant blockage of the superficial femoral artery, suffered pain distal to the knee in the posterior compartment muscles.

Claudication

Claudication is defined as lower limb pain or discomfort while walking (from the Latin *claudicare*, meaning "to limp"). Commonly, this condition is symptomatic of peripheral artery disease in the vessels supplying the lower limb. The term *intermittent claudication* indicates that the pain is not constant but rather occurs during exercise of the lower limb. Typically, the compromised blood supply is adequate to sustain the lower limb muscles when they are at rest. However, when they are exercised, such as in walking, the increased metabolic demand of the muscles exceeds the ability of the artery to supply oxygenated blood. The resulting ischemic condition results in pain. When the patient stops walking and allows the muscles to rest, the demand for oxygen subsides and the pain is relieved. Because the calf muscles are particularly active in walking, these muscles are often the ones that become painful.

Another form of claudication is known as *neurogenic claudication*. The cause of this pain is not vascular but rather neurological. Spinal stenosis is a common cause of the nerve compression that results in neurogenic claudication.

The Iliac Arteries and Ureter

The abdominal aorta and its branches are in the retroperitoneal space of the posterior abdominal wall. Therefore, it is possible to gain surgical access to these vessels without entering the peritoneal cavity. The surgical approach used in this patient was one in which the skin, the superficial fascia, and the muscle layers of the abdominal wall were incised but the parietal peritoneum was not. The surgeon entered the extraperitoneal space of the anterolateral abdominal wall and then remained in this space to gain access to the posterior wall structures. Because the ureter is in the retroperitoneal space in close proximity to the vessels of interest in this procedure, it is essential to be aware of the ureter's location and to safeguard it from injury. As the ureter leaves the renal pelvis to begin its descent down the posterior abdominal wall, it assumes a position on the anterior surface of the psoas major muscle. When the ureter crosses the pelvic brim to reach the posterior pelvic wall, it passes immediately anterior to the bifurcation of the common iliac artery. The ureter crosses the origin of the external iliac artery. This landmark can be used by the surgeon to help locate the ureter.

The Femoral Artery and Femoral Sheath

The external iliac artery is between the transversalis fascia and the parietal peritoneum, and as the artery passes under the inguinal ligament to enter the thigh, it evaginates the transversalis fascia. This evagination of fascia which covers the artery is the *femoral sheath*. Also within the femoral sheath are the femoral vein and the femoral lymphatics. The femoral nerve is not within the femoral sheath because within the abdomen the femoral nerve is external to the transversalis fascia and therefore does not evaginate it. The femoral sheath is larger than necessary to accommodate the artery, vein, and lymphatics. The most medial part of the sheath does not contain any vascular structures and is called the *femoral canal*. The opening into the femoral canal is the femoral ring. This is the site of femoral hernias.

The Femoral Triangle

The femoral triangle is a region in the anterior compartment of the thigh that contains the femoral vessels and the branches of the femoral nerve. The boundaries of the triangle are the inguinal ligament superiorly, the medial border of the sartorius muscle laterally, and the medial border of the adductor longus muscle medially. The triangle is covered over by the deep fascia of the thigh, the fascia lata. The floor of this triangular region is composed of the iliopsoas muscle laterally, the pectineus muscle, and the adductor longus muscle most medially. The femoral nerve enters the triangle after passing deep to the inguinal ligament. The nerve lies on the anterior surface of the iliopsoas muscle. Medial to the femoral nerve, the common femoral artery enters the triangle within the femoral sheath. Medial to the artery is found the femoral vein, also within the femoral sheath. The artery and vein lie anterior to the pectineus muscle.

The femoral artery enters the femoral triangle lateral to the vein, but shortly after doing so, these vessels rotate medially 90 degrees so that the artery assumes a position anterior to the vein. This relationship is maintained for the remainder of the course of the vessels through the thigh. It can be inferred that this rotation is evidence of the medial rotation of the lower limb that occurs during embryonic development. The positions of the femoral nerve, artery, vein, and lymphatics immediately inferior to the inguinal ligament can be remembered by the mnemonic NAVEL (*n*erve, *a*rtery, *v*ein, *e*mpty *l*ymphatic space), which lists the structures from lateral to medial. Sometimes the femoral vein is used for venous access if other veins are not accessible. This vein can be easily found by knowing that it is immediately medial to the femoral pulse immediately below the inguinal ligament.

The Adductor Canal and Adductor Hiatus

At the apex of the femoral triangle, the sartorius muscle passes superficial to the adductor longus muscle. The fascial plane between these muscles is the adductor canal (also called the subsartorial or Hunter's canal). The walls of this canal are the sartorius anteriorly, the adductor longus and adductor magnus posteriorly, and the gracilis medially. The superficial femoral artery, the femoral vein, and two branches of the femoral nerve (the saphenous nerve and the nerve to the vastus medialis) enter this canal. The adductor canal extends from the apex of the femoral triangle to the adductor hiatus, an opening in the tendon of the adductor magnus. The artery and vein pass through this hiatus (the nerves do not). When these vessels pass through the hiatus, they emerge in the popliteal fossa and their names are changed to popliteal artery and vein.

Popliteal Fossa

The popliteal fossa is a diamond-shaped region behind the knee. The four sides of the fossa are composed of the biceps femoris muscle superolaterally, the semimembranosus and semitendinosus muscles superomedially, and the lateral and medial heads of the gastrocnemius muscle inferolaterally and inferomedially, respectively. The floor of the fossa is composed of the posterior surface of the femur, the posterior knee joint capsule, and the popliteus muscle, from superior to inferior. The fossa is largely filled with fat. The sciatic nerve typically divides into its two components near the upper apex of the fossa. The tibial nerve continues vertically down the middle of the fossa. The common fibular (peroneal) nerve lies against the biceps femoris muscle (the superolateral border of the fossa) and travels along with this muscle and tendon to the head and neck of the fibula, where it divides into the superficial and deep fibular (peroneal) nerves.

The popliteal artery and vein enter the fossa through the adductor hiatus. Near the inferior end of the fossa, they divide into the anterior and posterior tibial vessels. The tibial nerve, popliteal vein, and popliteal artery pass through the fossa in that order from most posterior to most anterior. Because the artery is the deepest structure in the popliteal fossa, it is close to the popliteal surface of the femur. The pulse of the popliteal artery can be felt by deep palpation into the popliteal fossa with compression of the artery against the femur. Fracture of the femur in this region or posterior dislocation of the knee endangers the popliteal artery and can compromise blood flow to the limb below the knee.

Saphenous Veins

There are two major superficial veins in the lower limb, the great and small saphenous veins. Both saphenous veins arise from the dorsal venous arch of the foot. The great saphenous vein arises from the medial side of the venous arch, passes within the superficial fascia anterior to the medial malleolus, continues upward passing posterior to the medial condyle of the femur, and reaches the proximal thigh superficial to the femoral triangle. There, it penetrates the fascia lata at the saphenous hiatus to reach the femoral vein, into which it drains. The small saphenous vein arises from the lateral side of the venous arch and passes within the superficial fascia posterior to the lateral malleolus. In the leg, it penetrates the crural fascia (the deep fascia of the leg) and passes between the two heads of the gastrocnemius muscle to enter the popliteal fossa, where it drains into the popliteal vein. There are multiple communications between the saphenous veins and between each of those veins and the deep veins of the lower limb. Because of the length and accessibility of the great saphenous vein, it is frequently used as a graft for bypass surgery (in the heart as well as the lower limb), as was done in this case. Because of the presence of valves in this vein, it is necessary to reverse the orientation of the vein (proximal to distal) when it is used for an arterial bypass graft, so that the orientation of the valves will be consistent with the direction of blood flow.

Reference

White C: Intermittent claudication. *N Engl J Med* 356:1241–1250, 2007.

50

Anterior Compartment Syndrome

A 20-year-old male college football player comes to the emergency department with the complaint of severe pain in his right leg. He reports that earlier in the day, while he was playing in a game, an opposing player tackled him and the player's helmet struck him forcefully in the front of the leg, about halfway between his knee and his ankle. He came out of the game briefly because of the injury. His trainer evaluated his leg and determined that there were no fractures and no ligament damage. Concluding that he had suffered only a bruise, he returned to the game. After the game, the leg pain continued and became more intense. The pain was much more severe than seemed consistent with the injury that he had suffered. He was seen again by the trainer, who advised him to come to the emergency room. He describes a deep, burning pain in his leg and says that his leg feels tight.

Examination

On physical examination, the patient's temperature is 100.2° F, his heart rate is 90 bpm, his blood pressure is 110/60 mm Hg, and his respiratory rate is 16 breaths/min. Results of the head, eye, ear, nose, and throat (HEENT) examination and examinations of the lungs, heart, and abdomen are all normal. On examination of the extremities, there is redness and swelling over the anterolateral aspect of his right leg. On palpation, this area is extremely tender, and it feels hard and warmer than other parts of the leg. The hardening extends from 5 cm below the tibial tuberosity to the junction of the middle and lower thirds of the leg, and it seems to correspond to the anterior compartment of the leg. Dorsiflexion of the foot and extension of the toes are severely limited. When the examiner plantar flexes the patient's foot, the pain increases in severity. The pulse in the dorsalis pedis artery is reduced compared with the other limb. Sensation along the anterior leg is somewhat reduced, and sensation in the region of the webspace between the great toe and the second toe is reduced.

Therapy and Further Course

It is necessary to decompress the anterior compartment of the leg because of concern for the neurovascular compromise that is evident on the physical examination. The patient is admitted and prepared for surgery. The skin, superficial fascia, and deep fascia over the anterolateral aspect of the leg are incised (fasciotomy) with the patient under general anesthesia. Obvious necrotic material is debrided, and the fascia is left wide open, but the skin over it is partially closed.

During the next few days, there is minimal discharge from the incision, and the pain and fever subside. Dorsiflexion of the foot and extension of the toes continue to be restricted, but the patient is able to walk and is discharged home on postoperative day 5 with the wound healing nicely. He will be evaluated in 1 week to decide whether a skin graft will be necessary.

Diagnosis

Anterior compartment syndrome is diagnosed. This is a surgical emergency.

Discussion

The condition is caused by an acute impairment of the blood flow to the muscles of the anterior compartment. To avoid permanent injury to the muscles of the anterior compartment, the compartment needs to be decompressed within about 6 hours. The initial injury caused swelling of the muscles of the anterior compartment. Because these muscles are within a space with fairly rigid walls, the increased muscle volume causes an increase in pressure within the compartment. When this elevated pressure becomes greater than the capillary perfusion pressure, it causes collapse of the capillary beds and compromises capillary perfusion within the muscles, leading to degeneration and necrosis of muscle fibers and further swelling. This sets up a vicious cycle in which further swelling of the muscle further compromises blood flow, which further injures the muscle and causes more swelling.

The muscles of the anterior compartment of the leg include the tibialis anterior (which is particularly affected in this syndrome), the extensor hallucis longus, and the extensor digitorum longus. The fibularis tertius may be considered a fourth muscle of this compartment; it is actually the lateral portion of the extensor digitorum longus, which inserts on the fifth metatarsal rather than onto a digit. The configuration of the anterior compartment of the leg makes this region particularly prone to an increase in intracompartmental pressure. The compartment is bounded by rigid or semirigid walls formed by the tibia, fibula, interosseous membrane, crural fascia, and anterior intermuscular septum (Fig. 50.1). The tibia, fibula, and interosseous membrane separate the anterior compartment from the posterior compartment, and the anterior intermuscular septum separates the anterior compartment from the lateral compartment. The crural fascia is the very dense deep fascia that encircles the entire leg and forms the semirigid anterior wall of the anterior compartment.

Involvement of the Deep Fibular (Peroneal) Nerve

The major nerves and blood vessels in the anterior compartment may also be affected by the elevation in pressure. The deep fibular (peroneal) nerve and the anterior tibial vessels are important structures in the compartment. The deep fibular nerve is a branch of the common fibular nerve, which in turn is a branch of the sciatic nerve. As the sciatic nerve approaches the popliteal fossa in the

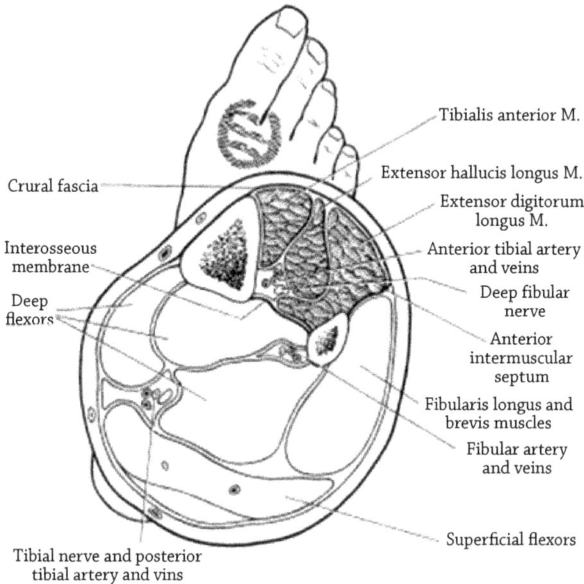

FIGURE 50.1

Cross section through the right leg at the junction of the intermediate and lower thirds of the leg. Notice the muscles, nerve, and blood vessels in the closed anterior compartment. Also notice the area of sensory loss on the dorsum of the foot resulting from the involvement of the deep fibular nerve. M., muscle.

posterior thigh, it divides into the tibial nerve (the medial branch) and the common fibular nerve (the lateral branch). The common fibular nerve wraps around the neck of the fibula, and there it divides into the superficial and deep fibular nerves. The superficial fibular nerve innervates the two muscles of the lateral compartment (the fibularis longus and brevis) and provides cutaneous innervations to the skin of the anterolateral leg and most of the dorsum of the foot. The deep fibular nerve enters the anterior compartment and innervates all muscles of that compartment; it then continues into the foot to innervate some small muscles on the dorsum of the foot and to innervate the skin in the webspace between the first and second digits.

In its course through the anterior compartment, the deep fibular nerve lies deep to the muscles of the compartment and on the anterior surface of the interosseous membrane (Fig. 50.1). With increased pressure in the compartment, the nerve can be compressed against this membrane. The integrity of this nerve can be evaluated by testing the cutaneous sensation in its region of distribution between the first two toes. Evaluation of muscle function in the anterior compartment would be difficult because of the effect of the compression on these muscles. This patient has diminished sensation in the space between the first two digits, suggesting that the deep fibular nerve is being affected by the pressure in the anterior compartment.

Arterial Involvement

The presence of a pulse in the dorsalis pedis artery, although weak, seems to prove patency of the anterior tibial artery in this patient. The anterior tibial artery is a direct branch of the popliteal artery, which is the distal continuation of the superficial femoral artery. The anterior tibial artery, after it branches from the popliteal artery, passes over the top of the interosseous membrane to enter the anterior compartment, where it is the major blood supply to the muscles of this compartment. It lies on the anterior surface of the interosseous membrane, along with the deep fibular nerve. When the anterior tibial artery crosses the ankle to reach the dorsum of the foot, its name is changed to *dorsalis pedis artery*. The patency of this artery can be evaluated by palpating the dorsalis pedis pulse, which can be found lateral to the extensor hallucis longus tendon on the dorsum of the foot. Branches from the posterior tibial and fibular arteries in the posterior compartment perforate the interosseous membrane to anastomose with the anterior tibial artery and provide a collateral pathway for supply of the anterior compartment.

51

Common Fibular Nerve Laceration

A 22-year-old man comes to the emergency department with concerns about his left lower limb. He reports that 2 days earlier, he and several companions were involved in a fight outside a bar where they had been drinking, and he received a knife wound on the side of his left knee. Although he bled from the wound, the bleeding was not extensive, and he was able to stop it with wrapping of the wound and direct pressure. He did not seek medical attention at the time because he was fearful of getting into legal trouble because of his involvement in a knife fight. When he got home, he applied an antiseptic solution to the wound and kept it wrapped with gauze bandage. He says that the next day he noticed that he had difficulty moving his foot properly; he had difficulty walking and repeatedly tripped over his left foot.

Examination

On physical examination, the man appears well nourished and in good health. His heart rate is 78 bpm, his respiratory rate is 12 breaths/min, his blood pressure is 118/74 mm Hg, and his temperature is 99.0° F. Examination of his lower limb reveals a 5-cm laceration on the lateral side of the proximal left leg in the region of the head of the fibula. The wound extends through the skin and subcutaneous fat, exposing the underlying deep fascia. The skin around the wound is slightly erythematous, but there is no exudate or other evidence of infection. Evaluation of sensation in the lower limb reveals diminished sensation on the lateral and anterior surfaces of the leg compared with the contralateral side. The dorsum of the left foot is almost entirely anesthetic with the exception of the fifth toe and the most medial side of the dorsum of the foot. Sensation to the posterior and medial surfaces of the left leg is normal. Evaluation of the motor function of the lower limb reveals an inability to dorsiflex the foot at the ankle and an inability to extend the toes. The patient can weakly invert the foot but is unable to evert it. The patient has a footdrop that causes him to elevate his limb abnormally high during the swing phase of gait, and he enters the stance phase with a toe strike.

Diagnosis

Lesion of the common fibular (peroneal) nerve is diagnosed.

Therapy and Further Course

The patient is referred to a neurosurgeon for evaluation of the common fibular (peroneal) nerve. Based on the presumptive diagnosis of a lesion of this nerve, he is scheduled for surgery later the same day. In the operating room and with the patient under general anesthesia, the wound is fully explored and damaged soft tissue is debrided. Careful examination reveals that the common fibular nerve is severed. The patient is prepared for surgical repair of the nerve.

He is placed in the prone position with padding under the ankle to keep the knee slightly flexed. Fascial extensions from the lateral head of the gastrocnemius that are covering the nerve are divided, and the proximal and distal stumps of the nerve are mobilized. Bleeding from small vessels is controlled by electrocautery. The posterior surface of the proximal fibula is shaved down to provide a less angulated course for the nerve and to reduce traction on it. Damaged tissue from the proximal and distal stumps is removed, and an end-to-end repair of the nerve is completed by suturing of the epineurium. The knee is placed in 15 degrees of flexion, and a plaster splint is used to maintain this position to minimize tension on the sutures. After 3 weeks, the splint is removed. With physical therapy, the knee is gradually extended.

After the surgery, it is explained to the patient that the nerve was completely severed and that it has been surgically joined. Because it takes time for nerve regeneration to occur, he should not expect return of sensory or motor function for many months. A schedule of electrical stimulation of the muscles of the anterior and lateral compartments is established in an effort to maintain the integrity of these muscles while they await reinnervation. He is fitted with an ankle-foot orthosis to stabilize the foot and prevent footdrop.

After 6 months, there is some restoration of sensory function on the anterolateral leg. Sensation on the dorsum of the foot begins to return after 9 months. Also after 9 months, motor function begins to be restored, first in the lateral compartment and then in the anterior compartment. During the following 6 months, increased motor function is observed, and with physical therapy, strength is restored, albeit not to the preinjury level. After 18 months, no further improvement is noted. Muscle strength is less than in the right leg, but the patient no longer has a footdrop. There continues to be hypesthesia in the leg and dorsum of the foot. He enters stance with a heel strike, and there is a noticeable foot slap on the left side during gait.

Discussion

The common fibular nerve is one of the two terminal branches of the sciatic nerve. (It should be noted that the common fibular nerve was formerly known as the common peroneal nerve, and it is still common to hear clinicians refer to it with that name.) The sciatic nerve typically divides at the upper end of the popliteal fossa, and the common fibular nerve lies against the medial edge of the biceps femoris muscle. It travels with the muscle across the knee toward the head of the fibula. At the head of the fibula, the tendon of the biceps femoris inserts onto the head of the fibula, and the common fibular nerve continues around the lateral aspect of the head and neck of the fibula. At that point, the nerve divides into the superficial and deep fibular nerves (Fig. 51.1).

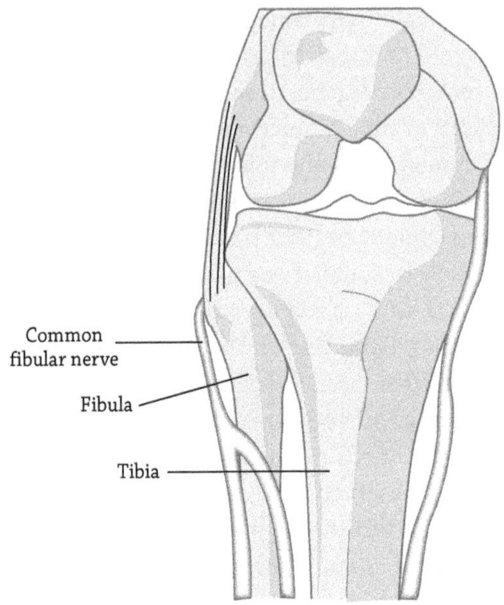

FIGURE 51.1

The common fibular nerve at the neck of the fibula.

The superficial fibular nerve enters the lateral compartment and innervates the two muscles in that compartment, the fibularis longus and brevis muscles, both everters of the foot. This nerve also provides cutaneous innervation to the anterolateral side of the distal leg and to almost all of the dorsum of the foot. The deep fibular nerve enters the anterior compartment and innervates the muscles of that compartment—the tibialis anterior, a dorsiflexor and invertor of the foot; the extensor hallucis longus, the extensor of the great toe and a dorsiflexor of the foot; the extensor digitorum longus, an extensor of digits II through V and a dorsiflexor of the foot; and the fibularis tertius, an evertor of the foot. The deep fibular nerve enters the dorsum of the foot passing deep to the extensor retinaculum. In the foot, it innervates the extensor digitorum brevis and the extensor hallucis brevis, two functionally unimportant muscles, and it provides cutaneous sensory innervation to the region of the webspace between digits I and II.

The other nerves that provide sensory innervation to the skin of the leg and foot are the saphenous nerve, the sural nerve, and the tibial nerve. The saphenous nerve is a branch of the femoral nerve, which provides sensory innervation to the anteromedial side of the leg and the dorsomedial surface of the foot as far distally as the head of the first metatarsal. The sural nerve receives contributions from the tibial nerve and the common fibular nerve, and it provides sensory innnervation to the skin of the posterior leg. The tibial nerve provides sensory innervation to the sole of the foot by way of two branches, the medial and lateral plantar nerves.

It is noteworthy that this patient did not suffer complete anesthesia of the anterolateral leg because of the overlap in distribution of the superficial fibular nerve with the saphenous nerve and the sural nerve. Most of the dorsum of the foot was anesthetic, but some sensation was retained on the medial and lateral borders of the dorsum, because in these regions there is some overlap with the innervation of the saphenous nerve and the medial and lateral plantar branches of the tibial nerve.

Injury to the Common Fibular Nerve

The common fibular nerve is the most frequently injured peripheral nerve in the lower limb. This nerve is easily traumatized as it passes over the head and neck of the fibula because it is in a very superficial position and is in contact with the firm fibula. The only structures covering (and protecting) the nerve in this position are the skin, the superficial fascia, and the deep fascia. The nerve can be injured by fairly superficial wounds, as in this case; by direct blunt trauma such as a blow to the side of the knee; or by a crush injury, such as from a car bumper. The nerve is also subject to being stretched, because it is tethered by the deep fascia covering the fibularis muscles. The deep fibular nerve is also tethered as it passes through the fibularis longus on its way to the anterior compartment. Because of its superficial position and the underlying fibula, the common fibular nerve can even be injured by compression of the nerve between a mattress and the fibula from the body weight of an ill patient who remains lying in bed on one side.

Superficial wounds that injure the nerve typically do not produce severe bleeding because the arteries and veins that supply this region do not take the same superficial course as the nerve. The posterior tibial artery and vein and their fibular branches are branches of the popliteal vessels, which are deeply placed in the popliteal fossa. The anterior tibial artery and vein, which supply the anterior compartment, enter that compartment by passing over the top of the interosseous membrane deep within the popliteal fossa; in contrast, the deep fibular nerve enters the anterior compartment by passing superficially around the fibula.

Nerve Repair

When a peripheral nerve is injured, the axons distal to the injury degenerate and the end organs innervated by these nerves are denervated. After a refractory period of about 2 weeks, the axons proximal to the injury attempt to regenerate and grow out toward the end organs. Among the factors that determine the success of this regeneration is the integrity of the pathway along which the axons will grow. If there is no physical disruption of the connective tissue sheaths of the nerve (i.e., epineurium, perineurium, and endoneurium), then the axons can regenerate along the pathways established by these connective tissue tubes. If there is physical disruption of the nerve sheath, as in this patient, then the connective tissue pathway must be surgically reestablished.

In this case, the proximal and distal stumps were near each other and could be sutured together. However, if there is significant damage to the nerve (e.g., bullet wound, complex penetrating wound), the removal of the damaged tissue may leave the two stumps too far apart to allow their union. In such cases, a nerve graft may be used. A common source of such a nerve graft is a large cutaneous nerve, such as the sural nerve. A segment of the sural nerve can be used as a "bridge" by suturing it to the proximal and distal stumps of the injured nerve. Although the axons in the grafted nerve degenerate, the connective tissue tubes left behind can be used by the regenerating nerve to reach the distal stump. As would be expected, the quality of restoration of function is greatest in those cases in which there is no physical disruption of the nerve sheath, less good if surgical union of the nerve is required, and least good if a nerve graft is required. The length of the graft is inversely related to the quality of restoration of function.

Gait Abnormalities

In normal gait, the stance phase of gait is entered with a heel strike and then the forefoot is slowly lowered to the ground. To enter stance with a heel strike, the foot must be dorsiflexed during the swing phase. Because the deep fibular nerve innervates the dorsiflexors, this patient was unable to dorsiflex during the swing phase and therefore had a footdrop that caused him to enter stance with a toe strike. Similarly, he brought his foot through the swing phase with a foot drop, which required him to elevate the foot away from the ground to avoid striking his toe. This is why he found that he was tripping over his toe and why he was elevating his foot unusually high by flexing his hip and his knee.

As he began to regain some muscle activity in the anterior compartment, he was able to dorsiflex his foot during the swing phase, and he therefore had a heel strike. However, to lower the foot slowly to the ground after heel strike requires forceful contraction of the anterior compartment muscles to resist the force of the ground against the calcaneus. Because his muscles were too weak to generate the required force, he had a foot slap, in which his forefoot forcefully struck the ground after the heel strike. This is to say, that although he had enough muscle strength to dorsiflex the foot during swing, when he only had to resist the gravitational force on his forefoot, he did not have enough strength to resist the force associated with his body weight striking the ground at heel strike.

Unit VII

Review Questions

The number in parentheses is a reference to the page on which information about the question may be found.

1. How does the sciatic nerve enter the gluteal region?
The sciatic nerve exits the pelvis and enters the gluteal region by passing through the greater sciatic foramen. Most of this foramen is filled with the piriformis muscle. In most cases, the sciatic nerve passes inferior to this muscle. However, in a common variation, the common fibular portion of the sciatic nerve passes above the piriformis muscle or through the muscle. (416)

2. What muscles are innervated by the superior and inferior gluteal nerves?
The superior gluteal nerve innervates the gluteus medius muscle, the gluteus minimus muscle, and the tensor fasciae latae muscle. The inferior gluteal nerve innervates the gluteus maximus muscle. (418)

3. Where is the cutaneous sensory distribution of the branches of the common fibular nerve?
The sural branch of the common fibular nerve provides sensory innervation to the skin of the lateral calf. The superficial fibular nerve provides sensory innervation to the skin of the lateral leg, the anterior leg, and much of the dorsum of the foot. The deep fibular nerve provides sensory innervation to the skin of the webspace between the first and second toes. (416)

4. What muscles are external rotators of the hip?
The largest of the external rotators is the gluteus maximus. Deep to this muscle there are several smaller external rotators. These include the piriformis, the obturator internus and externus, the superior and inferior gemelli, and the quadratus femoris. (425)

5. Why does a fracture of the femoral neck place the femoral head at risk of avascular necrosis?
The primary blood supply to the head of the femur comes from the medial femoral circumflex artery, which is most commonly a branch of the deep femoral artery. These branches pierce the fibrous capsule of the hip joint and run upward and medially along the posterior aspects of the neck. They course beneath the synovial membrane surrounding the neck to enter the head through bony foramina near the epiphyseal line. A fracture to the femoral neck can compromise these vessels, thus depriving the femoral head of its major blood supply. (426–428)

6. What nerves provide sensory innervation to the hip joint?
As is typical for other joints, the hip joint receives its sensory innervation from branches of the same nerve that innervate the muscles that cross that joint. The muscles that cross the front of the joint are innervated by the femoral nerve. The muscles that cross the medial side of the joint are innervated by the obturator nerve. The muscles that cross the back of the joint are innervated by the tibial nerve. Therefore, the hip joint receives its sensory innervation from these three nerves. (430)

7. What are the important structural differences between the medial meniscus and the lateral meniscus of the knee?
Both menisci are wedge-shaped, thicker at their peripheral margins. In contrast to its lateral counterpart, the medial meniscus forms a three-quarter segment of a larger circle; that is, it is more C-shaped than the lateral meniscus, which displays a sharper curve and approximates a more complete, smaller circle. The medial meniscus, in contrast to the lateral meniscus, is firmly anchored on its peripheral margin to the deep portion of the tibial collateral ligament, making it less mobile than its lateral counterpart. (442)

8. What are the functions of the anterior and posterior cruciate ligaments?
The cruciate ligaments lie inside the fibrous capsule but outside the synovial cavity of the joints. The anterior cruciate ligament (ACL) is attached superiorly to the lateral surface of the intercondylar notch; it is directed downward in a medial and anterior direction and inserts on the anterior intercondylar area of the tibia. The posterior cruciate ligament (PCL), which crosses the ACL posteriorly, also attaches to the intercondylar area of the tibia but behind the ACL. Both cruciate ligaments exert a stabilizing effect on all motions of the knee joint. They also limit anterior and posterior mobility of the tibia on the femur when the knee joint is in flexion. The ACL limits excessive anterior mobility, and the PCL limits excessive posterior mobility of the tibia on the femur. (441)

9. What muscle is responsible for "unlocking" the knee at the beginning of knee flexion?
The knee is "locked" at the end of extension by medial rotation of the femur on the tibia. To begin flexion of the knee, it must be "unlocked" by lateral rotation of the femur on the tibia. This motion is accomplished by the popliteus muscle. (439–440)

10. What are the origin and termination of the popliteal artery?
The popliteal artery begins as the superficial femoral artery passes through the adductor hiatus to enter the popliteal fossa. At the inferior end of the fossa, the artery terminates by dividing into the anterior and posterior tibial arteries. (447)

11. What arterial landmark at the pelvic brim can be used to identify the location of the ureter?
The ureter crosses the pelvic brim immediately anterior to the bifurcation of the common iliac artery into the external iliac and internal iliac arteries. The ureter crosses immediately anterior to the origin of the external iliac artery.(449–450)

12. What structures are within the femoral sheath?
The femoral sheath is an evagination of the transversalis fascia into the thigh posterior to the inguinal ligament. Within the femoral sheath are found the femoral artery, femoral vein, and femoral lymphatics. The femoral nerve is outside the sheath on its lateral side. (450)

13. What muscles are found in the anterior compartment of the leg?
The anterior compartment of the leg is bounded by rigid or semirigid walls formed by the tibia, fibula, interosseous membrane, crural fascia, and anterior intermuscular septum. The muscles of the anterior compartment of the leg include the tibialis anterior, the extensor hallucis longus, and the extensor digitorum longus. The fibularis tertius may be considered a fourth muscle of this compartment, but it is actually the lateral portion of the extensor digitorum longus. (456)

14. What nerve and artery are found in the anterior compartment of the leg?
The artery in the anterior compartment is the anterior tibial artery, which is a branch of the popliteal artery. This branch passes over the top of the interosseous membrane to enter the anterior compartment. The nerve in this compartment is the deep fibular nerve, which is a branch of the common fibular nerve. This branch passes around the neck of the fibula to enter the anterior compartment. (456–457)

15. How can the patency of the anterior tibial artery be assessed in a physical examination?
The anterior tibial artery continues onto the dorsum of the foot and changes its name to the dorsalis pedis artery. The pulse of this artery can be palpated on the dorsum of the foot immediately lateral to the tendon of the extensor hallucis longus tendon. The patency of the anterior tibial artery can be evaluated by palpation of this pulse. (458)

16. What are the motor and sensory distributions of the superficial fibular nerve?
The superficial fibular nerve is a branch of the common fibular nerve. It arises at about the level of the head of the fibula. The superficial fibular nerve innervates the muscles of the lateral compartment of the leg—the fibularis longus and fibularis brevis muscles. This nerve provides sensory innervation to the skin on the lateral and anterior sides of the leg and to the skin of most of the dorsum of the foot. (462)

17. What are the motor and sensory distributions of the deep fibular nerve?
The deep fibular nerve arises as a branch of the common fibular nerve at about the level of the head of the fibula. The deep fibular nerve innervates the muscles of the anterior compartment of the leg, the tibialis anterior, the extensor hallucis longus, and the extensor digitorum longus. It provides sensory innervation to the skin on the dorsum of the foot in the region of the webspace between the first and second toe. (462)

INDEX

Lightning Source UK Ltd.
Milton Keynes UK
UKHW020853130919
349684UK00006B/230/P